AF778715

Toxicological Aspects of Medical Device Implants

Toxicological Aspects of Medical Device Implants

Edited by

PRAKASH SRINIVASAN TIMIRI SHANMUGAM
HCL America Inc., Sunnyvale, CA, United States

LOGESH CHOKKALINGAM
HCL America Inc., Sunnyvale, CA, United States

PRAMILA BAKTHAVACHALAM
HCL, ELCOT-Sez Park, Chennai, India

ELSEVIER

ACADEMIC PRESS
An imprint of Elsevier

Academic Press is an imprint of Elsevier
125 London Wall, London EC2Y 5AS, United Kingdom
525 B Street, Suite 1650, San Diego, CA 92101, United States
50 Hampshire Street, 5th Floor, Cambridge, MA 02139, United States
The Boulevard, Langford Lane, Kidlington, Oxford OX5 1GB, United Kingdom

Copyright © 2020 Elsevier Inc. All rights reserved.

No part of this publication may be reproduced or transmitted in any form or by any means, electronic or mechanical, including photocopying, recording, or any information storage and retrieval system, without permission in writing from the publisher. Details on how to seek permission, further information about the Publisher's permissions policies and our arrangements with organizations such as the Copyright Clearance Center and the Copyright Licensing Agency, can be found at our website: www.elsevier.com/permissions.

This book and the individual contributions contained in it are protected under copyright by the Publisher (other than as may be noted herein).

Notices
Knowledge and best practice in this field are constantly changing. As new research and experience broaden our understanding, changes in research methods, professional practices, or medical treatment may become necessary.

Practitioners and researchers must always rely on their own experience and knowledge in evaluating and using any information, methods, compounds, or experiments described herein. In using such information or methods they should be mindful of their own safety and the safety of others, including parties for whom they have a professional responsibility.

To the fullest extent of the law, neither the Publisher nor the authors, contributors, or editors, assume any liability for any injury and/or damage to persons or property as a matter of products liability, negligence or otherwise, or from any use or operation of any methods, products, instructions, or ideas contained in the material herein.

British Library Cataloguing-in-Publication Data
A catalogue record for this book is available from the British Library

Library of Congress Cataloging-in-Publication Data
A catalog record for this book is available from the Library of Congress

ISBN: 978-0-12-820728-4

For Information on all Academic Press publications
visit our website at https://www.elsevier.com/books-and-journals

Publisher: Andre Gerhard Wolff
Acquisitions Editor: Kattie Washington
Editorial Project Manager: Anna Dubnow
Production Project Manager: Maria Bernard
Cover Designer: Mark Rogers

Typeset by MPS Limited, Chennai, India

Working together to grow libraries in developing countries
www.elsevier.com • www.bookaid.org

Contents

List of contributors

Sadasivam Anbumani
Ecotoxicology Laboratory, Regulatory Toxicology Group, CSIR-Indian Institute of Toxicology Research, Lucknow, India; Academy of Scientific and Innovative Research (AcSIR), CSIR-Indian Institute of Toxicology Research, Lucknow, India

Pramila Bakthavachalam
HCL, Chennai, Tamil Nadu, India

Jesudas Balasubramanian
HCL, Chennai, Tamil Nadu, India

Nobel Bhasin
Department of Medicine, University of Chicago, Chicago, IL, United States

Logesh Chokkalingam
HCL America Inc., Sunnyvale, CA, United States

Bhagyashree Choudhari
Department of Pathology, PRADO, Preclinical Research and Development Organization, Private Limited, Pune, India

Shreya Dwivedi
Ecotoxicology Laboratory, Regulatory Toxicology Group, CSIR-Indian Institute of Toxicology Research, Lucknow, India

Krishna Gautam
Ecotoxicology Laboratory, Regulatory Toxicology Group, CSIR-Indian Institute of Toxicology Research, Lucknow, India; Academy of Scientific and Innovative Research (AcSIR), CSIR-Indian Institute of Toxicology Research, Lucknow, India

Mounika Gudeppu
HCL, Chennai, Tamil Nadu, India

Praveen Kumar Gupta
Department of Toxicology, PRADO, Preclinical Research and Development Organization, Private Limited, Pune, India

Shobana Navaneeethabalakrishnan
Department of Endocrinology, Dr. ALM Postgraduate Institute of Basic Medical Sciences, University of Madras, Chennai, India

Nandakumar Palani
HCL America Inc., Sunnyvale, CA, United States

Somnath Pandey
Radiation Oncology, Massachusetts General Hospital, Harvard Medical School, Boston, MA, United States

S. Priya
Department of Pharmacology, Sathyabama Dental College and Hospital, Chennai, India

T. Pugazhenthan
Department of Pharmacology, AIIMS Raipur, Chhattisgarh, India

Manish Ranjan
Department of Surgery, Northwestern University, Chicago, IL, United States

V. Sajitha
Department of Microbiology, AIIMS Raipur, Chhattisgarh, India

Thamizharasan Sampath
ACSMCH, DRMGR Educational & Research Institute, Chennai, Tamil Nadu, India

Monisha Saravanan
IQVIA, Bangalore, Karnataka, India

M. Sathish Babu
Department of Biochemistry, JIPMER Karaikal, Puducherry, India

Prakash Srinivasan Timiri Shanmugam
HCL America Inc., Sunnyvale, CA, United States

Rajeev Sharma
Department of Toxicology, PRADO, Preclinical Research and Development Organization, Private Limited, Pune, India

Dhirendra Singh
Pathology Laboratory, Regulatory Toxicology Group, CSIR-Indian Institute of Toxicology Research, Lucknow, India

Karnika Singh
OSU Comprehensive Cancer Center, Columbus, OH, United States

Sandhiya Thamizharasan
SDC, Saveetha Institute of Medical and Technical Sciences, Chennai, Tamil Nadu, India

Priya Gupta Vajrapu
Boston Medical Center, Boston, MA, United States

A.R. Vijayakumar
Department of Pharmacology, JIPMER Karaikal, Puducherry, India

Pralhad Wangikar
Director, PRADO, Preclinical Research and Development Organization, Private Limited, Pune, India

About the editors

Prakash Srinivasan Timiri Shanmugam, PhD is currently contracted as an SME—Biocompatibility at Baxter International, Inc. in Round Lake, IL, United States. He was previously contracted at Johnson & Johnson Medical Device Sector. He has an MSc and a PhD in the specialization of Pharmacology and Toxicology with Chemistry (interdisciplinary) from the University of Madras, Chennai, India and completed his postdoctoral research at Tulane University and LSUHSC-Shreveport, Louisiana. He has authored a book, contributed several book chapters, and published research articles in various peer-reviewed international journals and conference proceedings/abstracts.

Logesh Chokkalingam is a Group Project Manager at HCL Technologies in Raynham, MA, United States. He has a bachelor's degree in Mechanical Engineering from Vellore Institute of Technology and earned a Diploma in Tool and Die Making from NTTF for passing a specialized course in the design and manufacturing of press tools, injection molds, jigs, and fixtures. He is a Mechanical Engineer with specialized knowledge on design development, program management, medical device regulations, supply chain integration, portfolio optimization, asset transfer, verification testing and validation, and value engineering.

Pramila Bakthavachalam, PhD, FASC (AW), MRQA is a Technical Manager for Medical Devices, Toxicology, and Biocompatibility at HCL Technologies PVT Ltd in Chennai, India. She has a Doctorate in Environmental Toxicology/Biotechnology and MPhil in Microbiology. She has experience in regulatory toxicology as a scientist and in quality assurance. She was instrumental in establishing a preclinical testing facility and GLP certification at Sri Ramachandra University. She has worked with pharmaceuticals, cosmetics, medical devices, agrochemicals, industrial chemicals, and veterinary drugs. She has numerous publications in both national and international journals in various disciplines such as environmental toxicology, toxicology, and pharmacology.

CHAPTER ONE

Introduction to medical implants

Nandakumar Palani*
HCL America Inc., Sunnyvale, CA, United States
*Corresponding author

Abstract

This chapter mainly focuses on the history and evolution of the medical implants, materials used in biomedical implantable devices, and consideration for medical implant materials that discuss the ease of fabrication, biocompatibility, and flexibility. It also discusses their characteristics such as electrical, chemical, thermal, and mechanical behaviors with a combination of different materials/alloys/prosthetics as composites. Implantable devices reside in the human body/biological medium either temporarily or permanently, for the purpose of diagnostics, monitoring, or therapeutic purposes. With the unique responsiveness and design in terms of clinical needs, responsive polymers have been used to facilitate the deployment or removal of the devices with minimum damage to the host tissue, support function of current devices to treat ailments, deliver drugs, control infection, or monitor physiological factors or biomolecules. This chapter also reviews the use of responsive polymers as various implants and devices, starting with addressing the biocompatibility issue of responsive polymers. Application of responsive polymers is based on the areas on which it is applied, including ophthalmic devices, surgical devices, cardiovascular devices, orthopedic dental, breast, respiratory devices, urogenital devices, and implantable biosensors. The biocompatible implants used for medical implants still have some chronic effects on the human body.

Keywords: Medical implants; generation/evolution of medical implants; silicone gel; inflammation; capsular contracture; rupture and deflation; implant materials; biological medium; tissues; alloys; polymers; temporary and permanent implants; biocompatibility; biosensors; chronic effects; implantable devices; standards

1.1 Introduction to medical implants

1.1.1 What is a medical implant?

Medical implants are planted into a human body by surgery or naturally formed cavity and are planned to retain over a short or long period

Toxicological Aspects of Medical Device Implants.
DOI: https://doi.org/10.1016/B978-0-12-820728-4.00001-0
© 2020 Elsevier Inc.
All rights reserved.

depending upon the type of surgery. FDA came up with the standards to classify the devices that are placed in the human body regardless of the location and period also called as medical implants.

Implantable devices are partly human-made implants or natural implants that are fully introduced into the subject and planned to retain after the surgery for a period of time depending on the need.

It has been observed that around 10% of the people in the United States and around 6% of the people in industrial revolutionized countries have gone through the surgically medical implants for reconstructing the human body functions and attaining a better standard of life or increasing life span.

1.1.2 History of medical implants

In the olden days (in the late 1880s), body anatomy was improved by changing the size and shape of the breast. The materials used to fill in the breast were different forms made of synthetic materials, oil, rubber, ivory, and glass. Then, silicone and even injections were used to augment the breast.

Injecting liquid substances are the most used technique to augment the breast shape and size by using substances such as paraffin wax or oil and petroleum jelly. Later, silicone fluid was injected into the breast by some illegal practitioners. These methods caused severe damage to the human body including pain, skin color changing, infection to other parts of the body, breast disfigurement and breast loss, respiratory issues and pulmonary issues, liver damage, and even unconsciousness or death.

When the first silicone gel breast implant was introduced, it became popular even though there were many disadvantages; the silica gel is a gum with amorphous silica, which has a high modulus. These olden day implants are made of gel and thick outer shell, whereas the modern-day silicone rubber shell has a smooth surface and inside fluid with a sturdy silicone gel. The burst rates were low compared to other breast implants because of the strong shell. However, when the capsule shrinks, tightens, and compresses the breast implant, seepage complications occur.

To avoid the seepage and leaks, the implant is manufactured with inside partitions; this keeps the implant to hold the gel from sagging, and the holes/slits and layers are sealed with patches, holes, or slits to avoid leaks during manufacturing.

With the advancement of technology, thin implant shells with no gaps between one part and another are manufactured. When the first saline-filled implants emerged, they were heavy and easy to break, with splashing noise that was audible, and the deflation rate was very high; the manufacturing process involves volcanization to strengthen the product.

Around the 1980s, the thick shell implants were replaced with thin shells, but this caused high burst rates and seepages that led to deflation. The next-generation implants were made with soft shells and different gel fluids that caused the burst rates and seepages to be high. Later, polyurethane foam, which was introduced in the market, reduced the burst rates and was increasingly popular among most women who underwent implant with this polyurethane foam shell. This foam shell implant was discontinued around the 1990s owing to inflammation, fluid buildup, swelling, pain, and infection side effects.

Breast implant types during these years evolved with different substances and shells; some of them were temporary or permanent. The burst rates or seepage frequencies for the implants vary in percentage based on the manufacturers with different generations.

The new-generation implants have improved silicone-gel implants and saline implants with less deflate rates with the help of stronger shells, partition layers, and textures. This type of implants comes with deflation and rupture rates and less gel diffusion or seepage. As there were no proper standards for breast implant manufacturing in America, more than 200 types of breast implant models were manufactured by different manufacturers with a difference in materials, shapes, sizes, and gels. It is also estimated that over 8000 types of breast implants are manufactured by different manufacturers with different materials over the years.

The major implant manufacturers today use single-lumen implants that are filled with silicone gel. The cover or shell is made of silicon rubber, which is a kind of elastic material called elastomer, and the inside partition is coated with fluorosilicone to prevent silicone gel seepage or bleeding from inside. The outer shell has a textured surface that allows the tissue to grow on its surface, causing an inflammatory reaction. The growth of fibrous scar tissue which is made of collagen that forms around the medical implant, tightens the capsule and squeezes the implant material leading to capsular contraction.

The modern-generation implants are not sure to be continued to use; the analysis and study results from the FDA will lead to a new generation of implants. The history of use and information is very less about the saline implants which was quickly evolved to silicone-gel implants. The saline implants history and usage information is very less which was quickly evolved to silicone-gel based implants.

1.1.3 Medical implant types and materials for implants

Natural as well as artificial medical implants are placed inside the body. Some of the artificial implants are made from prosthetics metal, ceramic, and plastic, which are placed inside the body for soft and hard missing body parts. The natural implants that are made from tissues, bone, and skin are used to support the human body to live a normal life. The implants are mostly used for medication, monitoring, and providing support to organs.

Implants can be temporary or permanent based on their use; some can be removed when the purpose is solved, or it can be placed permanently to provide life support to the human patient. For example, some of the tissues, skin, hip implants, and knee implants are intended to be permanent to support the human patient. In contrast, screws that are used to repair broken bones or metal plates are temporary, and they can be removed when no longer needed by the human patient.

Most surgical procedures have very less recovery time and very less risks, and the risks involved in medical implants are mostly related to the placement, infection, and implant failure; if the implant is not working as intended, then there is a high risk of operating again. Some implants are allergic and infectious to certain human patients and cause infections. The materials used to manufacture the implants can cause bruises, swelling, pain, and redness at the surgical site or even after recovering from surgery. Some of the implants are expected to have some common effects on the human patient like infections and bruises that will be reduced once the human patient's body adapts the implant, but some are very high risks that damage other parts of the body.

The implant life span is considered that, over time, they could break or are not working as expected. This could result in additional surgeries to repair or replace the implant in the human patient body.

1.1.4 Implant materials and purpose

Materials used for implants

- Alloys
- Biosensor
- Titanium
- Prosthetics
- Polymer
- Biocompatibility
- Biomaterials

- Protein
- Tissues
- Stent

Implants and prosthetics

- Implantable cardioverter defibrillators (ICDs)/heart pacemakers
- Artificial hips—metal-on-metal hip implants
- Metallic screws, rods, plates, and artificial discs (bone fracture repair)
- Knee caps
- Eye contact lenses—phakic intraocular lenses
- Breast implants
- Cochlear implants
- Birth control implants (permanent)
- Mesh implants
- Intrauterine devices—urogynecologic surgical mesh implants
- Dental implants

1.1.4.1 Implants categories and application

1.1.4.1.1 Physical Sensing and neurology

Physical sensing and neurological implants are used for making the body parts behave as expected and to fix the disorders affecting the brain and sensing capability also other neuro disorders. They are majorly used for eye diseases and other visual impairments; hearing issues, and otosclerosis, as well as neurological diseases. Some of the examples are intraocular lens, cochlear implant and neurostimulator.

1.1.4.1.2 Heart and blood vessels

Cardiovascular implants are used in the case where the heart, blood vessels and valves are in disorder like narrowed, blocked. They are used to treat heart disease such as heart attack, cardiac arrhythmia, ventricular tachycardia, valvular heart disease, angina pectoris, and atherosclerosis. Some of the examples include the artificial heart valve, defibrillator, pacemaker, and coronary stent.

1.1.4.1.3 Orthopaedic

Orthopaedic implants help to function the body part it is intended for. The implants here are used to treat dislocated bones, fractures, tissue tear, spinal stenosis, and chronic pain. Some of the examples are plates, pins, rods and screws used to anchor fractured bones while they heal.

1.1.4.1.4 Electric

Electrical implants generate electric signals and stimulate the nerves which are used to relieve pain and stimulate nerves to do its function properly. The electric implant is embedded in the human patients neck with rheumatoid arthritics and sends the electrical signals to electrodes in the vagus nerve.

1.1.4.1.5 Contraception

Contraceptive implants are primarily used to prevent pregnancy and treat conditions such as non-pathological forms of menorrhagia. Some of the examples are copper- and hormone-based intrauterine devices.

1.1.4.1.6 Cosmetic

Body anatomy implants which are used to enhance the body parts to an acceptable aesthetic norm. Some of the examples are breast implant, nose prosthesis, ocular prosthesis, and injectable filler.

1.1.4.1.7 Other systems

Other organ disorder occurring in the body system, includes gastrointestinal, respiratory, and urological systems. Medical implants used to treat this type of disorders such as gastroesophageal reflux disease, gastroparesis, respiratory failure, sleep apnea, urinary and fecal incontinence, and erectile dysfunction. Some of the examples are LINX, gastric stimulator, nerve stimulator, neurostimulator, surgical mesh, and penile prosthesis.

1.1.5 Medical implants design considerations

1.1.5.1 Design and structure of implantable devices

The human body is formed by numerous bones, organs, tissues, and cells. The human body system differs from individual to individual and with the same body with time. The body system is organized differently for each human based on different factors; this makes difficult to design the structure common for all the human body. The medical implant design requires a lot of research, studies, and data to benchmark with no substantial existence of the human body. During the research and development phase, the designer has to meet the systematic and medical criticality of the human body. For example the monitoring medical implant during a research and development phase is able to handle the data in transmitting and receiving, but if there is a mismatch of data occurs due to the integrated module, which needs a substitute module involving substantial rework and redesign.

Actively working implantable devices such as blood pressure monitoring devices require an energy source for driving, data processing, and wireless communication. The power requirement for operation needs to be available as a battery with the right capacity that needs to be the integrated part of the device. There are difficulties in finding a matching battery for commercial use.

In addition, the performance of medical implant devices is considered. Implantable devices are planted when the patient needs it to the most and the performance factor is the most critical part of the design.

1.1.5.2 Implantable medical device energy source

The designing of power budget and power management for the implantable medical devices is a challenge with considerations on the size, capacity, and performance.

The input power source to the implantable medical devices are of two types:

1. One-timer batteries (single use)
2. Rechargeable batteries.

Pacemakers, ICDs, and sensors/stimulators use single-use batteries that are high-risk implantable devices planting into the human patient. Cochlear implants, replacement heart implants, and retinal prostheses use rechargeable batteries.

The single-use battery makes the implantable device a very high-risk device when there is no enough charge to power the device and the battery is replaced with a new one by operating the human patient. The available charge of the battery for the single-use battery is checked on a regular basis and monitored. There were new advancements in the rechargeable battery-powered implantable device like pacemakers that also lead to new developments in charging the device by an external magnetic field called wireless telemetry. There were both advantages and disadvantages with the wireless telemetry powering of the implantable device; when the distance between the inner and outer magnetic coils is far or relatively long, there is a considerable amount of reduction in the induced current that makes the device to malfunction.

Recent research is more focused on power generation by using any of the human body parts, physical or chemical or electrical existence in the human body, to resolve the power issue for implantable medical devices.

1.1.5.3 Data transfer and monitoring

The implantable medical devices are very critical systems that help the human patient to overcome the hardships such as vision impairment, hearing aid, cardiac issues, and small pain. This makes the importance of closely monitoring the implantable medical device. The data transfer and signals are done with wireless at some distance without the help of a wire. Even though the transfer efficiency differs with the type of data and volume of data. The wireless communication techniques are active and passive wireless communication medical devices that are developed and comparatively efficient. The CardioMEMS implantable medical device used for monitoring the heart rate uses a pressure sensor to collect and transfer the data to an external storage or monitoring system using an external transmitting and receiving antenna which is mounted in a close distance with a sensor that is inductively coupled. There are a few factors that affect the data that are mainly contributed by noise, which is produced during inductive coupling with other devices or metal elements in the surrounding environment system. As the power to make the sensors work is made by inductive coupling, the device works without a battery source; however, it is hard to continuously monitor and transfer with the inductive coupling energy that is not stable or continuous sometimes.

1.1.6 Biological environment/medium

When a medical implant is placed in a body that is made of foreign elements, it will undergo a chain of events with the biological medium. The interaction between the biological medium and the foreign object creates different events within a fraction of seconds the implant is in contact. This is a known fact for understanding the events that need to be controlled to some extent understanding the effects it has on the human body. Some of the key observations are reliable implants and less adverse effects on the body. It is very hard for the human body to accept the foreign object, and it will affect even the most recovery materials. In addition, the chemical and physical property of a material plays a vital role in the interaction with the biological environment.

1.1.6.1 Biocompatibility and sterilization

The medical implants placed inside or on the surface of the human body quickly react to the outside and inside environment that responds to the material surface of the device when it comes into contact. During the initial stage of the implant, blood and tissue proteins stick to or break through the materials that cause the body to react. If the abiotic material does not adapt to the cells and tissues, it makes it difficult for the system to be in place for a long term and this could result in infection or affecting other parts of the body.

The surface of the material is also considered to be treated or sterilized before going for a medical implant because it may have microorganisms. Medical implant materials should be sterilized to remove all the harmful microorganisms. There are various types of sterilization processes for medical implants that include dry heat, vapor/steam and wet, ethylene oxide (EtO), formaldehyde, hydrogen peroxide gas plasma (H_2O_2), sporicidal chemicals, irradiation (gamma), and electron beam. The US FDA recommends EtO, gamma radiation, and electron-beam sterilization for the Class III medical devices. Some of the medical device implants such as pacemaker, ICD, and cochlear implants actively operated are sealed with biocompatible materials. The biocompatible materials used to seal the implants are selected based on the sealing feasibility. Some of the biocompatible materials are made with the purest form of materials and alloys (titanium, noble metals, cobalt-based, titanium–niobium, nickel–cobalt–molybdenum), stainless steel, fused silica, glass, and some biocompatible and biostable polymers.

The selection of appropriate materials and development processes of a medical implant is the first to account for biocompatibility, biostability, and biofouling. What makes the material to be appropriate for fulfilling biofouling, biocompatibility, and biostability is as follows:

1. The characteristics of considered materials.
2. The material application conditions.

To consider the appropriate material, the characteristics of the material alone are not enough for selecting as an implant. The implant material has to be accompanied by the information of the biological environment it is planned to be planted and how the human body responds to foreign material that is placed. This is because the response of the human body varies based on individual to individual and their biological medium to medium. Even it varies with time and other environmental factors.

Example: The use of rubber/plasters material inside or on the body causes different effects like skin allergies, and rubber/plasters produce coagulation of the blood, which causes the blood clot.

The way the body adapts to the placement of the implant material is referred to as biocompatibility, and the way the implant material trained without adverse effects with the biological medium is known as biostability.

These examples tell us that without taking its application into consideration, any materials cannot be classified directly as biocompatible or biostable. In addition, the implant materials placed are reactive and easily infectious; the factors we have to consider is whether the reaction is acceptable or manageable and whether the reaction can be resolved or brought to a acceptable state.

The accumulation of micro- and macroorganisms or unintended accumulation of biological material causing structural or other functional deficiencies on the medical implant is called biofouling.

The US FDA provides a list of raw components that, when combined, may lead to an "FDA compliant" material and it does not directly approve a material.

ISO 10993-5, the International Standard for cytotoxicity tests for the biological evaluation of medical devices, provides the contents that talk about biocompatibility.

1.1.6.2 Corrosion environment

The biological medium is reactive and complex that will affect the most inert materials. The issue faced is how to manage the chemical effect to the extent that it damages or impairs the medical implant functionality or causes damage to the human body.

The medical implants must be able to withstand the biological environment of the human body for a long term without any adverse effects. The medical implants will leach ions into the body and cause leaching. There are a few metals or alloys such as stainless steels, cobalt—chromium alloys, and nitinol are resistant against localized corrosion both in vitro and in vivo.

The chemical degradation of materials or corrosion is commonly associated with metals but affects all classes of materials, including polymers and ceramics. The medical implants that are placed inside react with the biological medium and make the material to corrode by affecting the surface of the material. Corrosion is caused as a result of electrochemical oxidation or the loss of electrons from one substance to an oxidizing agent.

Metals and alloys have been widely used as implants, most commonly in dentistry and orthopedic. The metals were slowly replaced with alloys over the years. Titanium is the purest and most resistive metal to corrosion, but still, it undergoes chemical reactions with very less impact either to the implant or the host.

The other mechanisms for corrosion resistance are passivation, which is applying oxide film on the material. The types of corrosion of the materials used are as follows:

1. Pitting corrosion
2. Crevice generation
3. Galvanic corrosion
4. Corrosion fatigue
5. Fretting corrosion
6. Stress corrosion
7. Intergranular corrosion

The polymers also undergo degradation in the human body. The most common one is hydrolysis. Polymers suffer degradation, and they do not lead to breakdown but cause effects in their mechanical properties. When the biological medium is in contact with the material, it absorbs water or other biological molecules and undergoes changes in elasticity or changes the implant performance.

Other than the reliability of the implant, there are other consequences to the host human body diffusion breakdown products called as leaching. Leaching is the diffusion of small molecules from the material. Leaching is closely related to corrosion; the by-products of the corrosion are released into the human body with adverse effects. Example: the release of iron, chromium, and nickel ions as a result of the corrosion of surgical stainless steel.

Leaching is a known problem in medical implants like breast implants, where silicone gel can seep through the small pores on the membrane. Although the effects are minor, it is important to identify the leaching and consider while designing for the implants. In addition, intentional leaching of drug additives can be used as a control tool for the inflammatory response.

1.1.6.3 Medical implant device stability

When a medical implant material does not undergo oxidation or reduction under operating conditions, it is said to be electrochemically stable. The electrochemical characterization is done using an electroanalytical method called cyclic voltammetry. This method consists of applying a voltage to the material with the reference electrode, and the resulting current is measured by a counter electrode. The voltammetry scan produces a current versus voltage plot and is plotted as a graph by checking the voltage for which the current is very low. This plot shows current peaks that correspond to the electron exchange seen in oxidation or reduction; the gap within which no peaks are seen and is therefore defined as the electrochemical window. The wider this window, the greater electrochemical stability the material possesses.

A pot (potentiostat) is used to scan the voltage applied, which is driven by an operational amplifier to minimize the voltage drop. Structural materials like packaging surfaces should do the work in avoiding these peaks for getting the stability.

The oxidation or reduction reactions are not avoided always. The material relies on oxidation or reduction reactions to solve the purpose in an implant: stimulation electrodes need to exchange electric currents with the ionic medium.

1.1.6.4 Inflammatory response and process

The injury caused by the medical implantation of a foreign object unfolds a chain of events and attempts to eliminate or neutralize the invader. In most cases, the implant introduction in the human body will disturb the vascular system, even if it happens at the capillary level and the blood–barrier interface level resulting in a host of defense agents.

When the implant placement is not accepted by the human body and it initiates acute inflammation reaction, this inflammatory response cause the cells significant damage.

It is possible to control to some extent the adsorption of proteins at the early stages of the inflammatory process. The polyethylene glycol has the effect to reduce the absorption of proteins. However, the polyethylene glycol easily tends to oxidize quickly upon implantation, and there are other robust solutions that are adopted during recent years, like tetraglyme, which yields a cross-linked structure similar to polyethylene glycol. This also has an important role in preventing the formation of biofilm.

Another way to prevent the early inflammatory response is through the elution of an antiinflammatory drug immobilized to the implant surface. This can be done by using corticosteroids (e.g., hydrocortisone), which are involved in the metabolism of carbohydrates, proteins, and fats, and have antiinflammatory activity.

The medical implant placement technique also has a significant impact on the inflammatory reaction. There are some good surgical technique needs to be followed during implantation to reduce the damage to the tissue as much as possible, and the blood–barrier interface has a very less impact.

1.1.6.5 Chronic inflammation and mechanical forces

Chronic inflammation generally develops as part of the sequence of cellular events following acute inflammation. Chronic inflammation is induced by mechanical stress from the implants, caused by the movement of the fibrous tissue on the implant or its parts.

The chronic inflammation is induced by mechanical stress from the implants. This stress releases inflammatory mediators and matrix enzymes and ends up degrading the extracellular matrix.

Mechanically stressed monocytes can induce other unstressed tissue and cells to undergo the remodeling of the structure. These changes will end up in the change of tissue framework with adverse effects to the implant and to the human body system.

Biological response to debris

1. Polyethylene debris
2. Metallic debris
3. Ceramic debris
4. Polymethylmethacrylate debris

The debris are the outcome of mechanical wear from the medical implant into the body.

The evolution of materials that are used to manufacture the medical implants uses different structures like highly texturized surfaces, by using materials such as carbon nanotube electrodes that have long-term outcomes. Debris by itself stimulates the inflammatory response, and the severity of the inflammation depends on the debris size, shape, and composition. Debris size ranges from 10 μm, and it will undergo phagocytosis by macrophages. In addition, they can also present antigens to T cells and initiate inflammation by releasing molecules (known as cytokines), leading to a more widespread reaction. This depends largely on the amount of debris.

1.1.7 Standards for medical implants

ISO 14708-1: 2014—Implants for surgery—Active implantable medical devices (ISO)

ISO 14708 specifies general requirements for active implantable medical devices to provide basic assurance of safety for both patients and users.

For particular types of active implantable medical devices, the general requirements can be supplemented or modified by the requirements of other parts of ISO 14708. A requirement of a particular part of ISO

14708 takes priority over the corresponding requirement of this general part of ISO 14708. Where particular parts of ISO 14708 exist, this general part of ISO 14708 is not intended to be used alone. Special care is required when applying this general part of ISO 14708 alone to active implantable medical devices for which no particular International Standard has yet been published.

ISO 14708 consists of the following parts, under the general title Implants for surgery—Active implantable medical devices:

- Part 1: Implants for surgery—Active implantable medical devices—Part 1: General requirements for safety, marking, and for information to be provided by the manufacturer
- Part 2: Cardiac pacemakers
- Part 3: Implantable neurostimulators
- Part 4: Implantable infusion pumps
- Part 5: Circulatory support devices
- Part 6: Particular requirements for active implantable medical devices intended to treat tachyarrhythmia (including implantable defibrillators)
- Part 7: Particular requirements for cochlear implant systems

ISO 8828:2014—Implants for surgery—Guidance on care and handling of orthopedic implants

ISO 8828:2014 specifies the recommended procedures for handling orthopedic implants, hereafter called as implants, from receipt at the hospital until they are implanted or discarded.

This guidance applies to implants (such as currently used metal, ceramic, or polymeric implants) and also to acrylic resin and other bone cement.

This guidance does not apply to the implant manufacturer. However, it contains references to the stocking of implants that can be useful for manufacturers and especially for third-party suppliers.

Some of the standards tested (Standards)

ISO 11135-1:2007 Sterilization of healthcare products—Ethylene oxide—Part 1: Requirements for development, validation and routine control of a sterilization process for medical devices

ISO 10993-4:2002 Biological evaluation of medical devices—Part 4: Selection of tests for interactions with blood

ISO 10993-5:2009 Biological evaluation of medical devices—Part 5: Tests for in vitro cytotoxicity

ISO 10993-6:2007 Biological evaluation of medical devices—Part 6: Tests for local effects after implantation

ISO 10993-10:2010 Biological evaluation of medical devices—Part 10: Tests for irritation and skin sensitization

ISO 10993-11:2006 Biological evaluation of medical devices—Part 11: Tests for systemic toxicity

Benefits to audience

This book helps to understand the significance of medical implants used in the human body and how it helps the human body to regenerate/restore the functionality. In addition, it helps the audience to understand the background of the medical implants' history and how they got evolved with electrical, mechanical, thermal, and natural implants that are used in today's modern world.

Further reading

[1] Greatbatch W, Holmes CF. History of implantable devices.
[2] Williams DF. On the mechanisms of biocompatibility. Biomaterials.
[3] Bruck SD. Biostability of materials and implants.
[4] <https://www.sciencedirect.com/topics/medicine-and-dentistry/implant>.
[5] <https://www.ncbi.nlm.nih.gov/pmc/articles/PMC3797898/>.
[6] <https://link.springer.com/chapter/10.1007%2F978-981-10-5607-9_8>.
[7] <https://www.sciencedirect.com/science/article/pii/B9781845699871500016?via%3Dihub>.
[8] <https://www.e-sciencecentral.org/articles/SC000000589>.
[9] <https://www.ncbi.nlm.nih.gov/books/NBK44775/>.

SECTION I

Toxicological Effects of Implants

CHAPTER TWO

Dermatology/cosmetics

Karnika Singh*
OSU Comprehensive Cancer Center, Columbus, OH, United States
*Corresponding author

Abstract

With increasing modernization, people's desire to be best in all fronts has led to a boom in the cosmetic implant industry. Earlier cosmetic implants were considered as an act of improving visual appeal for people in show business. However, today with increasing competition and the emphasis on overall personality, people are going for cosmetic implants as a measure to improve their appearance. These include subdermal or transdermal implants of substances like silicone or injections of silicone or body fat into body cavities for reshaping. The most common procedures for cosmetic implant surgery are pectoral and gluteal augmentation. However, it is recommended to consult a cosmetic implant surgeon before considering any cosmetic enhancements but with the upcoming body modification artists and their eccentric creativity, the range of body alterations has expanded. This has led to the repurposing of body modification from the improvement of appearance to create a statement in the most unusual way. Skin piercing and eyeball implants to wear decorative jewelry are just some of the examples. It should be highlighted that these procedures whether done for therapeutic purposes or for increasing aesthetic appeal have medical concerns that require consideration. The risks range from ordinary discomfort and swelling to more severe conditions like lung collapse and permanent tissue damage. Therefore expert consultation and heavy precautions are warranted to avoid any complications after surgery. However, changing oneself especially physically should be the last option in one's list, as loving yourself for what you are is the best approach to a healthy life.

Keywords: Dermal implants; breast implants; silicone implants; gluteal augmentation; body modification; hair transplant; magnetic resonance imaging

2.1 Introduction

The market for cosmetic implant procedures is as expanding as ever. According to 2018 estimates, 17.7 million cosmetic procedures were performed in the United States alone, which was 2% more than in 2017 and

Toxicological Aspects of Medical Device Implants.
DOI: https://doi.org/10.1016/B978-0-12-820728-4.00002-2
© 2020 Elsevier Inc.
All rights reserved.

163% more from 2000 [1]. It has been estimated that the cosmetic implant surgery market would grow up to 9–10 billion USD by the year 2022 [2]. These statistical figures indicate an increased interest of people in aesthetics. Besides common reasons like improving the appearance and boosting confidence, the FDA approved cosmetic enhancers like dermal fillers (Juvederm), botox injections, and breast implants have invigorated trust among the public for these procedures. In addition, body modification artists have started a new trend of creating designs under/on the skin using implant material that is attracting the attention of people as well. This chapter highlights key features about these implants and things to consider before going under the knife.

2.2 Dermal implants

The purpose of dermal implants is to give a body part more rounder or fuller appearance. This may be done for the purpose of reconstruction or increasing the aesthetic appeal. Pectoral and gluteal implants are popular in both males and females. The most common form of pectoral augmentation considered by people is breast implantation. In addition to improving one's appearance, medical reasons also prompt people to go for breast implantation. According to the American Society of Plastic Surgeons, 313,735 breast augmentation procedures and 101,657 breast reconstruction surgeries were performed in the United States amounting to a 48% and 29% increase in respective procedures as of 2000 [1]. In women, breast cancer is the most common motivator of breast reconstruction whereas in men some less commonly occurring congenital or acquired deformities of the chest wall like unilateral congenital absence of the pectoral muscle (Poland syndrome), pectoral denervation due to brachial plexus injury, sports muscle injury, pectus excavatum, and postsurgical chest wall deformities drive breast restoration. Today, the dermal implants comprise silicone and body fat. The silicone is an inert polymer made of repeating units of alternating silicon (Si) and oxygen (O) atoms. This repeating unit is known as siloxane (--Si–O–Si–O--), which has other organic elements like hydrogen (H) and carbon (C) bonded with Si. The presence of these organic elements actually allows silicone to be synthesized into a variety of forms such as liquid, gel, and rubber. The gel form is the one of which is widely used in medical science as a material for bandages and dressings, implants for breasts, testicle, chest, etc., and also in contact lenses. The first silicone implant was developed by Cronin and Gerow in 1961. Since then, the silicone implants have undergone considerable improvements as far as safety is concerned [3]. The FDA first approved the use of silicone breast implants in 2000. However, this approval was for the saline-filled implants for augmentation in women over the age of 18 and reconstruction in women of any age. The saline-filled breast implant contains sterile saltwater in a silicone shell. The water can actually be seen and felt under the thin skin that offers the advantage of postoperative adjustments. The silicone-based saline breast implants are also used in "revision surgeries" to alter the outcome of the initial surgical procedure. Later in November 2006, the FDA approved the silicone gel implants for breast augmentation in women of 22 years and above and breast reconstruction in women of all ages. Similar to saline-filled implants, these implants are filled with silicone gel. However, these implants can generate a more natural feel and look of the breast because of the viscous nature of this material. An image of breast implants is shown in Fig. 2.1.

Silicone implants have shown most use in breast reconstruction therapy done usually after tumor removal. This cosmetic procedure is employed to restore the patient's confidence and elevate their spirits. These implants are available in different shapes and sizes and can also be

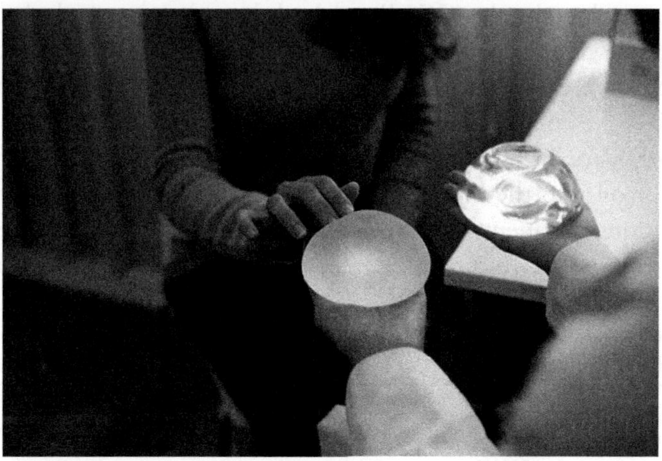

Figure 2.1 Silicone (left) and saline (right) breast implants. *Reproduced with permission from American Society of Plastic Surgeons.*

configured custom to suit patient needs. Pectoral implants can also be made of silicone rubber with a soft and spongy appearance. These are preferred for use in chest augmentation of men [4]. The pectoral augmentation can cause seroma, hematoma, implant displacement, infection, capsular retraction due to allergic reactions, conspicuous implant edges, or imprecise correction. However, hollow implants or implants with a textured surface or surgical stitching have been reported to have less implant rearrangement.

Gluteal augmentation is another popular application of silicone implants. FDA has approved only the solid silicone elastomer implants for buttock augmentation. Solid silicone elastomer possesses the capability to increase gluteal tone in patients with ptosis, congenital or acquired gluteal deformities, and asymmetry. However, in Mexico and South America, cohesive silicone gel is more favored than solid silicone elastomer. Surgery is the favored method of inserting implants into the gluteal region. Four sites are commonly known for implant placement: subcutaneous, subfascial, intramuscular, and submuscular regions. Surgical complications vary by the site of implantation. Seroma, dehiscence, infection, implant visibility, and implant displacement are associated with superficial implant placement. Submuscular implants contain the risk of damaging the sciatic nerve and is therefore rarely put. In addition, because of limitations accompanied by the submuscular anatomy, only small implants are placed in this location that should not extend beyond the lower edge of the pyramidal muscle, usually causing a "double-buttock" appearance. Intramuscular placement is done by the "XYZ" method these days in which the gluteus maximus muscle is split into two equal halves for ideal implant placement. This procedure is known to have the lowest complication rate. Table 2.1 summarizes the complication rate associated with each site [4].

In early days, breast augmentation was done by injecting materials like paraffin or oil into the breast tissue. Obviously, the use of paraffin led to complications in patients after 5–10 years of use. These ranged from pulmonary embolism, ulceration, infection, necrosis, etc., which often

Table 2.1 Complication rate at each site of gluteal implantation.

Site	Percentage
Intramuscular	18
Subfacial	55
Intramuscular XYZ	13
Submuscular	18

culminated in breast amputation. This led to the usage of other fascinating substances such as ivory, glass balls, and rubber for implantation in the early and mid-1900s. Later, injectable liquid silicone and polyacrylamide hydrogel came into practice. Liquid silicone was injected in combination with olive oil (popularly known as "Sakurai formula" in Japan) to minimize complications. However, the FDA banned the use of injectable silicone in 1992 due to its lack of effectiveness and safety concerns. Interestingly, due to significant improvements in silicone implants, they have become one of the most widely used materials for dermal implantation, as discussed earlier. The hydrophilic polyacrylamide gel was designed in Ukraine around the 1980s. It is an atoxic and stable material, made of a nonabsorbable sterile watery gel composed of 2.5% cross-linked polyacrylamide and nonpyrogenic water. Hydrophilic polyacrylamide is still used today in China and Iran for facial and breast augmentation even though they cause some serious cutaneous complications like skin induration and chest pain. Other associated problems include infection, chemical migration, granular atrophy, and necrosis [5].

Another method to alter body appearance is to utilize body fat as a dermal implant. In this procedure, the adipose tissue from the fat rich parts of the body (like thigh) is collected (termed as lipoaspirate) and used to reshape another area. This process is known as the autologous fat transfer or lipofilling. In 1893, Neuber used the fat grafts to fill the scars on the face. Czerny described the use of fat tissue in breast reconstruction after tumor removal in 1895. Van der Meulen first treated diaphragmatic hernia by autologous fat grafting in 1889. Soon many reports followed addressing the use of fat grafts for treatment and reconstruction of different body parts. Arpad and Giorgio Fischer developed the procedure of liposuction in 1975, which utilized a blunt hollow cannula and suctioning from multiple incision sites. This technique was later modified by Illouz in 1977 to decrease the hemorrhagic risk associated with it. The autologous fat transfer has undergone improvements over time in its safety and technique. Since then, it has found use in both aesthetic and medical procedures making them popular in plastic surgeons especially from the 1980s [6,7]. The body fat can be considered an "ideal dermal filler" because of its ready availability, ease of collection, little donor-site morbidity, repeatability of use, and economical and biocompatible at the same time (as it comes out of the person's own body). In 2018 alone, 45,360 cases of fat fillers were recorded in the United States (16% more than 2017). The clinical applications of autologous fat transfer range from breast reconstruction, clearance of painful scar contractures, and treatment of burn scars and radio dermatitis, cleft lip and palate surgery, orbital reconstruction, and treatment of painful neuromas. It has also been useful in the surgery of temporomandibular joint, for treatment of ankylosis and preventing the fibrosis and heterotopic ossification around total joint prosthesis; in neurosurgery for spine and skull base, treat or prevent CSF leakage, for obliteration of ear, frontal sinus cavities, and vocal cord augmentation. In aesthetic surgery, it is utilized in facial and hand revival, rhinoplasty, and breast and gluteal augmentation.

Although fat transfer seems safe from medical point of view, it can lead to some minimal complications such as bruising, swelling, pain, infection, necrosis, and calcification. It has also been reported that the fat grafts tend to get reabsorbed to about 70% of their volume in about a year's time. This has led to the lower success rate of the autologous fat grafting and caused reservations among the physicians about the whole methodology of fat grafting. Coleman's studies are considered a landmark in the field of autologous fat transfer. His studies reported that the success of fat grafting depends on the technique employed. According to his research, harvesting, refinement, and transfer of subcutaneous tissue to provide pure and undamaged fat parcels are important for successful fat grafting. The surgeon must also infiltrate the processed fat parcels into the recipient site so that they survive conclusively and evenly integrate into the host tissues and provide the asked structural adjustment. All these can be achieved by applying a small amount of fat tissue, as duly noted by Neuber in 1893 where he observed that small and sufficient grafts produced exceptional aesthetic outcomes [8].

2.3 Body modifications by implants

As can be gleaned from the term "body modification," the application of implants in this context is purely aesthetic. The idea is not just to look good but stand out in the most unforgettable way. This is an upcoming application of dermal implants where these materials are exploited for decorative purposes. These implants are placed in either subdermal or transdermal manner and are usually made of silicone or metals. These procedures are usually performed by the body modification artists but sometimes cosmetic surgeons may also be involved. Body piercing and tattoos are other known ways of body modification but "dermal implants" are going to be the focus of this section.

2.3.1 Subdermal implants

Subdermal body implants are placed under the skin through a minimally invasive procedure. Pacemakers and long-acting contraceptive implants are some known examples of subdermal implants that are introduced under the skin for respective medical conditions. Many tribes are also known to put stones or metals under the skin for ritualistic reasons. Similarly, the material for body modification is placed under the skin such that it can heal around the implant strengthening the foundation, giving rise to a pushed-up design. Steve Haworth is considered to be the pioneer of creating the 3D design by dermal implants. He created his first design in 1994 at his shop in Phoenix, AZ. His initial choice of material was surgical steel, later Teflon and carved silicone. However, now he uses implant grade silicone produced as injectable created by him. Although the procedure of subdermal implantation is well established, the lack of certified personnel to perform body modification poses a risk. Usually, these procedures are performed in poorly sterilized conditions that prompt infections. In addition, lack of training can cause nerve damage, bruising, and fluid retention at the site of implant. Other complications like implant rejection can also happen if the implant grade silicone is not used. Allergic reactions and tissue resorption can also occur. Some examples of dermal implants are shown below (Fig. 2.2).

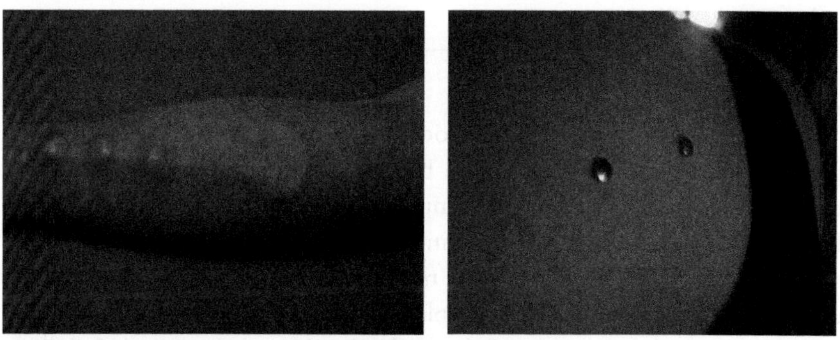

Figure 2.2 A subdermal implant (left): balls under the skin and a transdermal implant (right): beads on the back. *Courtesy Wikimedia commons.*

2.3.2 Transdermal implants

In this kind of implant, the object is inserted halfway below the skin and the rest half is visible from outside (Fig. 2.2). These types of implants are more commonly seen and resemble piercing. The procedure is known as dermal punching such that the stud or other jewelry material is placed inside the skin by digging a hole and then exposed by the dermal puncher. The tissue is then allowed to heal around the metal for proper placement. Because of this reason, the embedded jewelry item (studs, pins, rings etc.) usually have a hole in it for skin to grow through it providing a proper grip. As can be expected, this procedure requires skill and therefore can lead to complications if not done properly. It is not surprising that this procedure is banned in certain countries. Healing in this kind of implantation can be lengthy and the person has to take great care for it to work. First transdermal implant is reported to be done again by Steve Haworth in 1996. His famous creation is known as the "metal Mohawk," which his client carried for almost a decade. Infections are the commonest side effects associated with transdermal implants as the site of the implant is exposed to the environment. Other drawbacks are implant rejection, muscle and bone damage, scarring, bubbling, bruising, migration, and allergic reactions. Needless to say, the transdermal implants have to be removed at some point in person's life because of the body's ever-changing physiology and aging. Interestingly medical conditions, which prompt magnetic resonance imaging (MRI), could also initiate a compulsory implant removal. This may require a major surgery to remove all the scarred tissue near the implant, leaving a noticeable scar behind.

2.4 Hair transplant

As the name suggests, the procedure of hair transplant entails transplanting hair from one part of the body to another. It is often confused that in hair transplant fake hair is implanted into the scalp. The fact is that hair from one part of the body is "implanted" into another part (often the scalp) to achieve fuller hair in that region, and this cosmetic procedure is discussed in this chapter. Hair transplant is a surgical procedure that is performed to populate an area of the body that is experiencing hair loss to make that part of the body look hairy. Hair transplant is very common among men who have male pattern baldness. It is a genetic condition in which hair loss starts from the temples or the crown of the head. Complete hair loss is rare, and hairs at the rear and side of the head remains. Female pattern baldness also exists but is fairly uncommon. Other conditions like thinning of hair, lowering of hairline, etc. also inspire hair transplantation.

In brief, hair transplant entails removing small or large pieces of hair containing scalp to be used as grafts later. These grafts are then inserted onto the bald areas of the scalp or the part where hairs are thin. There are two common procedures that are followed for hair transplantation: follicular unit strip surgery (FUSS) and follicular unit extraction (FUE). In the FUSS process, a strip of skin containing hair, usually 6–10 inches in size, is removed from the back of the head. This strip is then divided into tiny grafts before insertion. This division depends on different factors such as hair type, quality, color, and size of the area to be implanted. The FUE procedure requires shaving of the back of the head, and hair follicles are isolated one by one. The sites of graft isolation that remain covered by the existing hair, therefore, are not visible. After the isolation of grafts, they are placed into the holes created in the area of interest. It should be noted that the procedure of hair transplant is long and therefore can take from 4 to 8 hours depending on the size of the transplant. In addition, it should be kept in mind that multiple sittings might be required to achieve complete coverage of the target area. In addition, the results of hair transplant are visible only 6 months after the procedure. Recently, eyebrows have emerged as another popular site for hair transplantation. In this case, hair from the patient's leg, beard, or chest are utilized as donors.

As can be expected, after hair transplant, the scalp is left tender and therefore the surgeons prescribe pain medications after this procedure. It may also require for the patient to take antibiotics or antiinflammatory medication as well. This is further supplemented with a hair-growing drug minoxidil (Rogaine). As this procedure is tricky and costly, it should be performed only by skilled and experienced surgeons. Although hair transplant is a relatively low-risk procedure, there are still several risks associated with it. Bleeding and infection are some general complications along with scarring and abnormal hair growth. Hair loss of the already existing hair is also noticed, but they usually reappear. Numbness of the treated areas of the scalp is also observed. More severe side effects include folliculitis, that is, inflammation of the hair follicles. This condition can be treated with medication. It is recommended to discuss the possible risks of hair transplantation with your surgeon, as each person is different in their requirements and conditions prompting hair transplant.

2.5 MRI as a tool for imaging implants

The need for MRI can arise anytime, whether it is due to an illness or the need to remove or readjust the cosmetic implant itself. Interestingly, sometimes the latter is necessary to achieve the former. Most of the implants used today are compatible with imaging as long as the manufacturer's conditions are met. The patients with implants can be imaged after changing the imaging conditions or just switching the implant to the setting specific to MRI. Companies like Medtronic and Boston Scientific manufacture implants that are MRI grade and provide guidelines for MRI scanning conditions for their implants. FDA has also published guidelines for imaging of implants; first, the process of screening at the site of implant needs to be followed; second, the manufacturer and model of the implanted device needs to be identified before the imaging; third, the MRI safety information on the device label needs to be understood. There are three kinds of safety warnings associated with implants: MR safe, MR conditional, and MR unsafe (Fig. 2.3). The MR safe devices have no scanning restrictions whatsoever. The MR conditional devices, however, require the MRI machine to meet certain conditions to scan the implant-bearing patient. The MR unsafe devices as the name suggests cannot and should not be scanned. Usually, the devices for which this safety information is unavailable are considered MR unsafe by default.

Figure 2.3 The MR safety signs on implants. *From FDA.*

The technologist usually collects information on the patient's implant and ensures that all conditions are met. After MRI, the patient is assessed for any discomfort or injuries and the device is checked for its function.

In cosmetic implants, female breast reconstruction is studied mostly by this technique [9]. The MRI is performed on a high field strength magnet because it can improve or reduce the signal strength from silicone, water, or fat. The silicone-saturated images usually produce a hyperintense water signal with suppressed silicone. Intravenous contrast is preferred when the integrity of the breast implant is being evaluated. There are several signs of definitive implant rupture that can be seen on MRI. First signs are the subcapsular lines, which signify intracapsular rupture. They look like definite hypotenuse lines that are outlined by silicone signals in continuation with the implant shell. Extravasation of silicone into the neighboring tissues can be visualized as free silicone, which happens when the integrity of the capsular shell is lost. Another sign is known as the "linguine sign," which represents the collapse of the silicone elastomer in the implant shell. It is composed of floating low-intensity curvilinear lines resembling the linguine noodles hence the name. Railroad track sign is other sign that looks like paired parallel lines in the subcapsule of the silicone gel.

2.6 Cosmetic surgeon as a career

Plastic surgery has been around since ancient times. The first record of plastic surgery comes from India where the Hindu surgeon Susrata performed rhinoplasty (nose reconstruction) in around 500 BCE where he used a flap of the forehead skin and created a new nose. This method was later adapted in the Arabic in CE 700 and English in the 1700s. This procedure was first repurposed for cosmetic improvements in 1898. Today, this "nose job" is very popular not only in the entertainment industry but also in the general public. With the recent boom in the cosmetic industry, cosmetic surgeon is a career path that is gaining popularity among medical personnel. It is not only in high demand but also provides an opportunity to showcase your creativity. Although the term plastic surgeons and cosmetic surgeons are used interchangeably, it should be noted that not all plastic surgeons are cosmetic surgeons. A doctor needs to be highly specialized in specific cosmetic procedures to perform a respective cosmetic surgery. The 2-year fellowship program in cosmetic surgery is considered critical in this field as it provides the doctors with the opportunity to get the required clinical exposure and training. After performing 50 or so documented cosmetic procedures, the plastic surgeons can get their certification from the American Board of Cosmetic Surgery by giving an exact 2-day test. Once the certification is obtained one can go for either private practice or join an established surgeon. Another benefit of cosmetic surgeries is that they do not demand emergency services thus allowing for flexible working hours for the surgeon.

2.7 Considerations before cosmetic procedures

In the earlier sections, the complications associated with various procedures have been specified. They suggest that as appealing these cosmetic procedures are, they possess health risks that can be permanently harmful. They not only lead to health problems but also can ironically deform the body in an irreversible way. Therefore careful considerations are warranted before undertaking any such procedure. It cannot be more emphasized that these processes are meant for extreme conditions such as accidents and should be opted only when no other options are left. However, in current times, changing appearance has just become another accessory where people either get their body parts altered or create a new one altogether (through body modification). Cosmetic surgery provides an easy path to the desired body image.

However, there are several ways that can be attempted before going under the knife. One is obviously exercise; by this way, one can shape and tone their calves, buttock, chest, etc. This takes a longer time but it makes you healthier in the process. Other way is weight gain; thin people have a thinner face and, small buttocks and chest. Eating the right food can lead to weight gain in the right areas making your body look more full and curvy. However, the easiest way of all is accepting yourself as it is and embracing the way God has made you. It means that one should not worry about the cosmetic looks but at the same time maintain a healthy lifestyle. This can be exemplified by the recent inclusion of plus-sized models in the modeling industry. These models are neither size 0 nor possess the perfect figure, but they are equally pretty and fit. They have even appeared on the cover of fashion magazines and are considered to be the ambassadors of an alternate body image.

To summarize, cosmetic surgeries should be considered as the last resort and before doing so all the risks should be weighed and understood.

References

[1] 2018 Plastic Surgery Statistics.

[2] Global Cosmetic Implant Market 2019 Industry Size, Growth, Segments, Revenue, Manufacturers and 2025 Forecast Research Report 2019. Available from: <http://www.industryresearch.co/enquiry/request-sample/13992136>.

[3] Gabriel A, Maxwell GP. The evolution of breast implants. Clin Plast Surg 2015;42(4):399–404.

[4] Yahyavi-Firouz-Abadi N, Menias CO, Bhalla S, Siegel C, Gayer G, Katz DS. Imaging of cosmetic plastic procedures and implants in the body and their potential complications. AJR Am J Roentgenol 2015;204(4):707–15.

[5] Chopra S, Marucci D. Cutaneous complications associated with breast augmentation: a review. Int J Womens Dermatol 2019;5(1):73–7.

[6] Bellini E, Grieco MP, Raposio E. The science behind autologous fat grafting. Ann Med Surg (Lond) 2017;24:65–73.

[7] Zielins ER, Brett EA, Longaker MT, Wan DC. Autologous fat grafting: the science behind the surgery. Aesthet Surg J 2016;36(4):488–96.

[8] Simonacci F, Bertozzi N, Grieco MP, Grignaffini E, Raposio E. Procedure, applications, and outcomes of autologous fat grafting. Ann Med Surg (Lond) 2017;20:49–60.

[9] Wiedenhoefer JF, Shahid H, Dornbluth C, Otto P, Kist K. MR imaging of breast implants: useful information for the interpreting radiologist. Appl Radiobiol 2015;10(44):18–24.

CHAPTER THREE

Ophthalmology and Otorhinolaryngology

A.R. Vijayakumar[1,*], T. Pugazhenthan[2], M. Sathish Babu[3] and V. Sajitha[4]
[1]Department of Pharmacology, JIPMER Karaikal, Puducherry, India
[2]Department of Pharmacology, AIIMS Raipur, Chhattisgarh, India
[3]Department of Biochemistry, JIPMER Karaikal, Puducherry, India
[4]Department of Microbiology, AIIMS Raipur, Chhattisgarh, India
*Corresponding author

Abstract

The medical device implants play an important role in the eye as well as ear, nose, and throat in physiological as well as pathological conditions. In ophthalmology, right from the external structure of the eye to the interior, various implants were used. They are the intraocular lens, corneal implants, glaucoma surgical implants, orbital implants, implants used in the posterior chambers, diagnostics, lasers, solution-filled containers, surgical instruments, stents, silicon tubes, and tubes in lachrymal structure for dry eye. Similarly, a wide range of Ear, Nose, Throat (ENT) implants was used in the external, middle, and inner ear pathology correction and for replacing the destroyed bony structures. Some were Grommet, Teflon Grommet, Teflon Ventilation Tube, Titanium Grommet, Titanium Ventilation Tube, T Tube Ventilation Tube, T Tube Grommet, Kurz Clip Piston, Kurz Soft Clip Piston, Soft Clip Piston, Grace Medical Piston, Gyrus Piston, Kurz Torp, Kurz Porp, Ossicular Prosthesis, Smart Piston, Malleus Piston, Teflon Torp, and Teflon Porp. With all the above specialization, plastics and metals were used. They create toxicity when they come in contact with the human body for many unknown and known reasons. Even though all the medical devices and implants undergo extensive toxicity studies, still there are regular cases reported regarding their ill effects on humans. Therefore, detailed information on the commonly used devices/implants and their toxicity studies will be discussed throughout the chapter with special emphasis on the most commonly used materials.

Keywords: Intraocular lens; Ocular diagnostics; Teflon Grommet; Smart Piston; Device-induced side effects

Toxicological Aspects of Medical Device Implants.
DOI: https://doi.org/10.1016/B978-0-12-820728-4.00003-4
© 2020 Elsevier Inc.
All rights reserved.

3.1 Ophthalmic implants

3.1.1 Introduction

The eye is a very sensitive and precious organ in human and animal beings. Vision is an essential process in day to life. Once the eye is affected physiologically, pathologically, or pharmacologically, other factors result in vision deterioration or blindness on either one eye or both eyes. Different types of implants are available in the market to restore or regain the deteriorated vision of the eye. The treatment of cytomegalovirus retinitis, posterior uveitis, vitreoretinopathy, and postcataract surgery complication requires a long term of medication therapy. Traditionally, long term used in topical agents are often compliant with the patients. Using a powerful systemic steroid, immunomodulatory agents, and antibiotics most often penetrates into the anterior and posterior chambers and may precipitate unwanted systemic side effects. Implants offer an alternative therapeutic approach to treat the many conditions and may produce safety rather than side effects.

3.1.2 Implants

Generally, implants are used to deliver high drug concentrations to provide sustained medication release or to the area surrounding the target tissue for systemic therapy [1]. In 1992, for the first time, an implantable device was developed for clinical uses and later different implantable devices are available in the market [2]. Ocular implants and inserts are such novel strategies that are designed to bypass blood–aqueous and blood–retinal barriers and facilitate the drug molecules to the posterior chamber of the eye. Advanced drug-delivery techniques to anterior segments such as cul-de-sac inserts, contact lens, subconjunctival/episcleral implants, and punctual plugs and to posterior segment implants such as dexamethasone intravitreal implants, and injectable particulate systems as cortiject implants have revolutionized the ocular drug delivery and overcome the traditional ocular dosage forms [3].

3.1.3 Corneal implants

3.1.3.1 Keratoprosthesis

Restoration of corneal opacity is challenging in the ophthalmic industry to overcome the reversible blindness worldwide. Corneal implants and corneal transplantation techniques are restoring the corneal opacity. Keratoprosthesis (KPro) is an artificial cornea that is available in various styles and designs with different types of materials, either biointegrated (hydroxyapatite (HA), porous polyethylene, and their composites) and nonbiointegrated (polymethyl methacrylate (PMMA)/acrylic and silicon).

Dohlman and his associates designed a prototype device, which uses a nut and bold model and other recent types available in the suture to the cornea [4]. Recently, a different category of keratoprosthesis is available in which a PMMA cylinder is placed in the cornea through the center opening.

A number of devices are available in the market, which are mainly used in two types of devices, namely Boston type-1 keratoprosthesis and osteo-odonto-keratoprosthesis (OOKP). An OOKP device contains the tooth, which is used as a carrier for the cylinder, and the device was designed by Strampelli and improved by Falcinelli.

The previous devices are synthetic in nature, and the current devices are available in semibiological materials. In humans, Boston type-1 KPro and OOKP produce a more successful outcome than other available devices. In wet blinking eye condition mainly used in Boston type-1 KPro and advantage of easy repeatability in case of device failure. Similarly, dry blinking eye and defective eyelids condition widely used in OOKP, which is golden standard KPro produce long-term success [5,6].

The success rate of KPro surgery mostly depends on the selection of a suitable patient to a suitable device. There is a possible complication to agree to the patient using this device such as further operations and the number of visits to the hospital for regular follow-up. After implantation, switching one device to another device may cause more complications in patients, and further surgical procedures will be needed to retain the prosthesis and again to treat may precipitate the complications. Utilizing the KPro device is till not consider for a permanent restoration of vision due to it may affect the long term visual outcome for the patient. The PMMA material has compensated the need for a stable and biocompatible optical component of KPro. David [7] suggested that using the porous and or nonporous implant is up to the decision of the operating surgeon and his or her patient.

AlphaCor design contains a soft material used intracorneally, and it is alternate to corneal graft in those who repeated corneal graft failure. Schellini et al. [8] suggested that only three published randomized controlled trials produce very low certainty evidence and did not show acceptable evidence to assess the effect of integrated and nonintegrated material orbital implants for using the anophthalmic sockets.

3.1.3.2 Intracorneal ring segments

Intracorneal ring segments are small devices made of synthetic material, which are implanted within the corneal stroma to induce a change in the geometry and the refractive power of the tissue. Prof. Joseph Colin proposed the use of such a medical device for the treatment of keratoconus for the first time in the year 2000 [9]. The first intracorneal ring design was composed of a 360-degree ring that led to several complications after the surgery like wound healing-related problems at the incision site; it was the main reason to abandon the 360-degree ring design and change it for the ring segments that we use today [10]. During the 1980s and at the beginning of the 1990s, the design of ring segments was extensively investigated as an alternative for the correction of refractive errors, specifically myopia. Intracorneal ring segments act as spacer elements between the collagen fibers of the corneal tissue. This will induce an arc-shortening effect thus flattening the central area of the cornea. Some theoretical models based on finite element analysis have shown that the flattening effect observed after intracorneal ring segment implantation is directly proportional to the thickness of the segment and inversely proportional to the corneal diameter where it is implanted. The thicker the segment and the smaller the diameter in the cornea where the device is implanted, the higher the flattening effect will be achieved [11]. The intracorneal ring segment is one of the most effective treatment alternatives in the management of keratoconus patients. It is a safe and reversible technique, which regularizes the morphological alterations present in the cornea, thus improving the visual function and the quality of life of patients with keratoconus. The stability of the results will depend on the progressive nature of the disease at the moment of the surgery; this way, Intracorneal ring segments provide long-term stability of the outcomes in those patients with no clinical signs of progression [12].

3.1.4 Orbital implants

3.1.4.1 Anophthalmic implants

Anophthalmic implants are widely used in the treatment of an anophthalmic socket or cavity to restore the lost volume after enucleation or evisceration due to congenital and acquired anophthalmic conditions [13]. There are mainly two types: integrated or nonintegrated implants.

The orbital volume is replaced using autologous or homologous tissues or implants using different types of materials such as PMMA (porous orbital) and silicon (solid silicon sphere) [14]. These material implants are very popular due to their smooth, nonporous, and nonintegrated characteristics, which are inert, and may cause a mild side effect in the host. Perry [15] used natural hydroxyapatite, which can screw the implant to the external prosthesis, to better transmit the movement of the extraocular muscles to the external prosthesis as a result of the fine finishing of the cosmetic.

The main advantage of using an integrated implant with a coupling system between the using implant and external prosthesis is allowed to improve mobility. Dehiscence is one of the main complications due to exposure to the implants [16]. Currently, surgeons favor the use of porous implants because they believe that fibrous ingrowth affords protection against migration [17]. Porous and nonporous implants are seeming to be well tolerated and major complications (like infection and extrusion) rates of both implants were low.

PMMA and silicon implants are having the lowest rate of complication when used as primary anophthalmic implants. The porous polyethylene-coated implants are just as effective as nonporous implants. Patients who undergo implant surgery may experience complications many years later, and longer-term follow-up may identify greater differences in complication rates related to implant type.

Two pediatric population studies have reported the incidence of extrusion of nonporous implants that ranges from 0% to 7.1%. In the adult population, the exposure rates are very low for porous implants, which range from 0% to 5.6% and the extrusion rates that ranged from 0% to 1.3% were reported [18]. Most of the pediatric case studies did not evaluate postoperative motility, and they address the only outcome of using porous implants to the child. Among the porous implants, the motility was very beneficial.

The incidence of infection rates was low in nonporous and less than 1% for porous implants. Some studies showed that, after enucleation, there may be complications many years later. A long-term follow-up may give clarity of the complication rates to both types of implants.

3.1.4.2 Hydroxyapatite orbital implant

HA orbital implant used in seven patients for postevisceration. The size of preoperative axial-length measurement was ax-2 mm, subtract 1 mm for evisceration and hyperopia, except for two patients with buphthalmos where 20 mm implant was used. The implant wrapped in sclera papillary area was turned anteriorly. The implant was pushed into the orbit with the help of malleable retractors. Extraocular muscles were sutured in their anatomic position. Two patients had granuloma before the pedicle division, which was removed and the area was healed, and there was no evidence of further exposure in any patient and all were able to wear orbital epiprosthesis. Tarsoconjunctival pedicle flap method is a safe procedure to cover the exposure of the HA orbital implant. The main disadvantage of this method is the limited size of the flap and the need for temporary tarsorrhaphy [19].

There is no significant difference between using HA and acrylic implants with clinical outcomes reported by patients and surgeons [20] and reassuring among patients and surgeon outcomes of low complication rates and high levels of satisfaction of the enucleation with either of HA and acrylic implants. Cochrane review of integrated versus nonintegrated implants showed that only 3 of 338 studies met the inclusion criterion for randomized or quasirandomized clinical trials [8], and the quality of the included studies was low. Another study showed only 2 of 25 studies met the level I rating like well-designed, well-conducted randomized clinical trials [21]. Moreover, the additional research with well-designed clinical studies would be a benefit to further assessment of implant types, and this is used to explore the role of the implant type on the outcomes of clinical relevance in the future.

3.1.5 Extraocular implants (eyeball jewelry)

In the western world, permanent jewelry has become very popular. From a cosmetic point of view, the eye is most intimately involved in social interactions and it can be positioned inside the conjunctiva. Five women (mean age of 31.5 years + 8.4 (SD)) involved in this study, with no ocular or medical history, were enrolled. A superficial tunnel was made toward the lower conjunctival area. A custom-made, 3.5-mm, curved platinum cosmetic extraocular implant (CEI) (Jewel Eye, Hippocratech Inc.) was inserted through the tunnel and positioned in the lower temporal quadrant. The unsutured incision was covered by upper eyelid and chloramphenicol was applied three times a day after implant incision.

After implantation, the following questions were asked to patients, especially any sensations associated with using CEI, "any temporary changes in visual performance", "do you feel the temporary double vision", "noticing of any other ocular side effects" and "whether you recommend to this implant to any persons". All the five women felt a slight discomfort during the first postoperative days but they did not feel the CEI or have any changes in the vision. Among the five, only in two patients, the CEI position was too high in the interpalpebral space. All of them reported recommending the CEI to others.

Implantation within the conjunctiva was more difficult, and the tunnel of the conjunctiva had to be approximately twice as wide as an implant diameter because of the elasticity of the conjunctiva and Tenon's capsules. This study recommended that a relatively short tunnel for implantation and marking the cornea instead of the conjunctiva as a reference point during the implantation may improve accuracy. The main risk factor of the conjunctiva piercing is that infection may occur in minor lacerations at the skin entry site. The study showed that the CEI implants are completely covered by conjunctival tissue to reduce postoperative infections; moreover, the implant materials are well tolerated by the human tissues that may reduce the risk of conjunctival damage or hypersensitivity reactions of the eye [22].

3.1.6 Intraocular lenses

Opacification is one of the major drawbacks of intraocular lens (IOL) implants. In MHRA (The Medicines and Healthcare products Regulatory Agency, UK), it has been notified that around five reports of the opacification of hydrophilic acrylic IOLs from one of the UK-based hospitals used intracameral of Alteplase (recombinant tissue plasminogen activator, r-tPA) to treat those who had fibrinous uveitis after cataract surgery. Alteplase (r-tPA) causes corneal edema, band keratopathy, anterior chamber turbidity, and hyphemia (hemorrhage into the anterior chamber of the eye).

Different types of contact lenses are available in the market. Soft contact lens-based drug-delivery devices are developed to enter the multicenter Phase III clinical trials for a contact lens presoaked to release antiallergic medications like ketotifen and for a disposable soft contact lens to release incorporated sodium cromoglycate for 1 day to prevent allergic conjunctivitis in contact lens wearers [23].

3.1.6.1 Multifocal IOL

The multifocal IOLs available are often able to restore visual function and allow spectacle independence after their implantation with great levels of patient satisfaction. The factors associated with the postoperative success include the careful selection of the patient, the knowledge about the IOLs' design, and their visual performance added to the proper surgical technique and management of possible complications as demonstrated by the evidence available. Multifocal IOLs are good options to correct pseudophakic presbyopia as they achieve spectacle independence in the majority of the cases with high levels of patient satisfaction. The visual needs of each patient should be carefully analyzed to choose the multifocal model that best fits their lifestyle [24].

3.1.6.2 Aspheric IOL

Aspheric lenses are designed to avoid adding positive spherical aberration to an optical system. Standard aphakic intraocular lenses increase the positive spherical aberration of the visual system, which has already been increased by the aging of the crystalline lens. Implanting an aspheric IOL avoids increasing this aberration and an IOL with negative spherical aberration may even return the optical system to zero spherical aberration by offsetting the cornea's slight positive aberration [25].

3.1.6.3 Anterior chamber IOL

Anterior chamber lens is fixed with the support of iris. It is primarily used as a backup lens when there is damage to the posterior chamber. Anterior chamber IOL (ACIOL) is also used in refractive surgery—implanting a lens in the phakic eye to correct the refractive power [26]. In 2003, Michael Wagoner led an American Academy of Ophthalmology (AAO) meta-analysis that found that ACIOL, iris-sutured IOL, and scleral-sutured IOL were equivalent [27]. Shortly thereafter, a study comparing ACIOLs with iris-fixated intraocular lenses in the setting of poor capsular support confirmed the findings of the AAO meta-analysis, stating that there were no significant differences in outcomes (specifically visual acuity and postoperative complications) between the two groups. However, a study conducted in response to these reports comparing primary scleral-fixated IOLs with primary anterior chamber IOLs in complicated cataract surgery found visual acuity to be significantly more favorable in the primary ACIOL group [28].

3.1.6.4 Scleral-fixated IOL

Options for IOL implantation in the absence of capsular support include ACIOLs, iris-fixated IOLs, and scleral-fixated IOLs. The choice of the

IOL and implantation technique depends greatly on patient age, comorbid ocular conditions, and the patient's ocular anatomy. Surgical options for patients with inadequate capsular support include alternative placement in the ACIOLs, fixation to the iris, or fixation to the sclera [29]. The surgical techniques for each of these approaches have improved considerably over the last several decades resulting in improved visual and ocular outcomes. If no capsular or iris support exists, the surgeon can fixate an IOL to the sclera or the patient can remain aphakic. IOLs can be fixated to the sclera using sutures or by tunneling the IOL haptics into the sclera without suture [30].

3.1.6.5 Phakic IOL

Phakic IOLs are clear implantable lenses that are surgically placed either between the cornea and the iris (the colored portion of your eye) or just behind the iris, without removing your natural lens. It enables light to focus properly on the retina for clearer vision without corrective eyewear. Implantable lenses function like contact lenses to correct nearsightedness [31]. The difference is that phakic IOLs work from within your eye instead of sitting on the surface of your eye. Phakic IOLs offer a permanent correction of myopia unless the lens is surgically removed [32]. The Visian ICL (Implantable Collamer Lens) marketed by Staar Surgical is a posterior chamber phakic IOL, meaning it is positioned behind the iris and in front of your natural lens. It received Food and Drug Administration (FDA) approval in 2005 for correcting nearsightedness ranging from −3.00 to −20.00 diopters (D). Because the Visian ICL is placed behind the iris, it is undetectable to the naked eye and can only be seen through a microscope. The Visian ICL is made of a soft, biocompatible collagen copolymer. Due to its flexibility, the lens can be folded during implantation, requiring only a small surgical incision. The Verisyse (Abbott Medical Optics) is an anterior chamber phakic IOL, meaning it is positioned in front of the iris. In 2004, the Verisyse phakic IOL received FDA approval for correcting moderate-to-severe nearsightedness within the range of −5.00 to −20.00 D. It is made of medical-grade plastic (PMMA) and is rigid in form.

3.1.7 Implants used in the posterior chambers

The drug is transporting to posterior chamber eye diseases very difficult to reaching to the vitreous, retina and choroid. Due to the limitation of the different types of transporter present in the blood–retinal barrier (BRB), there is difficulty in achieving the therapeutic dose reach this area. To achieve the therapeutic dose of the medication in the posterior chamber needed the implants, which are mainly in two types: biodegradable and nonbiodegradable polymer implants. Using this, both biodegradable and nonbiodegradable polymers have produced advantages and disadvantages to the treatment as well as to the patients. These both implants are inserted via ocular *pars plana* to vitreous humor to avoid the entry or diffusion of drug molecules to the blood–retinal barrier and at the same time enhance the drug to reach the specific area and also reduce the undesirable side effects. Other possible sites for an implant include the topical, sub-Tenon, intrascleral, subconjunctival, and suprachoroidal area [33].

3.1.7.1 Biodegradable implants

It contains biodegradable polymers, which are mainly in two types such as matrix or monolithic and reservoir systems. In the monolithic matrix system, the polymer degrades slowly by physiological conditions and drug molecules are released during polymer degradation due to diffusion through the matrix pores. In the reservoir system, the membrane is slowly degraded than the drug molecules and get them into the diffusion process [34].

The development of implants used a broad range of natural and synthetic biogradable polymers. Natural polymers such as bovine serum albumin, human serum albumin, gelatin, and collagen and similarly synthetic polymers such as poly(orthoesters), poly(amino acids), poly(esters), poly (amides), poly(urethanes), and poly(alkyl-α-cyano acrylates) are used in a wide variety of development of drug-delivery system. Due to the cost and percentage of purity of the natural polymers, they are limitedly used in the development of implants [35].

Poly(ε-caprolactone) is a semicrystalline and hydrophobic polyester, which degrades through hydrolysis due to ester bonds. The degradation rate is slow, that is, around 2–3 years [36,37]. As it is having slow degradation, high biocompatibility, and high permeability, it is widely used in ophthalmic drug-delivery devices [38–41].

Poly(ortho ester) (POE) is a hydrophobic biodegradable polymer, which consists of four families. POE I and POE II families are not used in ophthalmology. POE III has highly flexible chains that form a gel at room temperature and viscous in nature; therefore, POE III polymer incorporation with medicinal substances without the use of organic solvents. It can be injected directly into the eye using appropriate needles

[36,37]. POE III does not produce ocular toxicity and an increase in intraocular pressure (IOP). In intravitreal (IVI) administration of biodegradable polymer produces well-tolerated and polymer where degraded slowly in the vitreous chamber and there is no inflammatory process occurred [42]. Subconjunctival injection of POE IV produces complete degradation that occurred within 5 weeks. However, after intravitreal and suprachoroidal administration, degradation occurred within approximately 3 and 6 months, respectively. POE III and POE IV in the ocular application are more advantageous in the laboratory scale level and limited in an industrial scale.

3.1.7.1.1 Biodegradable implants for IOL drug delivery

The posterior segment of eye disorders is very complicated to treat because drug molecules can enter this region after topical instillation. An alternative of topical, intraocular injections is preferable to treat, but the disadvantages of this region have rapid clearance rates due to fast-flowing blood supply and suddenly fall in a therapeutic level of drug concentration. To achieve the study state concentration over a longer time in the posterior chamber using the polymer sustained—drug-delivery system implants are introduced into the vitreous. The polymers obtained from the lactic acid and glycolic acids are more capable of the drug-delivery system owing to their excellent biocompatibility and biodegradation [34].

3.1.7.1.2 Biodegradable implants used in postcataract surgery

After cataract surgery, patients may suffer due to inflammations and infections. To avoid this complication, eye drops containing antiinflammatory and antibiotics, which do not reach the exact region, are recommended. To avoid the use of eye drops, using implants that are rod-shaped and biodegradable with a controlled-release intraocular drug-delivery system containing dexamethasone, a monolithic system containing polylactic-coglycolic acid polymer with hydroxypropyl methylcellulose and 60 μg of homogeneously dispersed dexamethasone, were used. Initially, it was demonstrated preclinically, where it controlled release in drugs over a period of 7–10 days. Later, the performance of Surodex against eye drops containing 0.1% of dexamethasone was compared with those who underwent cataract surgery and received an intraocular lens. The results were more effective and showed reduced postsurgical inflammation [43]. Later, the safety and efficacy of biodegradable implants with a controlled-release intraocular drug-delivery system containing dexamethasone versus 0.1% of dexamethasone eye drops were performed against in patients who suffered from inflammation after cataract surgery, and the results were more effective in controlling intraocular inflammation [44].

3.1.7.1.3 Biodegradable implants used in uveitis

A rod-shaped polylactic-coglycolic acid biodegradable device incorporated with a dose of 0.7 mg dexamethasone, which provides peak doses for the first 2 months followed by lower doses for up to 6 months. It is mainly used in diabetic macular edema following branch retinal vein occlusion and central retinal vein occlusion and noninfectious posterior uveitis. An increase in IOP, conjunctival hemorrhage, eye pain, conjunctival hyperemia, cataract, vitreous detachment, and headache are causing the use of this device [45,46].

3.1.7.1.4 Advantages and disadvantages of using biodegradable implants

Biodegradable implants are mainly used in the sustained release of drug and drug stabilization. There is no need for the removal of the implants more than a week to months. The disadvantage is the requirement of the surgery or IVI to insert an implant as a result of the risk of complications. If, the breakdown of the implant may possibility to produce the toxicity. May chance to initial and final burst in drug release.

3.1.7.2 Nonbiodegradable implants

It is a polymeric implant that consists of a matrix (monolithic) or reservoir systems. The drug molecule is dispersed homogeneously in the polymer matrix or adsorbed onto the surface. The matrix controlled or sustained the drug by slow diffusion. In the reservoir-type system, the drug is surrounded by a permeable, nondegradable membrane, whose thickness and permeability properties can control the diffusion of the drug molecule into the body. The drug-release rate is determined by different factors such as the release area, thickness of the polymeric membrane, an implant form, as well as drug solubility [36]. Polyvinyl alcohol (PVA), silicon, and ethylene-vinyl acetate (EVA) are used in nonbiodegradable implants. Polyvinyl alcohol and silicon are easily absorbed in lipophilic drugs due to the polymer hydrophobic nature. Ethylene-vinyl acetate is not absorbed in most of the drugs and is used as a membrane around the reservoir to reduce the rate of drug diffusion through the implant [33,36,47].

3.1.7.2.1 Nonbiodegradable implants for cytomegalovirus retinitis

Vitrasert is a nonbiodegradable implant device, which contains a PVA/EVA reservoir incorporated with ganciclovir (4.5 mg) and magnesium stearate (0.25%) and which is placed in a vitreous cavity, and the ganciclovir-release rate is 1 μg/h for over the period of 5–6 months. It is removed, usually, after 6 months, if necessary, to place in another ganciclovir implant or if there are any complications like endophthalmitis, severe vitreous hemorrhage, or retinal detachment [2,48].

The systemic administration seems to be more effective in the dissemination of the cytomegalovirus and survival improvement than the intravitreal ganciclovir implant [49–51]. Vitrasert was voluntarily withdrawn from the market and also discontinued by the FDA at the moment.

3.1.7.2.2 Nonbiodegradable implants for uveitis

An intravitreal implant device is used for the treatment of chronic and noninfectious posterior uveitis. It is composed of a central core consisting of fluocinolone acetonide (0.59 mg) with silicone/polyvinyl alcohol and it is releasing the drug up to 2.5–3 years. The device was withdrawn from the market in 2007 because the implant did not suppress the reoccurring of the disease longer compared to the standard administration and also showed side effects such as cataract, eye pain, and elevated IOP [52,53].

3.1.7.2.3 Nonbiodegradable implants for diabetic retinopathy

An intravitreal implant contains fluocinolone acetonide (0.19 mg) with polyimide or PVA (with silicone bioadhesive in low dose version). It is used in the treatment of diabetic macular edema, age-related macular degeneration (approved in Phase II), and posterior uveitis (approved in Phase III). After IVI administration, drugs are sustained to deliver around 18–36 months [54,55]. Still, very limited data are documented about implant removal; in one case report, it was published that the implant migrated to the anterior chamber and it was removed and inserted back into the posterior chamber for two patient's eyes [56]. After the decentralized procedure, this implant was accepted for clinical use in 17 European union (EU) countries.

An intravitreal delivery technology consists of titanium helical coil coated with triamcinolone acetonide (925 μg), and nonbiodegradable polymers such as poly(methyl methacrylate) and ethylene-vinyl acetate possess a sustained delivery drug for a minimum period of 2 years.

This implant is mainly used in the treatment of diabetic macular edema and it causes the development of cataract and elevated IOP. Phase IIb trials were terminated, and no further clinical trials have been completed [45,57–59].

3.1.7.2.4 Advantages and disadvantages of using nonbiodegradable implants

Controlled drug-release rate, drug stabilization, and prolonged duration of action for a month to years are possible advantages in nonbiodegradable implants. The disadvantage is the requirement of surgery or IVI to insert an implant as a result of the risk of complications.The breakdown of the implant may cause reactions and toxicity. May chance to initial and final burst in drug release.

3.1.8 Implants for glaucoma surgery

3.1.8.1 Glaucoma valve implants

Implantation of the glaucoma valve is an effective surgical technique to reduce intraocular pressure in patients affected with glaucoma. The device works by bypassing the trabecular meshwork and redirecting the outflow of aqueous humor through a small tube into an outlet chamber or bleb [60]. The IOP generally decreases from around 33 to 10 mmHg by removing aqueous on average 2.75 mL/min. Although in the past, the use of this device was reserved for glaucoma refractory to multiple filtration surgical procedures, up-to-date mounting experience has encouraged its use as a primary surgery for selected cases. Implantation of glaucoma valve can be challenging, especially in patients who already underwent previous multiple surgeries. Several tips have to be acquired by the surgeon, and a long learning curve is always needed. Although the valve mechanism embedded in the glaucoma valve decreases the risk of postoperative hypotony-related complications, it does not avoid the need for a careful follow-up. Complications related to this type of surgery include early and late postoperative hypotony, excessive capsule fibrosis around the plate, erosion of the tube or plate edge, and very rarely infection [61].

3.1.8.2 Implants for nonpenetrating glaucoma surgery

The concept of nonpenetrating glaucoma surgery originated in 1964 when Krasnov published his first report on sinusotomy. This operation consisted of removing a lamellar band of the sclera, opening the

Schlemm's canal over 120 degrees from 10 to 2 o'clock position. The inner wall of the Schlemm's canal was untouched and the conjunctiva was closed. To avoid the secondary collapse of the superficial flap, a space maintainer implant is placed in the scleral bed [62]. The first to be used was the collagen Aquaflow implant, a highly purified porcine collagen dehydrated into a cylinder (4 × 1 × 1 mm). It swells rapidly once exposed to the aqueous humor and is resorbed within 6–9 months after surgery. Another device that has been proposed to maintain the intrascleral space is the reticulated hyaluronic acid implant, which is an equilateral triangle 3.5 mm long and 500 μm thick or an isosceles triangle of 4.5 × 3 mm at the same thickness. The advantage of this implant is that it occupies a large volume in the filtration area while allowing for sufficient circulation of the aqueous humor, and it does not need to be sutured at the sclera. More recently, a hydrophilic acrylic implant that is nonabsorbable has been developed. It is a T-shaped implant that creates an evacuating canal along the foot and each arm of the T shape and is inserted into one of the surgically created openings of the Schlemm's canal. New implants have been developed in the past few years with promising results, such as the 2-hydroxyethyl-methacrylate implant and a cross-shaped rigid nonabsorbable implant made of PMMA. Other low-cost implants such as chromic suture material and autologous scleral implant have been used in deep sclerectomy. Amniotic membrane has also been tried as an implant. Further studies are needed to evaluate the role of these implants [63].

3.1.9 Scleral buckle

Scleral buckling (SB) is a surgical technique that is employed successfully to treat rhegmatogenous retinal detachments (RRD) for more than 60 years. With the introduction of pars plana vitrectomy (PPV), there is a growing trend toward the use of PPV for the treatment of retinal detachment. There is a reluctance to perform scleral buckling in RRD due to the perceived steep learning curve, declining mastery over indirect ophthalmoscopy, and poor ergonomics associated with SB. In this chapter, we discuss the surgical challenges and tips to overcome these in four headings: localization of the break, retinopexy, SB, and subretinal fluid (SRF) drainage. Localization of the break can be performed by the use of forceps or illuminated scleral depressor. It can be facilitated by prior drainage of SRF in cases with bullous RRD. Chandelier with a wide-angle viewing system can be used for easier localization of break and cryopexy.

Sutureless buckling and suprachoroidal buckling are easier and faster alternatives to the conventional technique. Reshaping the silicone segment helps in accommodating the wider circumferential band. Modified needle drainage, laser choroidotomy, and infusion-assisted drainage can make SRF drainage easier and safer [64].

3.1.10 Intubation in lacrimal surgery

Lacrimal drainage obstructions causing epiphora is a common lacrimal disorder. Depending on the age of the patient and the pathophysiology of the condition, the disorder can either be relieved by simple probing or by a dacryocystorhinostomy. In certain conditions, the success rates of the treatment can be improved by intubating the lacrimal system. Canalicular intubation is also indicated in the management of lacerated canaliculus. Intubation is achieved commonly by placing a silicone stent in the lacrimal passages. The silicone stent maintains the passages where it is present and is also believed to allow tissue healing around itself thus maintaining lacrimal patency [65].

3.1.11 Glaucoma surgical implants/glaucoma drainage device

A glaucoma drainage implant is a type of medical shunt used to help lower your eye pressure. The shunt consists of two parts: a small tube and a plate. The small tube is inserted into your eye to let the fluid drain out. The plate is attached to the tube. It is placed beneath the skin of the eye to form a small pool, where the fluid will drain, called a bleb. This allows the fluid to drain out of your eye through your shunt instead of draining through your eye's natural drain. In glaucoma, the eye's natural drain does not work very well. This surgery helps bypass the natural drain and lower the eye pressure. The modern glaucoma drainage implant era was initiated with implantation of a plate posterior to the limbus connected to the anterior chamber by a long silicone tube. Nonrestrictive and flow-restrictive implants were developed. With increased clinical experience, variables influencing success and failure of glaucoma drainage implant surgery were better understood. In an iterative process, complications were reduced and indications for drainage implant surgery were broadened. The growth of the utilization of glaucoma drainage implants has dramatically increased in recent years. Glaucoma drainage implants have improved the prognosis for surgical success for refractory glaucoma and have a well-established role in the surgical treatment of glaucoma [66].

3.1.12 Ocular stents

Aqueous shunts and stents for the treatment of glaucoma create an alternative path for aqueous humor to leave the anterior chamber of the eye and thus lower the IOP. They are intended for use in individuals with inadequately controlled glaucoma. Aqueous shunts drain aqueous humor away from the anterior chamber by a variety of surgical installation details (e.g., canals, filters, valves). The incisional approach cuts through the conjunctiva and sclera *(ab externo)* and complications include corneal endothelial failure, infection, and erosion of the overlying conjunctiva [67].

3.1.13 Silicon tubes

Many substances, such as silk, nylon, plastic, and other suture materials, have been used as temporary stents to correct various acute and chronic disorders of the lacrimal drainage system. Henderson (1950) reported the use of polyethylene tubing placed at the time of a dacryocystorhinostomy to correct the concurrent canalicular obstruction. Huggert (1959) and others used polyethylene tubing to correct acute and chronic canalicular problems. In some of these cases, a surgical opening of the tear sac was necessary to place the tubing. Malleable metal rods have been advocated in the repair of lacerated canaliculi. Others have attempted more radical grafting procedures to produce a patent inferior canaliculus. More recently, silicone tubing has become popular because it reduces the frequency of problems caused by the stiffer polyethylene, such as punctual erosion, corneal irritation from kinking of the tubing, and even slitting of the canaliculi. Quickert and Dryden (1970) described a probe as well as a procedure for passing silicone tubing through the lacrimal drainage system. The probe, tubing, and technique have been modified by others to facilitate passage and retrieval [68].

3.1.14 Conclusion

Systemic administration of the drug-delivery molecules is very difficult to reach to the posterior segments of the eye. However, the drug is not effective before high doses, toxicity, Blood Retinal Barrier (BRB) and Blood Aqueous Barrier (BAB) and need the novel technology to provide sustained drug delivery, improving more bioavailability, reducing the patient compliance and unwanted effects. Drug-delivery developments in the fields of biomedical engineering, nanotechnology, and noninvasive techniques are future possibilities to the posterior segments of the eye.

3.2 Medical implants in Otorhinolaryngology [Ear, Nose, Throat (ENT)]

3.2.1 Grommets

Grommets are devices used to drain fluid from the middle ear by making a hole in the tympanic membrane during myringotomy (Fig. 3.1). This helps in equalizing air pressure and prevents further fluid accumulation. The operation lasts for approximately 20 minutes. As most of the patients are children, general anesthetic is used instead of local anesthesia. The grommets stay in place up to a year after which they are removed. The tympanic membrane heals on its own with time. About half the children treated require reinsertion of the grommets due to the recurrence of suppurative otitis media [69]. Simultaneous removal of adenoids is usually done during myringotomy to reduce the probability of upper respiratory tract infections that are often associated with otitis media with effusion (OME). Recent Scottish guidelines have included the treatment and management of childhood otitis media in primary care. In the early 1990s the number of surgeries shot up rapidly when the question against the necessity of the procedure has raised. A period of watchful waiting (regular monitoring of hearing level without other intervention) before surgical intervention has been adopted in recent guidelines [69,70]. Most nonsurgical interventions including the noninvasive technique of unknown

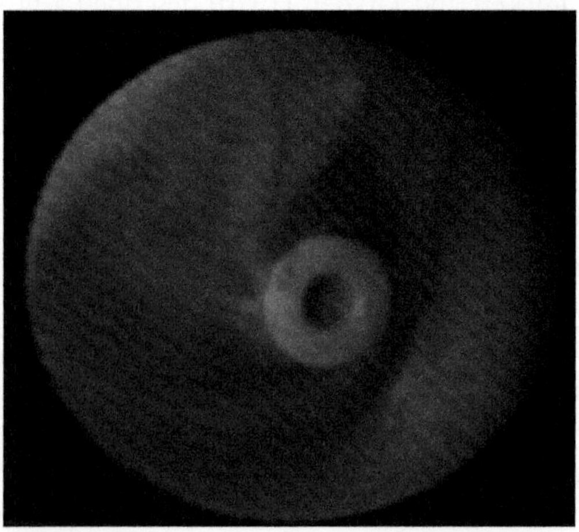

Figure 3.1 Grommet inserted. *courtesy: www.kidshealth.org.nz.*

efficacy a decongestant, antihistamines, mucolytic, steroids, and antibiotics are ineffective or have short-lived benefits that are either ineffective, of unknown effectiveness or of limited short-term benefit [71]. Hearing aids and autoinflation (blowing up a balloon through a nostril) are others being used [72].

3.2.2 Epidemiology

Otitis media can sometimes be asymptomatic middle ear inflammation, which can occur with or without symptoms [70]. Acute otitis media can manifest purulent middle ear effusion (pus), earache, and fever and is frequently associated with upper respiratory tract infections. Otitis media with effusion is also known as "glue ear," and it refers to a chronic disease state with the accumulation of fluid in the middle ear that is usually (but not always) absent of the signs and symptoms of an acute infection. The main symptom associated with OME is hearing loss. If this occurs during the course of OME, it is hard to differentiate. OME is common in young. It has been estimated that 80% of children have had at least one episode of OME by the age of 4, and 15%–20% of children aged between 2 and 6 suffer from this condition at any point in time [73,74]. The prevalence and incidence drop substantially afterward. The duration of OME is generally short, but 5%–10% of OME last 1 year or longer [69]. Resolution of OME in preschool children is quite fast 3 prime concern of OME in children if persistent (≥3 months), bilateral hearing loss of ≥25 decibels (dB), which could affect the children's language and social development and lead to learning and behavioral difficulties (eg. a hearing loss of 30 dB can mean that a normal conversation sounds like a soft whisper) [75]. The effect of OME in congenital defects has still not been established [76].

3.2.3 Effectiveness based on clinical evidence

The most recent systematic review on the use of grommets for OME is a Cochrane review by Lous and colleagues [77]. Evidence presented in this section is based on this review (literature search to March 2003) and supplemented by evidence published since from randomized controlled trials (RCTs) and other reviews covering the general management of OME that have applied complex methodology for evidence synthesis [71,75,78].

The efficacy of grommets in terms of correcting hearing loss has been demonstrated in early RCTs in which a grommet was inserted into one ear of a child who suffered from bilateral OME while the other ear of the same child was served as the control. Using grommets has improved the hearing level from 7 to 9 in contrast with surgeries done without using them [77,79].

Significant differences exist in the magnitude of observed improvement between some of the trials at 4–6 months (range 5–19 dB). Differences between treated and untreated ears appeared to decrease with time across studies, with an average difference of approximately 4 dB at 2 years and no significant difference at 5 years. Combining adenoidectomy with grommet insertion in myringotomy has only a little more benefit with regard to hearing than simple myringotomy with grommet [75,78]. The advantages of combining adenoidectomy have not been practically proved. More recent RCTs have randomized children rather than ears and have compared bilateral insertion of grommets (without adenoidectomy) to watchful waiting [77]. The watchful groups in RCTs have shown improvement in hearing in proportion if time with effusion in addition to hearing ability language development behavior and quality of life have also been assessed. The outcomes of both the trials cannot be summarized combined as they used a different study. Through screening, infants and children under 3 years old with chronic OME were picked through screening; a significant difference between grommet groups and watchful waiting groups was not found in any measures of language, quality of life [77,80], cognitive or psychosocial development, and behavior or academic achievement throughout long-term follow-up (to 9–11 years old in one of the studies) [81,82]. It has been shown that there was a delay in language development in the watchful group compared to the grommet group at 9 months and it was not observed at 18 months when the children of the watchful group had their grommets inserted [83].

Hence, the age at which the grommet is inserted does not affect a long-term language development. Myringotomy alone was less efficacious than myringotomy with grommet insertion in the RCT in children with persistent bilateral OME. This is consistent with the findings from a previous review [75]. A further UK-based RCT (TARGET trial) comparing nonsurgical management, bilateral grommets, and bilateral grommets plus adenoidectomy in children aged 3–7 has been completed but the full results have not yet been published [84,85]. Trails comparing grommets with hearing aids or auto inflation have not been done.

3.2.4 Safety

The events succeeding in the surgical insertion of grommet have been studied as randomized studies and case series [86]. Common sequelae included otorrhea (discharge from ears) during the postoperative period (16% of patients) and beyond (26%), tympanosclerosis (scarring of the tympanic membrane, 32%), and focal atrophy (25%). Less often seen but more complicated sequelae include perforation of tympanic membrane and cholesteatoma (abnormal growth of skin and accumulation of debris in the middle ear), both of which are more frequently associated with long-term tubes than short-term tubes. The risk of tympanosclerosis increased by three times with grommet insertion. Tymapanosclerosis if it occurs may or may not be associated with hearing loss [87]. The usage of antibiotics has been increased in children less than 3 years due to the high rate of otorrhea.

3.2.5 Hearing aid (Cochlear implants)

3.2.5.1 Introduction

There is an increased recognition of the global prevalence and the impact of hearing loss on health and function. According to the World Health Organization, hearing impairment stands as the third highest cause of years lived with disability in adults worldwide [88]. This is a major cause of concern regarding the health of the elderly population. As age increases, the incidence of hearing loss increases. Overall, in adults older than 75 years, more than 70% have some degree of hearing problems [88,89].

Most of these people have severe hearing loss, and they cannot be treated with conventional amplification of hearing aids. These people with profound sensorineural hearing loss require cochlear implantation (CI). The CI sends electric signals directly to the spiral ganglion cells of the cochlear nerve without the involvement of inner hair cells and with the help of surgically implanted intracochlear electrode (Figs. 3.2 and 3.3). For the functioning of CI, we need a flawless auditory pathway from spiral ganglion cells to the auditory cortex. The once considered barriers to implantation like age-related degeneration of the peripheral and central auditory pathways, long-term auditory deprivation, cognition, and neural plasticity are now areas of the active research. For the patients suffering and its relief, the patient is further evaluated on numerous aspects along with age, for the patient to be considered as a candidate for CI. Only 5%–10% of adult CI candidates are able to avail this benefit because of the above-mentioned constraints [90].

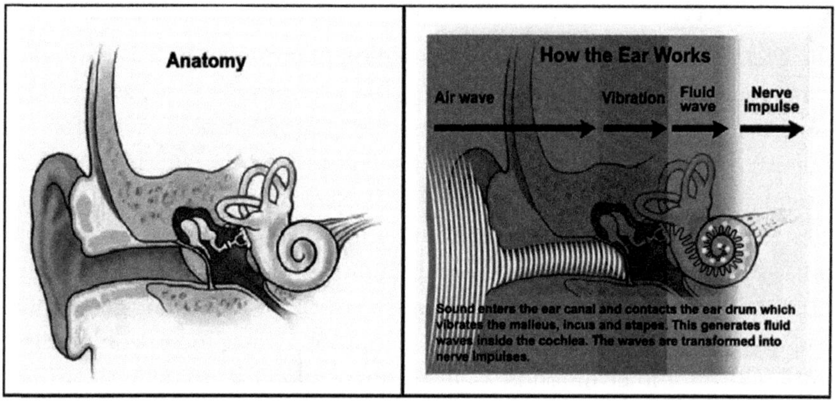

Figure 3.2 Anatomy and physiology of functioning normal ear. *courtesy: US FDA, 2019.*

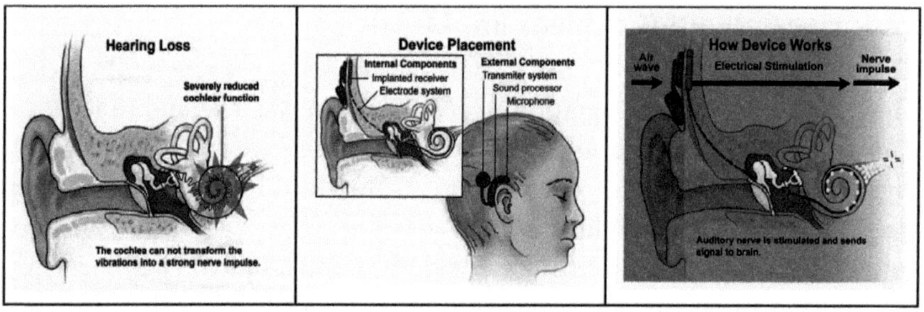

Figure 3.3 Cochlear implantation function. *courtesy: US FDA, 2019.*

3.2.5.2 Safety of cochlear implants and complications

It is important for us to review the safety profile of CI and perioperative morbidity for the veterans especially as they are vulnerable to poorer outcomes. It has been shown that the elderly population tolerated risks of both major and minor complications quite well. Meningitis, permanent postoperative facial nerve paralysis, device failure, flap dehiscence or wound breakdown, implant migration, or extra cochlear insertion are the major complications of CI. Minor complications include dizziness or imbalance, temporary facial nerve stimulation, tinnitus, and dysgeusia. The complications are not unique to elderly patients. The major complications are seen in 5% of older CI patients and minor complications are seen in 9.2%–16.7%. Dizziness, imbalance, or vertigo is the frequently observed postoperative complications of CI [91–95]. The predisposing factor for postoperative imbalance in elderly is the increased rates of cognitive decline and neurologic impairment in their retrospective cohort of 445 patients older than 60 at a single institution, 3.8% required implant removal for reasons such as nonuse or secondary to other major complications, such as infection, device failure, and flap dehiscence. Among these patients, 88.2% underwent subsequent reimplantation. At 5 and 10 years postimplantation, 95.4% and 93.1% of all elderly CI patients retained their original implant, respectively [93]. Thinning skin and decreased vascularization with age are a prime concern in the elderly [96]; flap thinning is seen in 13% of elderly CI patients but not serious enough to require removal of the implant. Meningitis is a rare but fatal postsurgical CI complication. CI vaccination protocol is important at all ages [97]. CI effectively improves hearing loss in patients with sensorineural hearing loss. Worldwide, there are 3,00,000 CI recipients and more are adding to the list. Undergoing magnetic resonance imaging (MRI) can be troublesome for CI recipients. Magnetic fields produced in MRI interfere with CI and can cause their dislodging. In addition, internal magnets in CI can induce artifacts in MRI scans. The major concern for CI candidates who undergo MRI is the exposure of internal magnet to a strong electromagnetic field that can induce notable magnetic forces and cause various problems. However, the US FDA has allowed the use of MRI on patients with CIs in specific cases under certain conditions of use [98]. For example, cochlear implants were approved for use with MRI instruments involving field strengths up to 1.5 T, as long as head dressings were used. Furthermore, CIs with removable magnets, such as the Nucleus Freedom, Nucleus 24, and certain Nucleus 22 models, were approved for the use with MRI systems up to 1.5 T following removal of the internal magnet.

The unpleasant events that have occurred in CI patients after MRI are magnet displacement and polarity changes. Hassepass et al. [99] have found that the use of compressive bandages during 1.5 T MRI does not eliminate the risk for dislodging of the internal magnet. On the other hand, Crane et al [100] reported that 16 patients with CI and head bandages safely underwent 1.5 T MRI and the images obtained were adequate. A separate case report detailed another CI recipient who safely underwent 1.5 T MRI without adverse effects. The safety of CI patients undergoing MRI has come into the limelight.

3.2.5.3 Regarding revision implantations

CI is a safe and effective treatment for children and adults with profound deafness. As CI is an electric device, it may undergo breakdown or failure.

Although the CI reliability rate is now very high, the continually increasing population of implant recipients will result in the continued occurrence of revision surgeries. The first report of a CI revision surgery occurred in 1985 by Hochmair-Desoyer and Burian. Since then, several reports have addressed the safety of this procedure [101].

3.2.5.4 Indications of cochlear implant revisions

They comprise two main categories: (1) device-related indications and (2) nondevice-related indications. The former has been responsible for 75% of cases of reimplantation where there were problems with either facial nerve stimulation or device failure or in cases that required device upgrade. The latter account for 25% of reimplantation complicated by scalp flap infections, allergic reactions, misplacement of the electrode array, and electrode extrusions.

In device-related indications, device failure is the most bothersome complaint associated with CI from patients as well as doctor's perspective. Furthermore, device failures can be classified as either hard or soft. A hard device failure is associated with significantly diminished or complete lack of auditory perception resulting from a confirmed malfunction of a component of the CI device that is more common in occurrence. It can be attributed to head trauma in children disrupting communication between the internal and external processors. Soft failures are suspected when there are abrupt deterioration and auditory skills as compared to the previous records. Hence, they become more challenging to recognize although many factors may affect the performance of a patient. Moreover, manufacture testing avails to know benefits when it comes to the detection of soft failures unlike hard failures. In the evaluation and amelioration of various contributing factors like electrode problems, external component upgrading is of more importance in case of CI failure. Symptoms of soft failure can be subtle and include decreased performance and speech perception, poor performance relative to expectations based on preimplantation characteristics, aversive stimuli causing subjective discomfort or pain especially at low stimulation levels, and hearing static while the device is off. A frequent need for reprogramming or difficulty programming often misattributed to complicated patients may be related to the device. A strong index of suspicion may be needed to detect accompanying signs [102].

Clinical documentation of signs such as changes in electrode impedances and inability to maintain a consistent connection with the internal receiver as well as reduced clinical benefit forms an important component of the diagnosis of malfunction of CIs. When a device failure is suspected, the manufacturer is contacted and in vivo integrity testing is performed. Objective measures that may be performed include impedance telemetry, electrically evoked stapedial reflexes, electrically evoked auditory brainstem response, and electrically evoked compound action potentials. When concerns arise regarding device function, tests are performed to obtain information that can be compared to baseline measurements. A computed tomography or even a plain radiograph to document the position of the electrode array within the cochlea is quite valuable associated with the benefit of low radiation dosage. Such imaging studies give information regarding electrode placements and identify problems such as a kink, a tip fold over, misplacement, over insertion, or partial insertion of the electrode array. Meticulous consideration of all factors responsible for reduced performance other than device malfunction should be done with the intention that reimplantation may result in no change or even a decline in performance. The last resort would be an explanation of the device followed by a complete analysis by the manufacturer when integrity tests are inconclusive. In rare cases, the analysis of explanted devices from a patient with clinical improvement subsequent to reimplantation may not identify the cause of the malfunction. For time-to-time evaluation of various reasons and conditions causing implant failure, a European consensus statement and explanation was put forward in 2005 comprising the following recommendations.

3.2.5.5 Principles of reporting on device failure

- All device failures must be reported to the competent authority (i.e., usually the implant manufacturer), with a calculated cumulative survival rate. The manufacturer's reports of device failure should comprise information containing the source data, sample size, and the time period over which the failure rate is being observed historic data and technical modification of a given device should be included in reports of survival rate. The complete dataset of the manufacturer's product should be supplied in situations where a change has been made. In the case of the electrodes or the electronic that has been labeled with its own European Conformity (CE) mark, a new device category may be assigned. European conformity mark is a certification mark that indicates conformity with health, safety, and environmental protection standards for products sold within the European Economic Area (EEA), which can also be found on products sold outside the EEA that

are manufactured in, or designed to be sold in the EEA. (A valid CE marking affixed to a product indicates that it complies with the relevant European product safety directives.)
- Cumulative survival rates should be separated for adults and children, with 95% confidence intervals reported
- Device survival time should start being tracked at the closure of the CI incision.

Replacement of a CI is done when it fails to function or if there is a need to upgrade the internal component of the device. Revision for upgrade purposes remains a controversial issue because the surgery beers risks of damage to the surviving auditory nerves and the outcome cannot be accurately predicted preoperatively [103]. Multichannel processing has enabled a higher level of speech recognition. Replacing an implant with an advanced version is still a debate of discussion as the postoperative results are unpredictable. The upgrade from single to multichannel has not shown any significant improvement in speech recognition because of binaural hearing. However, some patients might not want an implant in the contralateral ear, as they prefer using a more advanced CI that may come in the future [104]. Replacement of an implant carries a risk of damage to the cochlea while placing the intracochlear electrode that has been proved by preclinical experiments. Hochmair-Desoyer and Burian successfully implanted a scala tympani electrode of their own design in two patients [105]. Lindeman et al. [106], Chute et al. [107], and Economou et al. [108]. reported replacement of a single-channel House/3M implant with a Nucleus 22-channel implant. Gantz et al. [104]. reported on five patients who underwent successful revisions of CIs of various designs. These authors agreed that replacement of the implants did not cause deterioration of hearing and enabled the restoration of a similar or better auditory experience than the previous devices allowed. The audiological performance of patients was also comparable with those obtaining new devices. Facial nerves electric stimulation may occur as a complication in 1%–15% of patients [109]. Possible explanations of this adverse effect are leakage of currents caused by a change in the electric properties of the bone or close proximity of the facial nerve to the outer wall of the cochlea, together with the need for high electric current to stimulate the auditory nerve (i.e., malformations or ossified cochleae). Patients with osteosclerosis involving the otic capsule bone are particularly at high risk of facial nerve stimulation. Burmeister et al. [110] suggested that, in these scenarios, electrical discharge from CI electrodes through normal use causes twitching of the face; this symptom can range from mild irritation to an inability to use the implant entirely as a result of excessive facial pain. Kelsall et al. [111]. reported a study that consisted of 14 patients with facial nerve stimulation after placement of the Nucleus 22-channel CI. Records were reviewed retrospectively, and patients were studied with three-dimensional computed tomography scanning techniques. Electrical testing was performed, and various CI programming strategies were evaluated. Important clinical features were reviewed. The radiographic and anatomical relationships of the facial nerve to the cochlea were evaluated, and the programming strategies used to effectively control facial nerve stimulation were reviewed. The prevalence of facial nerve stimulation in population was 7%. The most common cause was osteosclerosis. Anatomical data confirmed the close proximity of the basal turn of the cochlea and the labyrinthine segment of the facial nerve. There was a high correlation between the electrodes causing symptoms, and those found radiographically to be the closest to the labyrinthine segment of the facial nerve. They were able to control facial nerve stimulation in all patients through programming mode changes. Familiarity with more elaborate programming techniques is critical to managing patients with this complication.

3.2.5.6 Complications

3.2.5.6.1 Bacterial meningitis

In the year 2002, a growing number of reports of bacterial meningitis were received by the US FDA in cochlear implant recipients. Irrespective of the manufacturer, the complications were found in almost all the cochlear implants. It was founded by authors Cohen and colleagues [112] that the number of meningitis cases was actually greater than as previously thought and reconfirmed that devices irrespective of the manufacturers were associated with bacterial meningeal infections. As per the existing protocol, the FDA put out an advisory notice in respect of minors. It throws a notification that all minors who were planned for cochlear implants should also be immunized. The vaccination against *Streptococcus pneumoniae* is advised [113,114]. Two factors that may contribute to the incidence of bacterial meningitis from a perspective of designing devices are electrodes that were at increased risk of development of biofilm and subsequent depression of immune cells. Another is the role of infection in those settings along with any trauma created during the procedure or by other means [115].

3.2.5.6.2 Safety considerations

The implants that are placed nearer to the brain should be absolutely safe. However, absolute implant product safety is almost impossible to achieve in human application procedures. Still, it should be a prime target for better efficacy and outcome. The safety of the patient should occupy the highest priority in case of cochlear implants or of any set of the product meant for this purpose. The four important categories that are purely considered for the safety of any implantable neural prosthetic device are the materials and their biocompatibility and toxicity followed by sterilization to eliminate the infection. The third is the mechanical design and its impact to cause structural tissue damage. The final is the energy exposure limits that are instrumental in the resulting tissue or neural damage or affections.

3.2.5.6.3 Risk management

It is important and critical to identify the interactions between the device, the recipient, and the environment it is being used. The US FDA has adopted a good human factors engineering approach for the above impact like to identify and to isolate these factors. They try to address the factors and help in the management of their risks [116].

To minimize the use-related hazards and to assure the recipient and the intended users to use medical devices very safely and effectively throughout the required timeline, the US FDA has set up the goal. This also facilitates the review of submissions for new devices and to design control in the documentation of materials.

3.2.6 Conclusion

From the available literature, it is concluded that the device-related complications were rare when compared to the surgical-related complications. However, still, device failure seen in cochlear implants by various factors has to be reported to the respective countries' medical device safety authorities.

References

[1] Pandit JK, Singh S, Muthu MS. Controlled release formulations in neurology practice. Ann Indian Acad Neurol 2006;9:207–16.

[2] Thomas JS, Andrew P, David LB, Joel DB, Kenneth AG, et al. Intravitreal sustained-release ganciclovir. Arch Ophthalmol 1992;110(2):255–8.

[3] Upendra N. Recent advances in ocular drug delivery system. J Adv Pharm Technol Res 2014;5(4):151.

[4] Dohlman CH, Schneider HA, Doane MG. Porsthokeratoplasty. Am J Ophthalmol 1974;77(5):694–700.
[5] Pintucci S, Pintucci F, Cecconi M, Caiazze S. New dacron tissue colonisable keratoprosthesis: clinical experience. Br J Ophthalmol 1995;79(9):825–9.
[6] Pintucci S, Pintucci F, Caiazza S, Cecconi M. The dacron felt colonisable keratoprosthesis: after 15 years. Eur J Ophthalmol 1996;6(2):125–30.
[7] David RJ. Porous versus Nonporous orbital implants: a 25-year retrospective. Am Acad Ophthal 2018;125(9):1317–19.
[8] Schellini S, El Dib R, Silva LRE, Farat JG, Zhang Y, Jorge EC. Integrated versus non-integrated orbital implants for treating anophthalmic sockets (review). Cochrane Database Syst Rev 2016;11 CD010293.
[9] Blevatskaya ED. Intralamellar homoplasty for the purpose of relaxation of refraction of the eye. Arch Soc Am Ophthalmol Optom 1968;6:311–25.
[10] Vega-Estrada A, Alio JL. The use of intracorneal ring segments in keratoconus. Eye Vis (Lond) 2016;15:3–8.
[11] Barnett M, Mannis MJ. Contact lenses in the management of keratoconus. Cornea 2011;30:1510–16.
[12] Colin J, Cochener B, Savary G, Malet F. Correcting keratoconus with intracorneal rings. J Cataract Refract Surg 2000;26:1117–22.
[13] Baino F, Perero S, Ferraris S, Miola M, Balagna C, Verne E, et al. Biomaterials for orbital implants and ocular prostheses: overview and future prospects. Acta Biomater 2014;10(4):1064–87.
[14] Levine MR, Fagien S. Enucleation and evisceration. In: Stuart WB, editor. Surgery of the eyelid, orbit and lacrimal system. San Francisco: American Academy of Ophthalmology; 1995. p. 84–108 [chapter 30].
[15] Perry AC. Integrated orbital implants. Adv Ophthal Plast Reconstr Surg 1990;8: 75–81.
[16] Yazici B, Akova B, Sanli O. Complications of primary placement of motility post in porous polyethylene implants during enucleation. Am J Ophthalmol 2007;143(5):828–34.
[17] Wells TS, Harris GJ. Direct fixation of extraocular muscles to a silicone sphere: a cost-sensitive, low-risk enucleation procedure. Ophthal Plast Resconstr Surg 2011;27:364–7.
[18] Tataru CP, Pop MD. Enucleation in malignant choroidal melanoma – results in 15 years of using a new material in the prosthesis of the orbital cavity. J Med Life 2012;5:185–8.
[19] Kuzmanovic ELabjer B, Petrinovic-Doresci J, Busic M, Henc-Petrinovic L. Our approach in the treatment of exposed hydroxyapatite orbital implant. Acta Med Cr 2006;60(2):141–4.
[20] Ho VMW, Hussain RN, Czanner G. Porous versus nonporous orbital implants after enucleation for uveal melanoma: a randomized study. Ophthal Plast Reconstr Surg 2017;33:452–8.
[21] Wladis EJ, Aakalu VK, Sobel RK, Yen MT, Bilyk JR, Mawn LA. Orbital implants in enucleation surgery: a report by the American Academy of Ophthalmology. Ophthalmol 2018;125:311–17.
[22] Melles GRJ, Ververs B, van der Linden JW. Cosmetic extraocular implant. J Cataract Refract Surg 2004;30:1595–6.
[23] Noriyuki K, Shinobu F. Recent advances in ocular drug delivery systems. Polymers 2011;3(1):193–221.
[24] Salerno LC, Tiveron Jr MC, Alió JL. Multifocal intraocular lenses: types, outcomes, complications and how to solve them. Taiwan J Ophthalmol 2017;7(4):179–84.
[25] Moshirfar M. Spherical aberration of intraocular lenses. J Ophthal Vis Res 2010;5 (4):215–16.

[26] Pineda R, Chauhan T. Phakic intraocular lenses and their special indications. J Ophthal Vis Res 2016;11(4):422−8.
[27] Wagoner MD, Cox TA, Ariyasu RG, et al. IOL implantation in the absence of capsular support: a report by the AAO. Ophthalmology 2003;110:840−59.
[28] Donaldson KE, Gorscak JJ, Budenz DL, et al. Anterior chamber and sutured posterior chamber intraocular lenses in eyes with poor capsular support. J Cataract Refract Surg 2005;31:903−9.
[29] Stem MS, Todorich B, Woodward MA, Hsu J, Wolfe JD. Scleral-fixated intraocular lenses: past and present. J Vitreoretin Dis 2017;1(2):144−52.
[30] Banaee T, Sagheb S. Scleral fixation of intraocular lens in eyes with history of open globe injury. J Pediatr Ophthalmol Strabismus 2011;48(5):292−7.
[31] Alio JL, Sanz-Diez P. Phakic intraocular lenses in keratoconus. Int J Kerat Ect Cor Dis 2015;4:103−6.
[32] Kamiya K, Shimizu K, Igarashi A, Hikita F, Komatsu M. Four year follow-up of posterior chamber phakic intraocular lens implantation for moderate to high myopia. Arch Ophthalmol 2009;127:845−50.
[33] Yasin MN, Svirskis D, Seyfoddin A, Rupenthal ID. Implants for drug delivery to the posterior segment of the eye: a focus on stimuli-responsive and tunable release systems. J Control Rel 2014;196:208−21.
[34] Fialho SL, Rego MGB, Cardillo JA, Siqueira RC, Jorge R, Silva-Cunha A. Biodegradable implants for intraocular administration. Braz Arch Ophthalmol 2003;66(6):891−6.
[35] Jain RA. The manufacturing techniques of various drug loaded biodegradable poly (lactide-co-glycolide) (PLGA) device. Biomaterials 2000;21:2475−90.
[36] Bourges JL, Bloquel C, Thomas A, Froussart F, Bochot A, Azan F, et al. Intraocular implants for extended drug delivery: therapeutic applications. Adv Drug Deliv Rev 2006;58:1182−202.
[37] Nair LS, Laurencin CT. Biodegradable polymers as biomaterials. Prog Polym Sci 2007;32:762−98.
[38] Dong X, Chen N, Xie L, Wang S. Prevention of experimental proliferative vitreoretinopathy with a biodegradable intravitreal drug delivery system of all-trans retinoic acid. Retina 2006;26:210−13.
[39] Fialho SL, Behar-Cohen F, Silva-Cunha A. Dexamethasone-loaded poly (ε -caprolactone) intravitreal implants: a pilot study. Eur J Pharm Biopharm 2008;68:637−46.
[40] Kimura H, Ogura Y. Biodegradable polymers for ocular drugs delivery. Ophthalmologica 2001;215:143−55.
[41] Peyman GA, Ganiban GJ. Delivery systems for intra-ocular routes. Adv Drug Deliv Rev 2006;16:107−23.
[42] Einmahl S, Behan-Cohen F, Tabatabay C, D'Hermies F, Heller J, Gurny R. A viscous bioerodible poly (ortho ester) as a new biomaterial for intraocular application. J Biomed Mater Res 2000;50:566−73.
[43] Tan DTH, Chess S, Lim L, Lim AS. Randomized clinical trial of a new dexamethasone delivery system (Surodex) for treatment of postcataract surgery inflammation. Ophthalmology 1999;106:223−31.
[44] Wadood AC, Armbrecht AM, Aspinall PA, Dhillon B. Safety and efficacy of a dexamethasone anterior segment drug delivery system in patients after phacoemulsification. J Cataract Refract Surg 2004;30:761−8.
[45] Dugel PU, Eliott D, Cantrill HL, Mahmoud T, Avery R, Erickson SR. I-VationTM TA: 24-month clinical results of the phase I safety and preliminary efficacy study. Invest Ophthalmol Vis Sci 2009;50:4332.
[46] Edelman JL. Differentiating intraocular glucocorticoids. Ophthalmologica 2010;224: 25−30.

[47] Yasukawa K, Ogura Y, Tabata Y, Kimura H, Wiedemann P, Honda Y. Drug delivery systems for vitreoretinal diseases. Prog Retin Eye Res 2004;23:253–81.

[48] Lim JI, Wolitz RA, Dowling AH, Bloom HR, Irvine AR, Schwartz DM. Visual and anatomic outcomes associated with posterior segment complications after ganciclovir implant procedures in patients with AIDS and cytomegalovirus retinitis. Am J Ophthalmol 1999;127:288–93.

[49] Daniel FM, David JP, Susan DM, Frederick LF, Christopher W, et al. Treatment of cytomegalovirus retinitis with intraocular sustained-release ganciclovir implant. Arch Ophtalmol 1994;112(2):1531–9.

[50] Jabs DA, Ahuja A, Van Natta M, Dunn JP, Yeh S, Studies of the ocular complications of AIDS group. Comparison of treatment regimens for cytomegalovirus retinitis in patients with AIIDS in the era highly active antiretroviral therapy. Ophthalmol 2013;120:1262–70.

[51] Kapel PJ, Charonis AC, Holland GN, Narayanan R, Kulkarni AD, Yu F, et al. Outcomes associated with ganciclovir implants in patients with SIDA-related cytomegalovirus retinitis. Ophthalmology 2006;113:673–83.

[52] Debra AG, David GG, Anthony H, David GC, Glenn JJ, Pearson PA, et al. Intraocular pressure in patients with uveitis treated with fluocinolone acetonide implants. Arch Ophthalmol 2007;125:1478–85.

[53] Jeffe GJ, Martin D, Callanan D, Pearson PA, Levy B, Comstock T. Fluocinolone acetonide implant (Retisert) for non-infectious posterior uveitis: thirty four-week results of a multicentre randomized clinical study. Ophthalmology 2006; 113:1020–7.

[54] Campochiaro PA, Brown DM, Pearson A, Chen S, Boyer D, Ruiz-Moreno J, et al. Sustained delivery fluocinolone acetonide vitreous inserts provide benefit for at least 3 years in patients with diabetic macular edema. Ophthalmology 2012;119:2125–32.

[55] Kane FE, Burdan J, Cutino A, Green KE. Iluvien: a new sustained delivery technology for posterior eye diseases. Expert Opin Drug Deliv 2008;5:1039–46.

[56] El-Ghrably IA, Saad A, Dinah C. A novel technique for repositioning of a migrated ILUVIEN® (fluocinolone acetonide) implant into the anterior chamber. Ophthalmol Ther 2015;4:129–33.

[57] Wang J, Jiang A, Joshi M, Christoforidis J. Drug delivery implants in the treatment of vitreous inflammation. Mediat Inflamm 2013;2013:780634.

[58] Xu X, Al-Ghabeish M, Rahman Z, Krishnaiah YS, Yerlikaya F, Yang Y, et al. Formulation and process factors influencing product quality and *in vitro* performance of ophthalmic ointment. Int J Pharm 2015;493(1–2):412–25.

[59] ClinicalTrials.gov. A study of MK0140 in diabetic patients with macular edema, <http: //clinicaltrials.gov/ct2/archive/NCT-00692614/>; 2015.

[60] Spiegel D, Kobuch K. Trabecular meshwork bypass tube shunt: initial case series. Br J Ophthalmol 2002;86(11):1228–31.

[61] Riva I, Roberti G, Oddone F, Konstas AG, Quaranta L. Ahmed glaucoma valve implant: surgical technique and complications. Clin Ophthalmol 2017;11:357–67.

[62] Krasnov MM. Sinusotomy in glaucoma. Vestn Oftalmol 1964;7737–41.

[63] Werner L, Apple D, Pandey S, Trivedi R, Izak A, Macky T. Phakic posterior chamber intraocular lenses. Int Ophthalmol Clin 2002;41:153–74.

[64] Shanmugam PM, Ramanjulu R, Mishra KCD, Sagar P. Novel techniques in scleral buckling. Indian J Ophthalmol 2018;66(7):909–15.

[65] Penttilä E, Smirnov G, Tuomilehto H, Kaarniranta K, Seppä J. Endoscopic dacryocystorhinostomy as treatment for lower lacrimal pathway obstructions in adults: review article. Allergy Rhinol (Providence) 2015;6(1):12–19.

[66] Ravi K, Srivastava P, Movdawalla M, Sen S, Kedia P. Implants in glaucoma: a minor review. Sci J Med Vis Res Foun 2017;XXXV:3–9.

[67] Wang J, Barton K. Aqueous shunt implantation in glaucoma. Taiwan J Ophthalmol 2017;7(3):130–7.

[68] Doganay S, Sarac K, Miman MC, Karadag N, Cokkeser Y. Polyurethane stent obstruction as a cause of recurrent epiphora. case report. Interv Neuroradiol 2006;12 (1):69–72.

[69] American Academy of Family Physicians; American Academy of Otolaryngology-Head and Neck Surgery; American Academy of Pediatrics Subcommittee on Otitis Media with Effusion. Otitis media with effusion. Pediatrics 2004;113:1412–29.

[70] Scottish Intercollegiate Guidelines Network. Guideline No. 66. Diagnosis and management of childhood otitis media in primary care. Edinburgh: Scottish Intercollegiate Guidelines Network. Available from: <http://www.sign.ac.uk/guidelines/fulltext/66/index.html/ > ; 2003 [cited 05.11.07]

[71] Williamson I. Otitis media with effusion in children. BMJ Clin Evid 2007;2007:502.

[72] Perera R, Haynes J, Glasziou P, Heneghan CJ. Autoinflation for hearing loss associated with otitis media with effusion. Cochrane Database Syst Rev 2006; CD006285.

[73] Zielhuis GA, Rach GH, van den Bosch A, van den Broek P. The prevalence of otitis media with effusion: a critical review of the literature. Clin Otolaryngol 1990;15: 283–8.

[74] Zielhuis GA, Rach GH, van den Broek P. Screening for otitis media with effusion in preschool children. Lancet 1989;1:311–14.

[75] Freemantle N, Long A, Mason J, Sheldon T, Song F, et al. The treatment of persistent glue ear in children. Leeds: University of Leeds; 1992. Effective Health Care. Number 4.

[76] Shekelle P., Takata G., Chan L., Mangione-Smith R., Corley P.M., *et al.* Diagnosis, natural history, and late effects of otitis media with effusion. Volume 1. Evidence report and evidence tables. Agency for Healthcare Research and Quality. AHRQ Publication No. 03-E023. Available from: <http://www.ahrq.gov/downloads/pub/evidence/pdf/otdiag/otdiag.pdf/>; 2003 [cited 22.11.07]

[77] Lous J, Burton MJ, Felding JU, Ovesen T, Rovers MM, Williamson I. Grommets (ventilation tubes) for hearing loss associated with otitis media with effusion in children. Cochrane Database Syst Rev 2005;(Issue 1) CD001801.

[78] National Collaborating Centre for Women's and Children's Health. Surgical management of otitis media with effusion (draft for consultation). London: RCOG Press; 2007[cited 10.12.07]. Available from. Available from: http://www.nice.org.uk/guidance/index.jsp?action = download&o = 38056.

[79] Koopman JP, Reuchlin AG, Kummer EE, Boumans LJ, Rijntjes E, Hoeve LJ, et al. Laser myringotomy versus ventilation tubes in children with otitis media with effusion: a randomized trial. Laryngoscope 2004;114:844–9.

[80] Rovers MM, Straatman H, Ingels K, van der Wilt GJ, van den Broek P, Zielhuis GA. The effect of ventilation tubes on language development in infants with otitis media with effusion: a randomized trial. Pediatrics 2000;106:e42.

[81] Paradise JL, Feldman HM, Campbell TF, Dollaghan CA, Colborn DK, Bernard BS, et al. Effect of early or delayed insertion of tympanostomy tubes for persistent otitis media on developmental outcomes at the age of three years. N Engl J Med 2001;344:1179–87.

[82] Paradise JL, Feldman HM, Campbell TF, Dollaghan CA, Rockette HE, Pitcairn DL, et al. Tympanostomy tubes and developmental outcomes at 9 to 11 years of age. N Engl J Med 2007;356:248–61.

[83] Maw R, Wilks J, Harvey I, Peters TJ, Golding J. Early surgery compared with watchful waiting for glue ear and effect on language development in preschool children: a randomised trial. Lancet 1999;353:960–3.

[84] Browning GG. Two-year outcome of ventilation tubes in a randomized controlled trial of persistent childhood otitis media with effusion. Clin Otolaryngol Allied Sci 2001;26:342–4.
[85] Medical Research Council Multicentre Otitis Media Study Group. Surgery for persistent otitis media with effusion: generalizability of results from the UK trial (TARGET). Clin Otolaryngol Allied Sci 2001;26:417–24.
[86] Kay DJ, Nelson M, Rosenfeld RM. Meta-analysis of tympanostomy tube sequelae. Otolaryngol Head Neck Surg 2001;124:374–80.
[87] Ingels K, Rovers MM, van der Wilt GJ, Zielhuis GA. Ventilation tubes in infants increase the risk of otorrhoea and antibiotic usage. B-ENT 2005;1:173–6.
[88] Cruickshanks KJ, Tweed TS, Wiley TL, et al. The 5-year incidence and progression of hearing loss: the epidemiology of hearing loss study. Arch otolaryngol Head Neck Surg 2003;129(10):1041–6.
[89] Sprinzl GM, Riechelmann H. Current trends in treating hearing loss in elderly people: a review of the technology and treatment options – a mini-review. Gerontology 2010;56:351–8.
[90] Sorkin DL. Cochlear implantation in the world's largest medical device market: utilization and awareness of cochlear implants in the United States. Cochlear Implants Int 2013;14(Suppl. 1):S4–12.
[91] Wong DJ, Moran M, O'Leary SJ. Outcomes after cochlear implantation in the very elderly. Otol Neurotol 2016;37:46–51.
[92] Carlson ML, Breen JT, Gifford RH, et al. Cochlear implantation in the octogenarian and nonagenarian. Otol Neurotol 2010;31:1343e1349.
[93] Chen DS, Clarrett DM, Li L, Bowditch SP, Niparko JK, Lin FR. Cochlear implantation in older adults: long-term analysis of complications and device survival in a consecutive series. Otol Neurotol 2013;34:1272e1277.
[94] Roberts DS, Lin HW, Herrmann BS, Lee DJ. Differential cochlear implant outcomes in older adults. Laryngoscope 2013;123:1952–6.
[95] Schwab B, Gandolfi M, Lai E, Reilly E, Singer L, Kim AH. The impact of age on cochlear implant performance. Int J Otolaryngol Head Neck Surg 2015;4:329–37.
[96] Spitzer JB, Cellum IP, Bosworth C. Stability of audiometric measures and challenges in long-term management of the elderly cochlear implant patient. Otol Neurotol 2013;34:1636–41.
[97] Wei BP, Shepherd RK, Robins-Browne RM, Clark GM, O'Leary SJ. Pneumococcal meningitis post-cochlear implantation: preventative measures. Otolaryngol Head Neck Surg 2010;143:S9–14.
[98] Azadarmaki R, Tubbs R, Chen DA, Shellock FG. MRI information for commonly used otologic implants: review and update. Otolaryngol Head Neck Surg 2014;150 (4):512–19.
[99] Hassepass F, Stabenau V, Maier W, et al. Revision surgery due to magnet dislocation in cochlear implant patients: an emerging complication. Otol Neurotol 2014;35(1):29–34.
[100] Crane BT, Gottschalk B, Kraut M, Aygun N, Niparko JK. Magnetic resonance imaging at 1.5 T after cochlear implantation. Otol Neurotol 2010;31(8):1215–20.
[101] Elgandy Mohamed Salah, Mobashir Mohammad Kamal, Ezzeddin EL Sheikh, Hansen Marlan, Tyler Richard, Dunn Camille, et al. Revision cochlear implant surgery. Int Tinnitus J 2018;22(2):188–97.
[102] Balkany TJ, Hodges AV, Gomez MO, Bird PA, Dolan AS, Butts S, et al. Cochlear re implantation. Laryngoscope. 1999;109 351-35.
[103] Balkany TJ, Hodges AV, Buchman CA, Luxford WM, Pillsbury CH, Roland PS, et al. Cochlear implant soft failures consensus development conference statement. Otol Neurotol 2005;26:815–18.

[104] Gantz BJ, Lowder MW, McCabe BF. Audiologic results following reimplantation of cochlear implants. Ann Otol Rhinol Laryngol 1989;98:12–16.
[105] Hochmair DI, Burian K. Re-implantation of a molded scala tympani electrode Impact on psychophysical and speech discrimination abilities. Ann Otol Rhinol Laryngol 1985;94:65–7.
[106] Lindeman RC, Mangham CA, Kuprenas SV. Single-channel and multichannel performance for reimplanted cochlear prosthesis patient. Ann Otol Rhinol Laryngol 1987;96(Suppl. 128):150–1.
[107] Chute PM, Hellman SA, Parisier SC, Tartter VC, Economou A. Auditory perception changes after re implantation in a child cochlear implant user. Ear Hear 1992;13:195–9.
[108] Economou A, Tartter VC, Chute PM, Hellman SA. Speech changes following re implantation from a single-channel to a multichannel cochlear implant. J Acoust Soc Am 1992;92:1310–23.
[109] Niparko JK, Oviatt DL, Coker NJ. Facial nerve stimulation with cochlear implantation. Otolaryngol Head Neck Surg 1991;104:826–30.
[110] Burmeister J, Rathgeb S, Herzog J. Cochlear implantation in patients with otosclerosis of the otic capsule. Am J Otolaryngol 2017;38:556–9.
[111] Kelsall DC, Shallop JK, Brammeier TG, Prenger EC. Facial nerve stimulation after nucleus 22 channel cochlear implantation. Am J Otol 1997;18:336–41.
[112] Cohen NL, Roland Jr JT, Marrinan M. Meningitis in cochlear implant recipients: the North American experience. Otol Neurotol 2004;25:275–81.
[113] Whitney CG. Cochlear implants and meningitis in children. Pediatr Infect Dis J 2004;23:767–8.
[114] Reefhuis J, Honein MA, Whitney CG, Chamany S, Mann EA, Biernath KR, et al. Risk of bacterial meningitis in children with cochlear implants. N Engl J Med 2003;349:435–45.
[115] Wei BP, Shepherd RK, Robins-Browne RM, Clark GM, O'Leary SJ. Effects of inner ear trauma on the risk of pneumococcal meningitis. Arch Otolaryngol Head Neck Surg 2007;133:250–9.
[116] Guidance for Industry and FDA Premarket and Design Control Reviewers: Medical Device Use-Safety: Incorporating Human Factors Engineering into Risk Management. U.S. Food and Drug Administration, July 18; 2000.

CHAPTER FOUR

Dental

Priya Gupta Vajrapu*
Boston Medical Center, Boston, MA, United States
*Corresponding author

Abstract

This chapter provides an overview of dental devices and classifies them based on FDA subpart C. A list of dental devices, their toxic effects, adverse effects, and side effects of the devices are discussed. The effects of the long-term placement of these materials in the oral cavity and possibly leading to unwanted reactions are further discussed.

Keywords: Dental devices; implant; root canal; dental filling material; dental cement; dental resin; dental X-rays; crowns; cytotoxic; corrosion

4.1 Introduction

All matter in the human mouth, be they naturally occurring or artificially implanted, continuously interact with a variety of substances ranging from slightly acidic saliva to highly acidic fruits, from hot coffee to cold ice cream, from soft bread to crunchy nuts. This constant interaction makes the oral cavity one of the most inhospitable environments in the human body [1]. Implantation of any materials for relatively long durations could potentially result in unforeseen and undesirable reactions.

These criteria make the selection of dental materials a meticulous process, and the people responsible have to be cautious in their choices. Factors such as corrosiveness, biocompatibility, cost, availability, mechanical properties, and aesthetic appearance should feature into these decisions. However discriminating these decisions may be, it just is not possible to eliminate risk. Accordingly, medical devices are categorized into three risk classes: class 1 (low risk), class 2 (moderate risk), and class 3 (high risk) based on the risk posed to the patient and practitioner and the level of experience and control needed to handle the device safely.

Toxicological Aspects of Medical Device Implants.
DOI: https://doi.org/10.1016/B978-0-12-820728-4.00004-6
© 2020 Elsevier Inc.
All rights reserved.

We will discuss these classes and some examples of the devices that fall into these classes in the following sections divided by device types:

1. Diagnostic
2. Prosthetic
3. Surgical
4. Therapeutic

4.2 Diagnostic dental devices

See Table 4.1.

Diagnosis in any medical field is the process of obtaining data from questioning, examining, and testing to ascertain any deviations from the normal to suggest a prognosis [2]. Equipment used to diagnose dental and oral health typically are safe to use and are not implanted. It does not spend an excessive amount of time in contact with biological fluids in the mouth, and as such are classified as class 1 and class 2 risks. Some dental diagnostic devices and their possible toxic side effects are discussed below.

Table 4.1 List of diagnostic dental devices.

Device name	Class	Description	Implanted
Gingival fluid measurer	1	Measures the fluid in the gingival sulcus	No
Electrode gel for pulp tester	1	For electrical activity	No
Dental X-ray exposure alignment device	1	To maintain the alignment of the X-ray	No
Dental X-ray film holder	1	To hold the film in position	No
Pulp tester	2	To test the vitality of the pulp	No
Caries detection device	2	Detects caries	No
Extraoral source X-ray system	2	X-ray source to take extraoral X-rays	No
Intraoral source X-ray system	2	X-ray source to take X-rays inside the mouth	No
Cephalometer	2	Device that measures the head diameter	No
Dental X-ray position-indicating device	2	Helps in positioning the X-ray	No

4.2.1 Pulp tester and electrode gel for testing

Dental pulp status diagnosis depends on prior history, clinical, and radiological examination. Vitality testing is an essential aid in the diagnosis of pulp disease and apical periodontitis.

Dentists should be vigilant while conducting the pulp testing procedure. An improper technique or procedure may cause the spread of electrical impulses to adjacent teeth or gingival tissue. Metallic restorations in the oral cavity act as a path of transfer of electric current between adjacent teeth [2]. It can lead to false positives and false negatives, causing difficulties in making a correct diagnosis. The inconsistencies encountered with the pulp tester could be due to several factors [3]:

1. The inaccuracy of the instrument
2. The unreliability of the instrument
3. Differences in each clinician's technique
4. Different electrode media
5. Various responses with different individuals

A false-positive response is said to occur when a nonvital tooth appears to respond positively to testing. This occurrence can be seen in anxious or young patients, as they are anticipating an unpleasant sensation. Examples of other false positives can include the ability to conduct electric currents to viable nerve tissue in the surrounding area through the necrotic breakdown products in the root canal system, metallic restorations that act as a path of transfer of the conduction of current to the periodontium and gingiva. Inadequately dried teeth could also result in false positives. Other factors that possibly play a role in generating inaccurate results are the effects of dental development, multirooted teeth, the influence of age, effects of drugs, trauma, and periodontal disease (Figs. 4.1, 4.2).

A little voltage or current does tend to pass even without an electrode medium. The electrode gel acts as a medium and efficiently disperses the electric stimulation to the target area. Potential health risks with the use

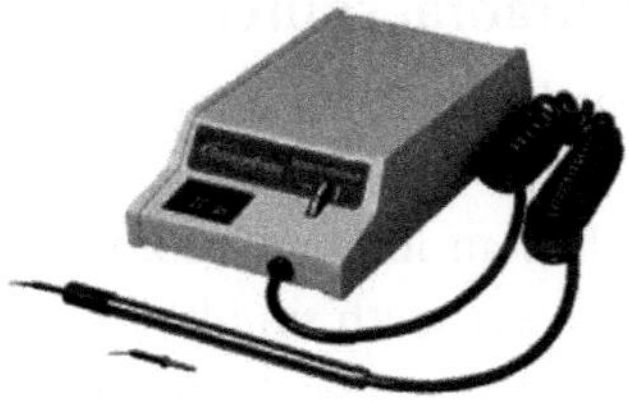

Figure 4.1 Vitality scanner.

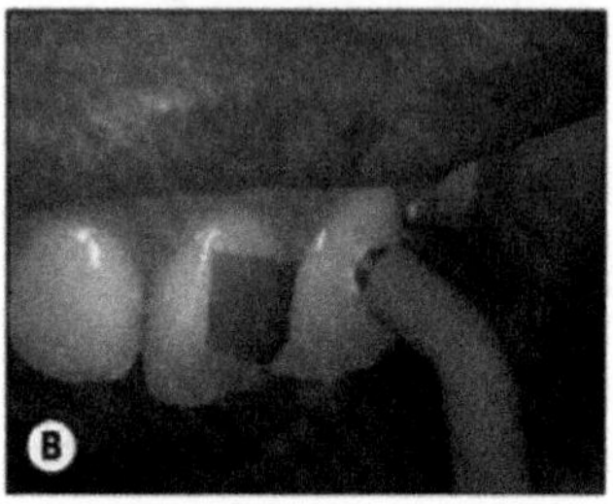

Figure 4.2 Pulp tester unit with two tips.

of electrode gels include irritation in the eyes and skin upon contact, and for large doses ingested, it can cause gastrointestinal tract irritation with thirst, nausea, vomiting, and diarrhea. It may also affect the central nervous system, the urinary system, the cardiovascular system, and the liver causing headaches, insomnia, toxic psychosis, muscle weakness, and elevated blood sugar levels.

4.2.2 Dental X-rays and their segments

One of the most vital tools used in the diagnosis of oral abnormalities and conditions is radiography. Even though the radiation levels involved in dental radiography are quite low, dentists should take care to minimize a patient's exposure to radiation. An example: taking multiple radiographs in a short time leads to a slight increase in the radiation dose absorbed by the patient and should be avoided. Shifted radiographs are taken during root canal treatments and other endodontic therapies to differentiate between the buccal and lingual canals. The process to obtain shifted radiographs while also trying to align the position-indicating device with the film is cumbersome at best. This often-frustrating task can potentially result in several technical errors, and lead to retakes and lower radiographic quality. Prolonged and consistent exposure to X-rays is associated with a higher risk of cancer as per the literature [4].

4.2.3 Intraoral and extraoral source system

Bitewing and digital dental panoramic radiographs play a significant role in dentistry.

A bitewing radiograph is an intraoral radiograph that shows images of crowns of the upper and lower teeth simultaneously.

The panoramic radiograph is an extraoral radiographic technique that captures both the maxilla and the mandible on a single exposure. This type of radiograph helps determine the development of the jaws of children and adolescents. It also provides information about the mixed dentition stages and the status of resorption of primary dentition. Children are vulnerable to a higher risk of genetic damage from radiation exposure as compared to adults, due to a higher degree of active cell division and having rapidly growing tissues that are more radiosensitive than mature tissue in adults. In both radiographic techniques, the oral-buccal epithelium is directly exposed to ionizing X-ray radiation. Even though X-rays are used extensively for diagnostic and therapeutic reasons, there is significant concern about the potentially harmful effects associated with radiation exposure. Ionizing radiation either acts directly on DNA or indirectly by synthesizing reactive compounds that interact with DNA causing cell cytotoxicity [5].

Bitewing and panoramic radiographs should be prescribed only when essential. There has been an uptick in the frequency of micronuclei post-exposure to both radiographic procedures. The micronuclei are extranuclear bodies that carry damaged chromosome fragments. These act as a sensitive biomarker for genotoxicity. Bitewing radiography creates a threefold increase in micronuclei frequency, and digital panoramic radiographs create a twofold increase in micronuclei frequency. Thus the increase in radiation exposure time increases the occurrence of micronuclei frequency (Figs. 4.3, 4.4).

Recurring exposure to dental X-rays can result in multiple head and neck cancers such as the brain, the parotid gland, the salivary gland, and thyroid cancer, and other systemic problems. Systemic health abnormalities, such as leukemia and low birth weight, were reported in the literature. Observational studies have found that X-rays exposure is often associated with the risk of meningioma [8].

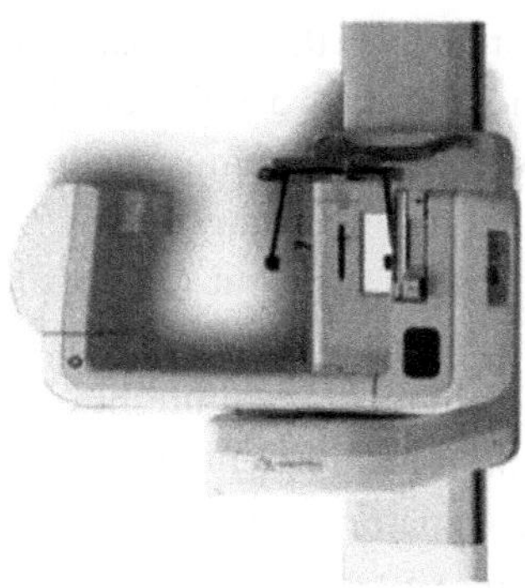

Figure 4.3 Extraoral X-ray machine [6].

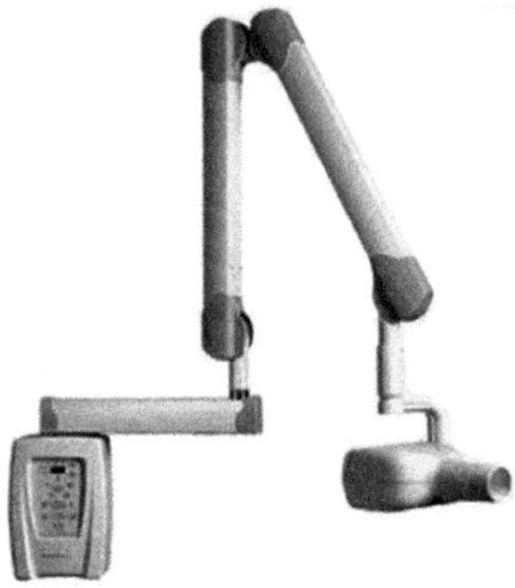

Figure 4.4 Intraoral X-ray machine [7].

4.2.4 X-ray position-indicating device and collimators

As has been discussed, the low doses of radiation from X-rays cause little damage, but it is not nonexistent. Biological damage inevitably occurs every time a photon delivers radiation. Consider the fact that just standing outside in the sun can cause sunburn without protection.

A collimator is a device that narrows down a beam of particles or waves. Collimators make use of two sets of lead shutters that absorb a significant percentage of photons, thus focusing the beam of particles on the desired area. The collimator is positioned at the tube head or the end of the beam-indicating device, that is, cone. In circular collimation, almost three times the area of radiation necessary to expose a number 2 film is delivered. However, in rectangular collimation, the beam is restricted to approximately the size of the number 2 intraoral film (3.2×4.1 cm). Consequently, this restricted beam size can result in exposure errors [9]. Nevertheless, the significantly reduced risk of radiation damage means that dentists prefer the use of rectangular collimators over their circular counterparts.

Rectangular collimation exposes a little less than half the area exposed by circular collimation, and there is a minuscule margin of error when using it. However, when a position-indicating device is used to align the film, there are higher possibilities for cone cut and misalignment errors resulting in retakes and leading to an increase in radiation exposure (Figs. 4.5, 4.6).

Employing the use of collimators diminishes image brightness, and this requires an increase in the radiation entrance surface dose [10]. Another disadvantage of using collimators is that it increases the kinetic energy released per unit mass, and so possibly inducing deterministic effects such as epilation and erythema.

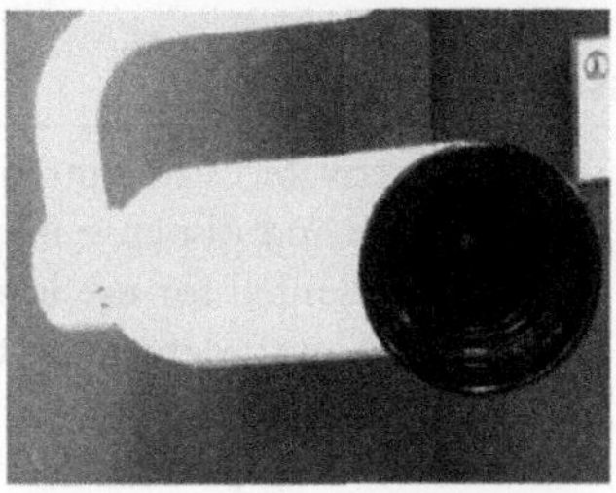

Figure 4.5 Circular collimator [9].

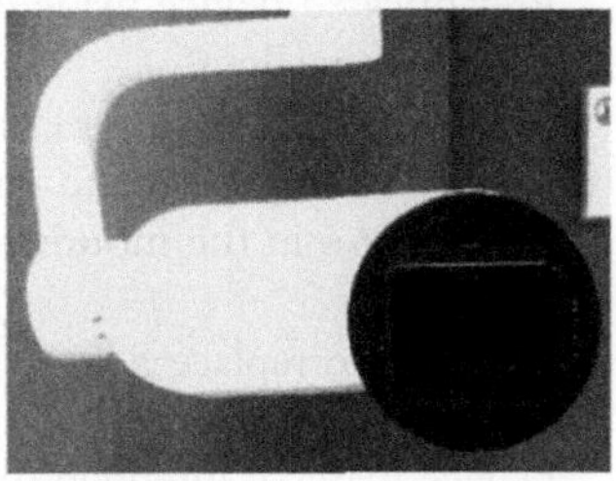

Figure 4.6 Rectangular collimator [9].

Radiation risk in dental radiography is mostly related to the radiosensitive structures in the head and neck area. Studies reported that the chances of one cancer fatality could be expected from 47,620 full mouth examinations made with D-speed film and circular collimation or from every 17,000 cone-beam computed tomography examinations. Even though the benefits of diagnostic imaging outweigh the risk, a dentist must always be conscious of the fact that imaging carries a risk.

4.3 Prosthetic devices

See Table 4.2.

Different varieties of dental cement have been widely used in various clinical applications as filling materials, protective cavity liners, luting materials for crowns, bridges, inlays and orthodontic appliances, root canal fillings, and pulp capping. Prosthetic devices are classified under class 1, class 2, and class 3 devices based on the amount of risk. Most of these devices can be temporarily or permanently implanted in the oral cavity. Some prosthetic devices and their possible toxic side effects are discussed below.

Table 4.2 List of prosthetic dental devices.

Device name	Class	Description	Implanted
Mercury and alloy dispenser	1	Spring-activated valve intended to measure and dispense mercury	No
Facebow	1	Device intended for use in denture fabrication to determine the spatial relationship	No
Denture relining, denture cushion or pad	1	Intended to replace a worn denture lining	Yes
Preformed crown	1	Prefabricated device made of plastic or austenitic alloys	Yes
Gutta-percha	1	Intended to fill the root canal of a tooth	Yes
Dental bur	1	Rotary-cutting device to cut hard structures in the mouth, such as teeth or bone	No
Denture cushion or pad	1	Intended to replace a worn denture lining	Yes
Calcium hydroxide cavity liner	2	Device material intended to be applied to the interior of a prepared cavity before insertion of restorative material	Yes
Endosseous dental implant	2	A prescription device surgically placed in the bone to provide support for prosthetic devices	Yes
Subperiosteal implant material	2	Device is intended to provide support for prostheses, such as dentures	Yes
Noble metal alloy	2	Device composed of noble metals for the fabrication of cast, crown, bridges	Yes
Dental cements	2	Device material intended to serve as a temporary tooth filling or as a base cement or to fix crowns or bridges	Yes
Root canal filling resin	2	Device used along with the core root canal filling material to fill any gaps provide an access route for bacteria	Yes
Dental amalgam/ mercury/amalgam alloy	2	Silver alloy is intended to be mixed with mercury to form a dental amalgam	Yes
Resin tooth bonding agent	2	Painted on the interior of the prepared cavity for retention	Yes
Denture adhesive	3	Intended to replace a worn denture lining	Yes

4.3.1 Dental amalgam

Dental amalgam is an alloy of the metal mercury (Hg). It is known for its versatility, strength and durability, low cost, and bacteriostatic effect. Dental amalgams appeared in Germany nearly 500 years ago and became the preferred dental restorative in the 1800s and are still widely used, though not without their share of controversy.

Amalgams are particularly durable, long-lasting, and least technique sensitive. Concerns, however, are being raised regarding mercury toxicity caused by the use of amalgam [11]. Maximum exposure to mercury in the amalgam occurs during the placement or removal of the restoration in the tooth. Once placed, this exposure is minimized to below the current health standard.

Dental amalgam is known to cause delayed hypersensitivity reactions in some people. These reactions are commonly observed with dermatological or oral symptoms. Some people are susceptible to oral lichenoid lesions, caused by sensitivity to mercury released from amalgam restorations [12]. Most restorations associated with lichenoid lesions are poorly contoured, corroded, and old. A person can develop hypersensitive reactions from the corroded amalgam restoration or the biofilm present on such restorations. Symptoms of amalgam allergies can include skin rashes in the head and neck area, itching, swollen lips, localized eczema-like lesions in the oral cavity [13]. These signs and symptoms usually disappear on their own and require no treatment. However, in a few people, removal of the amalgam restoration is the only way to treat the symptoms and an alternative material used in its place [14]. Mercury allergy may be rare, but hypersensitivity to it can lead to dermatitis or type IV delayed reactions most often affecting the skin as a rash.

4.3.1.1 Biocompatibility and mercury toxicity

Mercury is available in three forms: (1) elemental mercury (liquid or vapor); (2) inorganic compounds; (3) organic compounds.

Mercury, in the form of methylmercury, can cross the blood–brain barrier. It exists in the extracellular fluid of the brain and is slowly released into the blood. Mercury vapors can cause tremors, restlessness, and loss of concentration; however, at 4000 μg/kg, it causes impaired brain function, insanity, and death.

Inorganic mercury is naturally occurring, and its salts are used for cosmetic purposes. It can be corrosive to the digestive system. Exposure to inorganic mercury compounds for a prolonged period can result in effects similar to those seen in mercury vapor exposure and other effects such as skin rashes and kidney abnormalities.

Organic mercury can cause damage to the nervous system. Methylmercury is extraordinarily hazardous to a developing fetus. Babies of women exposed to methylmercury were born with developmental abnormalities and cerebral palsy [15].

The average daily dose of mercury released from amalgam restorations for patients with more than 12 restored surfaces is estimated at up to 3 μg. The lowest dose of mercury that can elicit a toxic reaction in the body is 3–7 μg/kg of body weight. The following are some toxic reactions and the doses of mercury that can trigger them (Table 4.3; Table 4.4).

4.3.2 Dental materials and cement

Dental materials such as fillings or cement are intended to be placed in the oral cavity for a prolonged duration. Biocompatibility requirements must be met when selecting the materials. A few types of dental cement contain chemicals that could induce allergic reactions in various tissues in the oral cavity. Common allergic reactions include stomatitis/dermatitis, urticaria, swelling, rash, and rhinorrhea. These may predispose to life-threatening conditions such as anaphylaxis, edema, and cardiac arrhythmias [16].

Table 4.3 Doses and toxic reactions.

Paresthesia	500 μg/kg body weight
Ataxia	1000 μg/kg body weight
Joint pain	2000 μg/kg body weight
Hearing loss and death	4000 μg/kg body weight

Table 4.4 Quantification of mercury.:Mercury release has been quantified for several procedures: [15].

Trituration	1–2 μg
Placement of amalgam restoration	6–8 μg
Dry polishing	44 μg
Wet polishing	2–4 μg
Amalgam removal under water spray and high velocity suction	15–20 μg

4.3.2.1 *Zinc oxide eugenol*

This type of cement is used for temporary and permanent cementation, cavity liners, base, pulp capping, and root canal material. In endodontic therapy, zinc oxide eugenol (ZOE) is used as a sealer. The ZOE remains inside the root canal, and at times is pushed beyond apical constriction. It is always in close contact with the surrounding soft and hard tissues for an extended duration. Localized inflammation with ZOE sealers has been seen, both in soft tissue and in the bone. ZOE has an antimicrobial effect when used with a thermoplasticized obturation technique. However, eugenol is found to leak from ZOE sealers, which is known to induce toxic effects and decrease signal transmission in nerve cells. The effect is persistent even after the setting of the material. ZOE sealer with *para*-formaldehyde is both cytotoxic and mutagenic [17].

4.3.2.2 *Composites*

There have been reports of gingival reactions following contact with composite materials. The inflammatory reactions adjacent to unfilled, cold-cured acrylic resin were intense compared to heat-cured resins. The permeability of the gingival epithelium allows penetration of leachable components and, thus, there is potential for toxic and allergic reactions with composite materials. Lichenoid reactions can occur in the oral mucosa, when in contact with resin-based composite materials. Such lesions usually heal spontaneously when the restoration is replaced with a different type of restorative material. White lichenoid lesions of the oral mucosa and gingiva have been reported in patients with amalgam restorations, composite resins, and cast alloys.

4.3.3 Metal crowns

Lichen planus and other metal allergies

Lichen planus appears at the oral mucosa attached to the metal restoration that contains the allergy-positive metal element. The lichen planus is mainly observed on the buccal mucosa. Histological findings reveal parakeratosis, liquefaction degeneration of the basal cell, and T lymphocyte infiltration under the epithelial tissue. Metal allergies are a suspected predisposing factor that can cause lichen planus (Fig. 4.7).

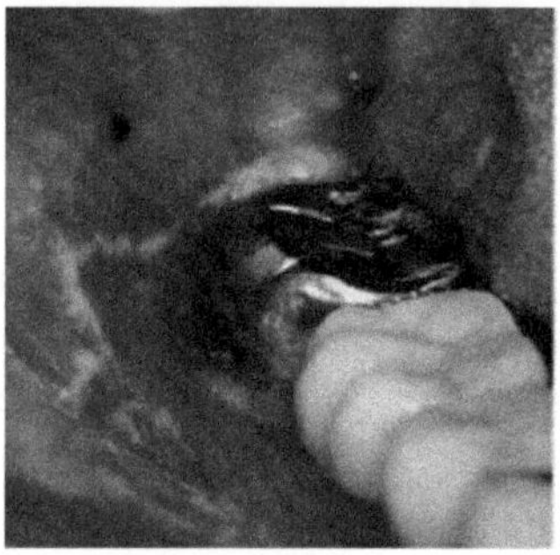

Figure 4.7 Lichenoid lesion adjacent to a high noble alloy.

4.3.3.1 Gold foil

Gold foil is one of the most stable and relatively insoluble materials. Patients sensitive to gold may have specific adverse reactions such as burning sensation of the oral mucosa, lichenoid lesions, and other general systemic reactions.

Other reactions in the pulp caused by forces of condensation of the gold foil, thermal conductivity, cavity prep, and dehydration of the cavity have been noticed. The most common toxic effect caused by these materials is microleakage. The toxicity of gold foil leads to pulpal inflammation, destruction of the odontoblasts, and hemorrhage [18].

4.3.4 Dental casting alloys

In dentistry, casting alloys are used in the fabrication of inlays, onlays, crowns, bridges, partial dentures, and porcelain-fused metal restorations. Most developed countries widely use cast gold alloy and all-ceramic materials; whereas, developing countries in the Middle East and South America use base metal alloys and prefabricated stainless-steel crowns. Prosthesis made of cast alloys are fixed in the oral cavity for an extended duration, and the patients cannot remove them [19].

4.3.4.1 Causes for alloy-related reactions

Biological interactions between dental cast alloys and oral tissue are one of the principal reasons for local adverse effects observed clinically. General diseases in the body like diabetes and vitamin deficiency, side effects of medications used for high blood pressure, and some sedatives are some nondental/nonoral causes of adverse effects. Dental/oral factors that cause adverse reactions include plaque, periodontal health, viral, and fungal infections. Tissue anomalies, inadequate tooth preparations, and biologic incompatibility of materials used in the fabrication of prosthesis are also common causes of adverse effects.

Dental alloys play a prominent role in dentistry, as pure metals lack appropriate physical properties required to function in different restorations. Base metal alloys are used to make most dental prostheses and nickel–chromium to make fixed dentures. Other materials may lack strength, wear resistance, and biologic compatibility required for the long-term survival of the material in the mouth as fixed prosthesis. Cobalt–chromium is more widely used for the manufacture of removable partial dentures.

Bacterial adhesion, toxic/subtoxic effects, and allergies are the basis for the biological incompatibility of materials. Cast alloys containing copper and silver have a rough surface with positive surface energy levels to promote bacterial adhesion.

Plaque accumulation is a significant cause of poor gingival and periodontal health. Due to the mechanical influences in the mouth, the buccal areas have a thicker bacterial layer than lingual areas, and so it is essential to maintain good oral hygiene that can significantly restrict plaque/bacterial adhesion.

Cytotoxicity is one of the most crucial factors used in evaluating the biocompatibility of a material. Placing a foreign material in the mouth creates an active interface at the point of contact. The body and the material affect each other through this interface. These interactions take place regardless of the material. Only the types and effects vary depending on the material, the host, and the forces and conditions placed on the material or the function of the material. Biodegradation is another factor used to assess biocompatibility. Biological processes can be harmful and destructive to dental materials; the process of destruction and dissolution in saliva, chemical/physical destruction, and wear and erosion are caused by food, chewing, and bacterial activity [20].

Metals like nickel and copper leach out from certain dental cast alloys and can cause toxic reactions such as gingival inflammation. Metals released from high noble and noble alloys cause discoloration and hyperplasia of the adjacent gingiva.

Nickel alloys are used in dentistry for restoration purposes and manufacturing endodontic instruments and orthodontic appliances. Leaching of nickel and chromium from dental restorations causes allergic reactions. The oral manifestations of the contact allergy to nickel used in

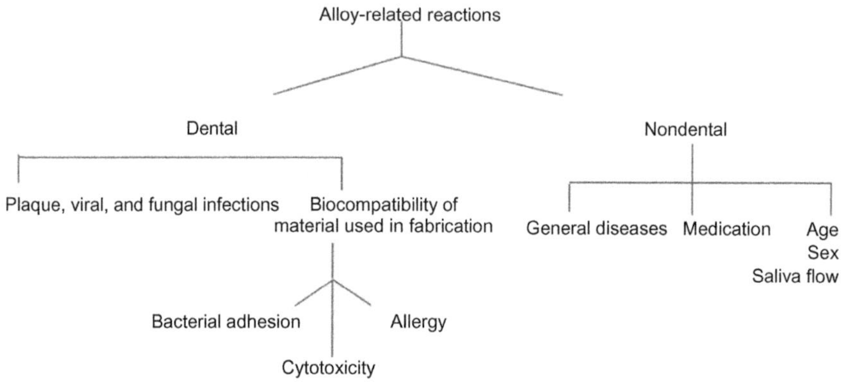

Figure 4.8 Flowchart for alloy-related reactions.

dentistry include lichen planus or stomatitis. There has been a notable increase in concentrations of these metals in the blood of patients with removable partial dentures made of nickel and chromium.

Nickel–chromium alloys may elicit adverse tissue and cellular reactions. Elements released from these alloys may subsequently interfere with many biochemical and enzymatic cellular reactions, resulting in necrosis (Fig. 4.8).

4.3.5 Dental implants

A dental implant is an artificial tooth root, embedded in the jaw bone that bonds with the natural bone. It provides a sturdy foundation for supporting one or more artificial teeth called crowns.

4.3.5.1 Endosseous implants

These are devices made of titanium or titanium alloys, intended to be surgically placed in the jaw bone to support prosthetic devices such as crowns, bridges, or dentures to restore the patient's chewing function.

Corrosion is said to occur when materials slowly degrade as a result of a chemical or electrochemical reaction. Fluorides and oral fluids, restorations, and galvanic action also cause corrosion. Titanium and its alloys corrode when they come into contact with biological tissues after implantation. During corrosion, ions from the metal get deposited into the surrounding tissue increasing cytokines and inflammatory reactions. These ions bind to the host proteins and initiate the degranulation of leukocytes, thereby causing a hypersensitivity reaction. Proinflammatory and proosteoclastogenic cytokines cause gum inflammation around the soft tissue of the implant called periimplant mucositis that in turn is a precursor to periimplantitis, which is gum inflammation with loss of bone. Either of these conditions can result in dental implants failing. Additionally, hypersensitivity reactions can also lead to implant failures and allergic reactions. Clinical conditions such as glottis edema, spontaneous exfoliation of implants, and eczema can also occur.

By-products of corrosion of dental implant surfaces can have toxic effects on the human body. Accumulation of these particles in the gingival sulcus and adjacent tissues can cause the blue-gray pigmentation of gingiva and root dentin [21]. If ingested, these nanoparticles can breach the blood–brain barrier and have a potentially toxic effect on the central nervous system (CNS) [22]. Systemically deposited titanium ions can lead to toxic reactions causing yellow nail syndrome. The most common symptoms found are postnasal drip and cough-associated sinusitis. A change in the growth, color, and thickness of the nails is the main characteristic of the yellow nail syndrome. Nails affected by this syndrome grow slow, thick, and are yellow [23].

4.3.5.2 Subperiosteal implants

The subperiosteal implant is designed to sit on top of the bone and beneath the periosteum. This design helps in distributing the stress created from the prosthesis to the larger area of supporting bone.

Cobalt–chromium alloy is the most commonly used material for subperiosteal implants. The alloy typically consists of the elements cobalt, chromium, nickel, and molybdenum. When the alloy undergoes corrosion, the subsequently released toxins that are carcinogenic can cause cancerous tumors. Although these tumors may be few at the site of the implant, there is a high chance for more tumors to appear in other parts of the body, due to the released ions (Table 4.5).

Table 4.5 Various metals and their effects on corrosion.

Metals	Effects of corrosion
Nickel	Dermatitis
Cobalt	Anemia
Chromium	Ulcers and CNS disturbances
Aluminum	Epilepsy and Alzheimer's
Vanadium	Toxic in elementary state

Table 4.6 Types of corrosion in dental implants [24].

Type of corrosion	Material	Implant location	Shape of the implant
Crevice	Stainless steel	Bone plates and screws	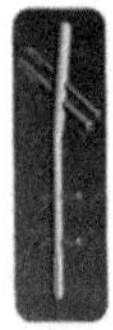
Galvanic	Stainless steel Cobalt–chromium Titanium Cobalt–chromium Molybdenum	Oral implants screws and nuts	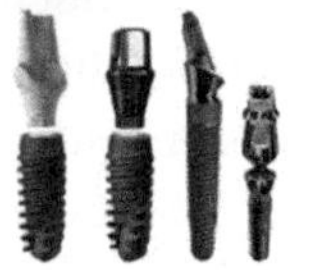
Selective leaching	Mercury from gold	Oral implants	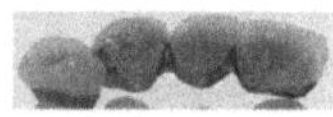

Metals corrode for several reasons; some of which include temperature, quantity, and quality of saliva, plaque, pH, protein, and the physical and chemical properties of food and liquids as well as oral health conditions. Galvanic corrosion is an electrochemical process frequently occurring in implants; the metal corrodes when in electrical contact with another and in the presence of an electrolyte. Galvanic corrosion commonly occurs in alloys of cobalt–chromium, nickel–chromium, silver–palladium, and in gold and titanium dental implants. Corrosion products from these metals cause discoloration of the soft tissue adjacent to the implants, allergic reactions, and rashes (Table 4.6).

The ions released from corrosion modulate tissue healing after the insertion of dental implants [25]. Wear particles from the implants also affect the functioning of the different types of cells involved (e.g., endothelial cells).

4.3.6 Resin tooth bonding agent

Dentin bonding agents (DBA) are designed to form strong bonds with dentin. These agents strengthen the bond between resin and the tooth structure, improve restoration retention, reduce microleakage, and diffuse the occlusal stress [26].

Irregular dentin formation and inflammatory changes of the dental pulp are seen histopathologically. These inflammatory changes are due to irritation by DBAs that are released after light curing, in cases of exposed pulp during cavity preparation. Some of the ingredients from the DBAs get leached out through the dentinal tubules injuring the peripheral pulp cells [27].

4.3.6.1 *Acrylic resins in denture reliners and cushion or pads*

Acrylic resins are most commonly used in the manufacture of denture bases, removable orthodontic appliances, temporary crowns, and denture relining. These temporary crowns are usually placed after tooth preparation using temporary luting cement.

Continuous interaction of human saliva with denture base acrylic resins causes some substances to leach out, the most common of which is the unreacted residual monomer. The saliva causes the openings between the resin's polymer chains to expand; the unreacted monomer leaks out and transfers to the surrounding oral structures, inevitably leading to cytotoxic effects and adverse allergic reactions. These include soreness in the mouth and burning sensation. Other areas in the mouth affected are the palate, tongue, oral mucosa, and the oropharynx [28].

4.3.7 Denture adhesives

Denture adhesives used to help dentures stay in place. Available in the form of pastes, powders, and pads, these adhesives provide temporary relief from loosened dentures by filling in the gaps caused by the shrinking of the bone [29].

Most denture adhesives contain zinc as an ingredient. Zinc improves the adhesive properties of the dentures but can become toxic when overused. When this zinc gets ingested into the small intestine, the intestine synthesizes a protein called metallothioneins to try and prevent the zinc's excessive absorption into the body by binding it; this attempt though, is ineffective. However, these proteins have a higher affinity for copper than zinc; dietary copper firmly attaches to the intestinal cells and is not absorbed into the body, and consequently, the metallothioneins bind to all the copper. The body purges this copper via excretion rather than being absorbed as it typically is in the absence of excessive ingested zinc, thereby lowering the copper levels in the body, causing hypocupremia [30]. Other adverse effects of denture adhesives include vertical dimension increase, mucosal hypersensitivity, and altered oral flora.

Copper is one of the most critical cofactors in enzymes required for nerve function, and its depletion causes abnormal nerve function. Symptoms of neuropathy include tingling numbness, loss of movement in the limbs, poor balance and coordination, decrease in walking stride, abnormal blood pressure and heart rate, reduced ability to sweat, constipation, and bladder dysfunction.

It also causes nerve damage in the hands and feet. This damage occurs slowly over some time and leads to bone marrow suppression and degeneration of the spinal cord resulting in a condition called "human swayback disease" [31].

4.3.8 Gutta-percha

Gutta-percha is the most common material used for the root canal filling in endodontic treatment. Gutta-percha is composed of zinc oxide powder or zinc ions, which cause cytotoxicity (Fig. 4.9).

Gutta-percha toxicity is attributed to the leaching of ions into the oral fluids leading to health issues. The addition of naturally treated material to gutta-percha did not lower its toxicity [32].

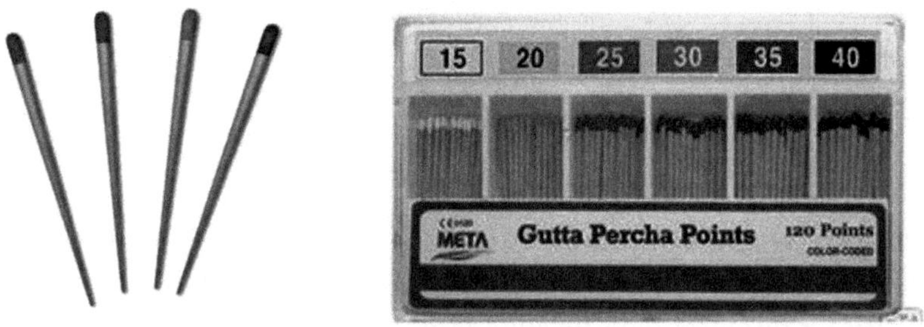

Figure 4.9 Gutta-percha.

4.3.9 Root canal filling resin

Core-filling materials for root canals is meant to be used alongside a root canal sealer (cement). The filling materials do not adhere to the canal walls and shrink after cooling down, resulting in gaps that provide an easy access route for bacteria. Root canal sealers are used to fill these gaps. The most commonly used resin-based sealer is AH 26, which consists of an epoxy resin base and an activator. This sealer initially causes a severe inflammatory reaction, which reduces after the periapical tissues well tolerate the material. The resin also has a strong allergenic and mutagenic potential. The AH Plus is a next-generation sealer that is less cytotoxic but still causes bacterial leakage. The epoxy resin sealer shrinks during the setting, which decreases its adaptation capabilities and causes it to debond from the root canal wall. Lack of adhesion between the sealer and the core-filling material can cause bacterial leakage [33].

4.3.10 Temporary crown and bridge resin

Several varieties of monomers, polymers, and additives are used in the fabrication of crowns and bridges. The monomers have a very complex composition, and after polymerization, several components leach into the oral cavity. Temporary restorations are used in the interim between tooth prep and a permanent restoration. The time lapse between a freshly cut dentine to the fabrication and the implantation of a permanent restoration is long enough for the saliva in the oral cavity to cause biodegradation of the composite resins.

The most commonly used monomers are polymethyl methacrylates, also called acrylic resins. However, more recently, bis-acryl composite resins, similar to resins used in direct restoration therapy are utilized. Acrylates, methacrylates, and monomers such as (bisphenol A-glycidyl methacrylate), Tri-ethylene-glycol-dimethacrylate (TEGDMA), and urethane dimethacrylate are cytotoxic. These resin monomers interfere with collagen proteins and intracellular glutathione affecting the pulp repair and regeneration. TEGDMA induces apoptosis in gingival fibroblasts, and BisGMA induces toxic reactions to the local and systemic cells and tissues [34].

The BisGMA interferes with the wound healing process by increasing the migration of keratinocytes. In sublethal concentrations, the BisGMA promotes the drop of tenascin glycoprotein in fibroblasts and keratinocytes, which is followed by a sudden increase in tenascin production after a prolonged period. BisGMA can also reduce the ICAM-1 gene, which is a surface glycoprotein expressed on endothelial cells. This, in turn, could reduce the attraction of leukocytes to the inflamed area and cause cell damage [35].

4.4 Surgical devices

See Table 4.7.

Table 4.7 List of surgical devices used in dentistry.

Device name	Class	Description	Implanted
Bone-cutting instrument and accessories	1	Device used in reconstructive oral surgery	No
Intraoral dental drill	1	Device attached to a dental handpiece to drill holes in teeth	No
Gas-powered jet injector	1	Syringe device intended to administer a local anesthetic	No
Spring-powered jet injector	1	Syringe device intended to administer a local anesthetic	No
Dental operating light	2	Device intended to illuminate oral structures and operating areas	No
Rotary scaler	2	Device to remove calculus deposits from teeth during dental cleaning	No

4.4.1 Gas powered jet injectors

Jet injectors are needle-free devices that push the liquid medication through a nozzle orifice. The medication is ejected through the nozzle as a narrow stream under high pressure. This medication stream penetrates the skin to deliver a drug or vaccine into intradermal, subcutaneous, or intramuscular tissues. Local reactions at the injection site such as pain, blood, redness, induration, and ecchymosis at the injection site are common [36] (Fig. 4.10).

4.4.2 Spring-loaded jet injector

This type of injector works on a spring mechanism. When triggered, the spring releases, generating a jet stream of medication for the delivery of a drug. The activated spring load must be redrawn manually for the next administration [37].

Because the jet injector breaches the skin barrier, there is a risk of the transfer of blood and biological material from one user to the next. As such, it is crucial to implement appropriate measures of sterilization are to avoid infection.

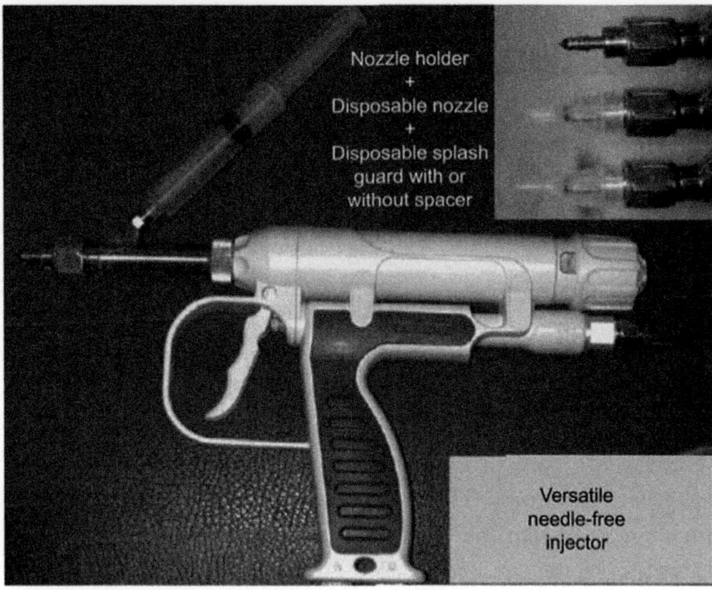

Figure 4.10 Jet injector.

4.4.2.1 Splash-back

In this case, the jet stream penetrates the outer skin at a high velocity causing a little of the stream to bounce backward resulting in nozzle contamination [38]. This forceful impact releases pressure, which expels the debris away from the site of impact and can transfer blood-borne viruses.

4.4.2.2 Fluid suck-back

When the blood left on the nozzle of the jet injector is sucked back into the injector orifice, it contaminates the next dose to be discharged.

4.4.2.3 Retrograde flow

In this case, the jet stream penetrates the skin and creates a miniature hole. The pressure of the jet stream causes the spray to mix with tissue fluids and blood, and then rebound back out of the hole, against the incoming jet stream and back into the nozzle orifice [39].

4.4.3 Dental diamond bur

The dental diamond bur is used to grind tooth tissue such as enamel. Using the bur usually results in creating a rough surface on the tooth. Multiple uses of the diamond bur can lead to a loss in cutting efficiency and result in the microleakage of composite restorations.

Prolonged usage of the bur on the tooth surface will redeposit the cutting debris on the prepared tooth surface that in turn becomes less adhesive, thereby decreasing the retention of the restoration and causing microleakage [40].

4.4.4 Dental operating light

High-intensity lights like light-emitting diodes (LEDs) are the most commonly used in dental setups. LED lights used in headlamps are of three types.

1. Neutral
2. Cool LED
3. Extremely cool

The neutral type emits in the blue spectrum similar to the green spectrum; whereas, the cool LED emits in the blue spectrum slightly stronger than the green spectrum. The extremely cool type of LED emits blue light much stronger than the green spectrum [41].

LED lights in dental setups are potential ocular hazards. Prolonged exposure to the LEDs may be harmful to the eyes, distorting colors, and retinal damage [42]. "Photo retinitis" means the retinal damage resulting from exposure of the retina to shorter wavelengths (400–500 nm) of violet and blue lights. These high intensities can destroy photopigments and release free radicals that can cause irreversible oxidative damage of retinal cells, eventually resulting in blindness.

In the elderly, the blue light absorbed by the retina causes immediate and irreversible retinal burning. Prolonged exposure to low levels of blue light causes accelerated retinal aging and degeneration, which results in photochemical injury to the epithelium. This phenomenon is called an age-related macular derangement.

4.4.5 Rotary scalers

Rotary scalers are sonic and ultrasonic scalers used in the treatment and prevention of periodontal disease. These scalers are power-driven, and the scaler tips are designed to remove plaque and calculus deposits from the dental surface. Disruption of the plaque is the result of the vibration of the scaler tip and the constant flushing of the water coolant used to cool the tips.

Potential hazards of scalers include thermal changes to the pulp, contamination of the blood and air with aerosols, and loss of cementum and bone from mechanical debridement of the root surface. The angulation of the tip of the scalers can cause cavitation of demineralized surfaces, eventually resulting in hypersensitivity. Dentinal exposure by the loss of enamel creates a direct path to the pulp for bacteria and their elements. This bacterial infection, in turn, results in increased sensitivity of exposed root surfaces to thermal, tactile, evaporative, and osmotic stimuli. Other disadvantages of scalers include pain, vibration, excessive noise, bad taste, and need for a high volume of water coolant [43].

Scalers can get heated up due to frictional contact between the scaler and the tooth or direct temperature application by the irrigation fluid. The rise in temperature can cause pulpal damage, which can promote vascular injury and tissue necrosis, causing irreversible pulpitis [44].

Cavitation is the formation of an air bubble inside a liquid, usually created by using high-intensity ultrasonic waves. Ultrasonic scalers help in the removal of the plaque deposits by fracturing the attached deposits by using ultrasonic waves. Naturally, this creates a risk of cavitation in the blood or plasma containing platelets. This vibrating activity can damage the blood cells, thereby forming a clot within the microvasculature of the pulp, leading to pulp death.

"White finger" is an adverse effect caused to the clinicians who use scalers frequently and for a prolonged period. The constant vibrations can cause repeated injury to the small nerves and blood vessels in the fingers. These blood vessels gradually go into spasm, causing a change in color and loss of feeling in the finger. The fingers go pale, bluish, and then dull red as the circulation returns [45].

4.4.6 Bone-cutting instruments

Some bone-cutting instruments used in dentistry are the Rongeurs side-cutting and end-cutting instruments, drills, surgical handpieces, piezosurgery devices, and lasers.

Rongeurs bone-cutting instruments are the most effective and commonly used for cutting the interradicular and alveolar bones in dentoalveolar surgeries. There are two types of Rongeurs instruments: side cutting and end cutting. Both types consist of a pair of sharp blades, squeezed together for cutting/pinching through bone (Figs. 4.11, 4.12).

There are a few drawbacks with these instruments: they cannot cut chunks of bone; only tiny bits repeatedly, they are made of carbon steel or stainless steel; easily corrodible materials that are very sensitive to chemicals.

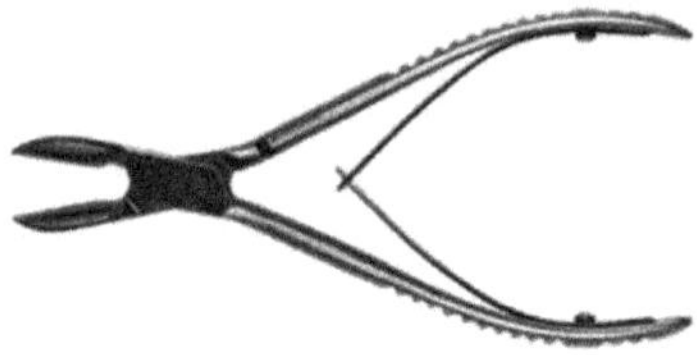

Figure 4.11 Rongeurs—side cutting [46].

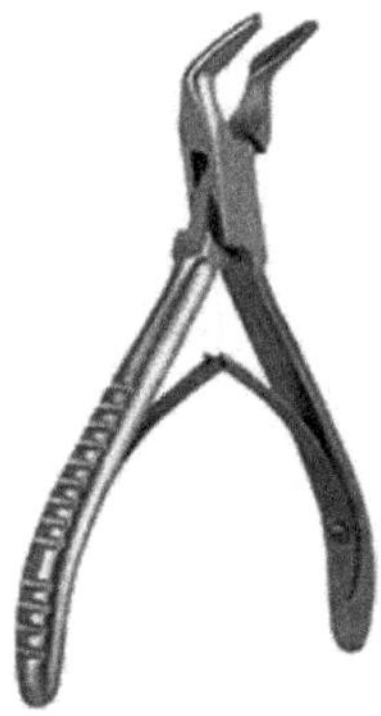

Figure 4.12 Rongeurs—end cutting [47].

4.4.7 Drill

During jaw correction surgeries, the bone site is fixed using immobilization screws, wires, and plates.

The jaw bone is drilled to fix the screws and plates. Consequently, there is an increase in the temperature of the bone; when it crosses, a threshold can result in its necrosis, that is, irreversible death of bone cells. Drilling can also cause micro damage to the bone. Small cracks start to develop in the bone matrix, leading to cell death of the osteocytes. The depletion of osteocytes can reduce blood flow, thereby increasing the risk of osteonecrosis that may further lead to the formation of a weaker bone, due to osteoclastic resorption that takes place [48].

4.4.8 Burs

Burs are the rotating, bone-cutting devices used primarily in orthodontics. The most common intraoperative complications with the use of burs include drill bit breakage. It occurs due to the application of excessive bending moment during the cutting of the bone. These drill bits, if left in the body elicit inflammatory reactions causing osteolysis [49].

Other types of bone-cutting instruments are the piezosurgery devices and lasers that are primarily used in osteotomy and osteoplasty cases. Piezosurgery was developed to achieve high levels of precision and intraoperative safety in bone surgery. However, the chief disadvantages with piezosurgery are that it has a low-grade cut precision, and it takes a long time to complete the procedure [50].

The Er:YAG (Erbium YAG) laser is now the most commonly used device in various branches of dentistry such as periodontology, oral surgery, and restorative dentistry, and in implantology. The emitted infrared radiation has a wavelength of 2.94 mm, can be entirely absorbed by water, and so can work on hydrated oral tissues. The irradiated bone tissue has an increased inflammatory cell filtration and faster revascularization. However, thermal damage to the margins of the osteotomies is possible, in case of inadequate coolant.

4.4.9 Intraoral dental drill

A dental drill or handpiece is a hand-held, mechanical instrument that plays a vital role in performing various dental procedures, including removing decay, polishing, fillings, and altering prostheses.

There are a few unexpected occupational hazards with the use of a dental drill. These could be physical, chemical, biological, mechanical, and psychological. Physical and mechanical hazards include cuts from sharp instruments or puncture wounds from needles or other sharp projectiles that can injure the eyes. Infectious diseases resulting from these injuries could be transmitted to dental workers [51].

The risk of cross-infection is another common hazard seen with the use of a dental drill. A dental drill or handpiece can consist of straight, contra angled, and prophy angles. These handpieces can be attached to the slow-speed and high-speed motors based on the requirement. These attachments are prone to contamination as they are used in the patients' mouths, from cleaning and polishing teeth, to drilling for cavity preparations. Significant amounts of biological residue that are not flushed out remain in the crevices of handpieces and open up a possibility for viral transmission. Most potential pathogens proliferate in waterlines to the dental handpieces. These waterlines to the high-speed handpieces provide a suitable environment for the formation of biofilm. The microorganisms from the biofilm may periodically shed pathogens during the high-speed handpiece operation [52].

4.5 Therapeutic devices

See Table 4.8.

Below are some of the therapeutic devices and their possible toxic side effects.

Table 4.8 List of therapeutic devices used in dentistry.

Device name	Class	Description	Implanted
Teething ring	1	Device intended for use by infants to soothe gums during the teething process	No
Extraoral orthodontic headgear	2	Device used with an orthodontic appliance to exert pressure on the teeth from outside the mouth	No
Oral rinse to reduce the adhesion of dental plaque	2	Device to reduce the presence of bacterial plaque on teeth and oral cavity	No
Intraoral devices for snoring	2	Devices that are worn during sleep to reduce the incidence of snoring	No

4.5.1 Teething rings

Teething rings are small rings for infants to bite on while teething. There are various types of teethers available in the market. The most common types are the gel and water-filled teethers. These teethers have some preservatives in them, such as paraben, which can affect the endocrine system. Different amounts of parabens and antimicrobials, including triclosan and triclocarban, leach out into the water from most teethers. People exposed to toxins during infancy often develop detriments later in life. They have been linked to developmental problems, reproductive interference, increased cancer risk, and disturbances in the immune and nervous system. Exposure to endocrine disruptors during childhood could lead to asthma, diabetes, neurodevelopment disorders, obesity, and reproductive abnormalities [53] (Fig. 4.13).

There is a possibility that liquid-filled teething rings can break open by the force of the baby's chewing, allowing the liquid to spill out. This liquid presents a potential choking hazard and may even be contaminated. Some liquid-filled teething rings have been recalled in the past due to bacterial contamination of the liquid. Teething rings with small parts also

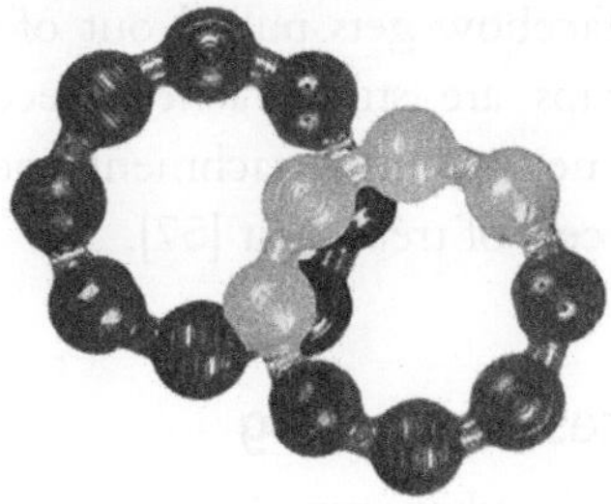

Figure 4.13 Infant teething rings.

present a choking hazard for babies. Some teething rings are decorated with beads, rattles, or other decorations, and while these are entertaining, they are also potentially dangerous [54].

4.5.2 Orthodontic headgear

This device is designed to correct severe bite problems. The headgear has attachments through which tension is exerted on the braces, which help in promoting jaw alignment (Fig. 4.14).

Displacement of the device during play or sleep can be damaging to the soft tissues in the mouth, causing minor lacerations. The bow of the headgear is sharp and has the same width as the eyes. There is a high possibility of the bow being covered in oral bacteria due to its placement in the mouth. There is a potential risk of a bilateral injury to the eyes with the facebow. An eye injury with the facebow might not cause immediate pain, but the oral bacteria on the bow can multiply within the eye, thereby causing an eye infection. Through a process called sympathetic ophthalmitis, infection from the eye can be transmitted to the other undamaged eye, eventually leading to temporary or permanent loss of vision [56].

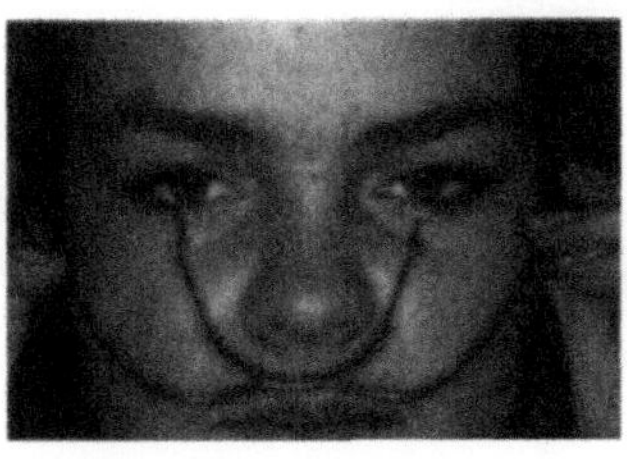

Figure 4.14 Orthodontic headgear [55].

In a few cases, the facebow gets pulled out of the molar tubes while the head and neck straps are still attached, recoiling and hitting the patient's face, head, or neck. This detachment and the resulting injuries can compromise the success of treatment [57].

4.5.3 Intraoral devices for snoring

Obstructive sleep apnea is when muscles around the tongue and throat relax to such an extent that tissues in the throat collapse and obstruct airflow to the lungs when sleeping. The most common dental devices used in the treatment of sleep apnea are the mandibular advancing device and tongue-retaining device (Figs. 4.15, 4.16).

The mandibular advancing device prevents the upper airway collapse by altering the position of jaw and tongue by protruding the mandible forward. Some side effects of using this device are excess salivation, dental

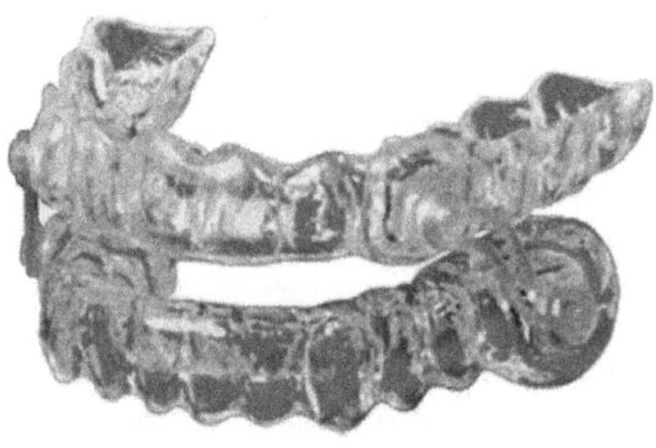

Figure 4.15 Silent Nite SL (mandibular advancing devices [58]).

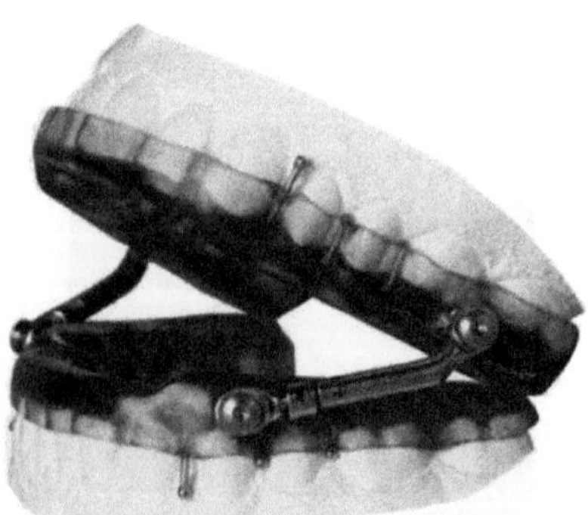

Figure 4.16 Herbst appliance (mandibular advancing devices [58]).

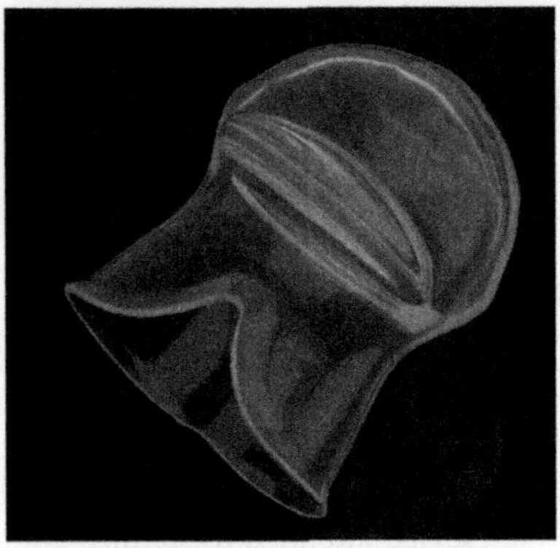

Figure 4.17 Mouthguard (tongue-retaining device [59]).

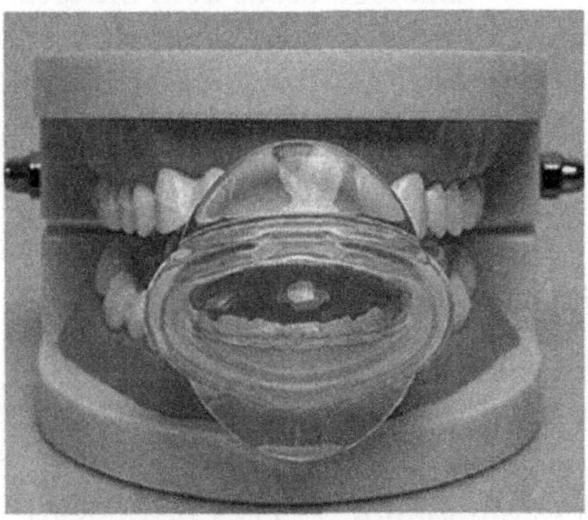

Figure 4.18 Tongue stabilizing device (tongue-retaining device [59]).

pain, gingival irritation, myofascial pain, dry mouth, and temporomandibular joint discomfort. Long-term side effects of using this device include dental changes such as overjet and overbite.

A tongue-retaining device restricts the tongue in an anterior position, thereby effecting moderate mandibular protrusion. Some side effects of using this device are discomfort, pain, excessive salivation, and excessive mouth dryness (Figs. 4.17, 4.18).

4.6 Miscellaneous devices

See Table 4.9.

Table 4.9 List of miscellaneous devices available in dentistry.

Device name	Class	Description	Implanted
Dental floss	1	String-like device made of cotton or other fibers intended to remove plaque and food particles from between the teeth	No
Endodontic dry heat sterilizer	3	Device intended to sterilize endodontic and other dental instruments by the application of dry heat	No
Manual toothbrush	1	Device composed of a shaft with either natural or synthetic bristles at one end intended to remove adherent plaque and food debris from the teeth	No
Dental operative unit and accessories	1	Devices intended to supply power to and serve as a base for other dental devices	No

4.6.1 Dental floss

Several types of dental floss are available in the market. Concerns have been raised about dental floss containing a PFHxS compound. Most varieties of floss contain fluorine in them. The presence of fluorine indicates the presence of PFAS compounds. PFHxS belongs to a large class of chemicals called PFASs. They have an immense area of applicability ranging from cookware, waterproof clothing, and food packaging to more exotic uses such as in firefighting equipment and military equipment. Exposure to these chemicals can result in liver damage, immunological problems, developmental issues, and cancer and can persist in a human body and the environment for many years [60].

Research indicates that adults with considerable levels of these chemicals in their systems are prone to renal problems, high cholesterol, issues with reproductive organs, and ulcerative colitis. Elevated PFAS levels are associated with thyroid disease, compromised immunity, low birth weights in newborns, and low sex and growth hormones in children. However, the research is still ongoing, and the data present are insufficient to support the conclusions presented [61].

4.6.2 Endodontic dry heat sterilizer

Dry heat sterilization is a technique used to kill all microorganisms, including bacterial spores. A significant disadvantage is that this process requires longer exposure times and higher temperatures when compared to other sterilization techniques. The high temperatures used in this process are not suitable for dental materials made of plastic and rubber; this may even result in destroying the materials.

4.6.3 Glass bead sterilizer

A glass bead sterilizer sterilizes endodontic files only up to 80%. A 100% sterilization was not obtained even at 240°C for 45 seconds. It is important to note that a glass bead sterilizer only sterilizes the working end. Nonworking ends such as the handle of the files are not sterilized. This is a reason for an increased risk of infection (Figs. 4.19, 4.20)

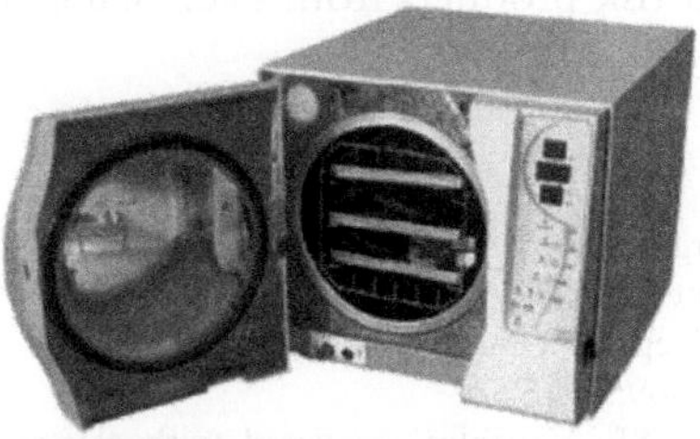

Figure 4.19 Dry heat sterilizer [62].

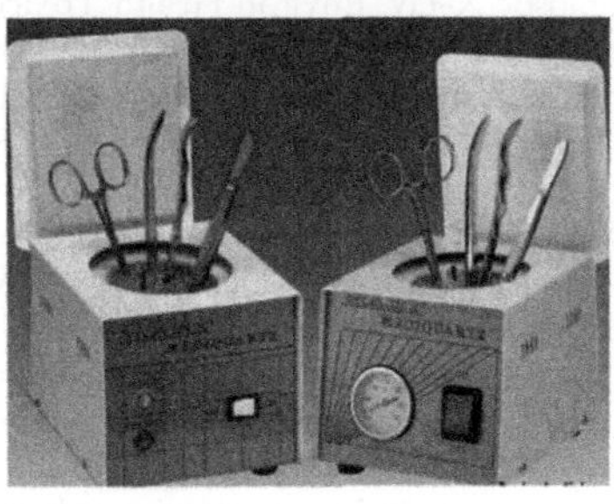

Figure 4.20 Glass bead sterilizer [63].

4.6.4 Manual toothbrush

A toothbrush is a device that is manually operated, used to remove plaque and debris from the teeth and the oral cavity. Brushing helps in maintaining a healthy oral cavity by preventing tooth decay, gum diseases, and ultimately loss of teeth. A disadvantage with manual toothbrushes is that they depend on the dexterity and thoroughness of the user. People with poor dexterity have difficulty using it effectively.

4.7 Conclusion

Everything we inhale or ingest interacts with the multiple systems, processes, and parts inside of a human body before eventually making its way out. This fact makes it crucial that we regulate the approval and promotion process of medical devices. We also need to demonstrate their safety and effectiveness to increase confidence in the same. Advancing toxicology assessment techniques and regulatory acceptance protocols will help in moving low-risk products to the market faster while also preventing high toxicological risk products from ever being released.

References

[1] Chaturvedi T. Allergy related to dental implant and its clinical significance. Clin Cosmet Investig Dent 2013;57–61.

[2] Gopikrishna V, Pradeep G, Venkateshbabu N. Assessment of pulp vitality: a review. Int J Paediatr Dent 2009;3–15.

[3] Cooley RL, Robison SF. Variables associated with electric pulp testing. Oral Surg Oral Med Oral Pathol 1980;66–73.

[4] Hwang S-Y, Choi E-S, Kim Y-S, Gim B-E, Ha M, Kim H-Y. Health effects from exposure to dental diagnostic X-ray. Environ Health Toxicol 2018;33.

[5] Preethi N, Chikkanarasaiah N, Bethur S. Genotoxic effects of X-rays in buccal mucosal cells in children subjected to dental radiographs. BDJ open 2016.

[6] Dental x-ray machines; 2006–2019. Retrieved from ASHTEL dental: <http://www.ashteldental.com/site/dental-x-ray-units-category.html/>.

[7] Provecta 70 intra oral dental X-ray machine; n.d. Retrieved from Dental Compare: <https://www.dentalcompare.com/4456-Dental-X-Ray-Machine-Dental-X-Ray-Generators/34163-Provecta-70-Mobile-Intraoral-X-Ray-Generator/>.

[8] Xu P, Luo H, Huang GL, Yin XH, Luo SY, Song JK. Exposure to ionizing radiation during dental X-rays is not associated with risk of developing meningioma: a meta-analysis based on seven case-control studies. PLoS One 2015.

[9] AlAli T. A comparison of rectangular vs. circular radiographic collimation during simulated endodontic therapy. A comparison of rectangular vs. circular radiographic collimation during simulated endodontic therapy. Virginia: Virginia Commonwealth University; 2013.

[10] Collimation effects, October 4; 2018. Retrieved from Upstate Medical University-Radiology: <http://www.upstate.edu/radiology/education/rsna/fluoro/collimation.php/>.

[11] Rathore M, Singh A, Pant VA. The dental amalgam toxicity fear: a myth or actuality. Toxicol Int 2012;81–8.

[12] Smart, Macleod, Lawrence. Resolution of lichen planus following removal of amalgam restorations in patients with proven allergy to mercury salts: a pilot study. Br Dent J. 1995. p. 108–12.
[13] McCullough M, Tyas M. Local adverse effects of amalgam restorations. Int Dent J 2008;3–9.
[14] Forte, Petrucci, Bocca. Metal allergens of growing significance: epidemiology, immunotoxicology, strategies for testing and prevention. Inflamm Allergy Drug Targets 2008;145–62.
[15] Mercury; November 2009. Retrieved from The Centers for Disease Control and Prevention (CDC): <https://www.cdc.gov/biomonitoring/pdf/Mercury_FactSheet.pdf/>.
[16] Hosoki M, Nishigawa K. Dental Metal Allergy. Intech; 2011.
[17] kaur A, Shah N, Lognani A, Mishra N. Biotoxicity of commonly used root canal sealers: a meta-analysis. J Conserv Dent 2015;83–8.
[18] Dental Amalgam; January 1993. Department of Health and Human Services.
[19] Elshahawy W, Watanabe I. Biocompatibility of dental alloys used in dental fixed prosthodontics. Tanta Dent J 2016;150–9.
[20] Schmalz, Garhammer. Biological interactions of dental cast alloys with oral tissues. Dent Mater 2002;396–406.
[21] Dental and orofacial implants. Mosby; 2012.
[22] Feng X, Chen A, Zhang Y, Wang J, Wei L, Shao L. Application of dental nanomaterials: potential toxicity to the central nervous system. Int J Nanomed 2015;3547–65.
[23] Kyeong TK, Mi YE, Thi HN, Soung M.K. General review of titanium toxicity. Int J Implant Dent 2019.
[24] Manivasagam G, Dhinasekaran D, Rajamanickam A. Biomedical implants: corrosion and its prevention – a review. Recent Pat Corros Sci 2010;40–54.
[25] Subperiosteal Implants. In: Misch CE, editor. Dental implant prosthetics. 2nd ed. Mosby; 2015. p. 315–39.
[26] Chen R-S, Liu C-C, Tseng W-Y, Jeng J-H, Lin C-P. Cytotoxicity of three dentin bonding agents on human dental pulp cells. J Dent 2003;223–9.
[27] Lee B-S, Jan Y-D, Huang G-S, Huang C-H, Chou H-Y, Wang J-S, et al. Effect of dentin bonding agent diffusing through dentin slices on the reactive oxygen species production and apoptosis of pulpal cells. J Formos Med Assoc 2015;339–46.
[28] Rashid H, Sheikh Z, Vohra F. Allergic effects of the residual monomer used in denture base acrylic resins. Eur J Dent 2015;614–19.
[29] Darwish M, Nassani MZ. Evaluation of the effect of denture adhesives on surface roughness of two chemically different denture base resins. Eur J Dent 2016;321–6.
[30] Singh VD, Misra SK, Singh V, Misra V, Yadav PK, Chaturvedi A. Denture adhesive and zinc toxicity. Int J Oral Health Med Res 2015.
[31] DeNoon DJ. Zinc poisoning linked to popular denture creams, February 15; 2011. Retrieved from Web MD: <https://www.webmd.com/oral-health/news/20110215/zinc-poisoning-linked-to-popular-denture-creams#1/>.
[32] Pascon EA, Spngberg LS. In vitro cytotoxicity of root canal filling materials: 1. Gutta-percha. J Endod 1990;429–33.
[33] Yanpiset K, Banomyong D, Chotvorrarak K, Srisatjaluk RL. Bacterial leakage and micro-computed tomography evaluation in round-shaped canals obturated with bioceramic cone and sealer using matched single cone technique. Restor Dent Endod 2018;43.
[34] Ulker M, Ulker HE, Zortuk M, Bulbul M, Tuncdemir AR, Bilgin MS. Effects of current provisional restoration materials on the viability of fibroblasts. Eur J Dent 2009;114–19.

[35] Engelmann J, Janke V, Volk J, Leyhausen G, Neuhoff N, Schlegelberger B, et al. Effects of BisGMA on glutathione metabolism and apoptosis in human gingival fibroblasts in vitro. Biomaterials 2004;4573–80.
[36] Jet Injector; 2018. Science Direct.
[37] Barolet D, Benohanian A. Current trends in needle-free jet injection: an update. Clin Cosmet Investig Dermatol 2018;231–8.
[38] Hoffmana, Abuknesha, Andrews, Samuel, Lloyde. A model to assess the infection potential of jet injectors used in mass immunization. Vaccine 2001;4020–7.
[39] Inherent problems with Jet Injectors; 2016.
[40] Fraunhoferm JA, Smith TA, Marshall KR. The effect of multiple uses of disposable diamond burs on restoration leakage. J Am Dent Assoc 2005;53–7.
[41] Mathew J, Nair M, Narayan, James B, Syriac G. Ocular hazards from use of light-emitting diodes in dental operatory. J Indian Acad Dent Spec Res 2017;28–31.
[42] Stamatacos, Harrison J. The possible ocular hazards of LED dental illumination applications. J Tenn Dent Assoc 2013;25.
[43] Thennukonda RA, Natarajan BR. Adverse events associated with ultrasonic scalers: a manufacturer and user facility device experience database analysis. Indian J Dent Res 2015;598–602.
[44] Kishida M, Sato S, Ito K. Comparison of the effects of various periodontal rotary. J Oral Sci 2004;1–8.
[45] Çiçek Y. Sonic and ultrasonic scalers in periodontal treatment: a review. Int J Dent Hygiene 2007.
[46] Rongeurs #5; 2019. Retrieved from Medical Supply Equipment & CO: <https://www.medical-supplies-equipment-company.com/dental-supplies-equipment/product/rongeur-5-65in-side-cutting_26930.html/>.
[47] 3H Dean Rongeurs; 2019. Retrieved from Hu-Friedy: <https://www.hu-friedy.com/surgical/rongeurs/3h-dean-rongeurs/>.
[48] Pandey RK, Panda S. Drilling of bone: a comprehensive review. J Clin Orthop Trauma 2013;15–30.
[49] Bertollo N, Walsh WR. Drilling of bone: practicality, limitations and complications associated with surgical drill-bits. London: IntechOpen; 2011.
[50] Romeo U, Vecchio AD, Palata G, Tenore G, Visca P, Maggiore C. Bone damage induced by different cutting instruments – an in vitro study. Braz Dent J 2009.
[51] Hailu K, Lawoyin D, Glascoe A, Jackson A. Unexpected hazards with dental high speed drill. MDPI; 2017.
[52] Lewis DL, Boe RK. Cross-infection risks associated with current procedures for using high-speed dental handpieces. J Clin Microbiol 1992;401–6.
[53] Baby teether study finds many contain potentially harmful chemicals, December 7; 2016. Retrieved from CBC NEWS: <https://www.cbsnews.com/news/baby-teether-study-bpa-endocrine-disruptors-chemicals/>.
[54] Teething ring safety tips; n.d. Retrieved from Colgate: <https://www.colgate.com/en-us/oral-health/life-stages/infant-oral-care/teething-ring-safety-tips-0915/>.
[55] Govindaraju R. Headgear. Health & Medicine; 2018.
[56] Meeran NA. Iatrogenic possibilities of orthodontic treatment and modalities of prevention. J Orthod Sci 2013;73–86.
[57] Samuels R, Brezniak N. Orthodontic facebows: safety issues and current management. J Orthod 2002;101–7.
[58] Sleep Apnea Guide. RSS feed; 2018.
[59] Exsnorer; 2018. Retrieved from: <https://www.exsnorer.org/top-snoring-aids-reviewed/>.
[60] Macmillan A. Is dental floss really toxic, January 11; 2019.

[61] American Dental Association News, January 21; 2019. Retrieved from American Dental Association: <https://www.ada.org/en/publications/ada-news/2019-archive/january/ada-questions-conclusions-in-study-linking-dental-floss-with-toxic-chemicals/>.
[62] Dry heat sterilizer; 2012. Retrieved from BeyondVet: <https://beyondvetstore.com/dry-heat/466-dry-heat-sterilizer.html/>.
[63] Desktop glass bead sterilizer; 2013. Retrieved from Monotaro.

CHAPTER FIVE

Cardiology

S. Priya*
Department of Pharmacology, Sathyabama Dental College and Hospital, Chennai, India
*Corresponding author

Abstract

Implants are man-made medical devices made of biomedical materials or electronic devices that are designed to substitute a missing biological structure, support a damaged biological structure, or enhance an existing one. They are classified based on their usage as sensory and neurological, cardiovascular, orthopedic, electric, contraception, cosmetic implants, etc. In recent years, the use of cardiovascular implants to improve both diagnosis and treatment of cardiovascular disorders such as heart failure, cardiac arrhythmias, ventricular tachycardia, valvular heart disease, angina pectoris, and atherosclerosis have become inevitable. Artificial heart, heart valve, cardioverter defibrillator, cardiac pacemaker, and coronary stents are some of the commonly used cardiovascular implants. Common complications of any implants that lead to implant failure including infection, inflammation, pain, rejection, coagulation, and allergic responses. As these cardiovascular implants are foreign materials to the human circulatory system, they pose a considerable risk of superficial thrombus formation and subsequent embolization and further organ injury. Even though cardiovascular implants possess numerous applications, managing adverse effects and complications to these implanted medical devices are considered the major challenges. These hindrances can be overcome through stringent regulations such as obtaining FDA approval or clearance for sale, premarket, postmarket reviews, tracking and monitoring efficacy, and patient safety of these implantable devices. This chapter will enlighten the readers on various cardiovascular implants their applications, toxicity, and regulations.

Keywords: Implants; FDA; IMD; cardiovascular; pacemaker; heart

5.1 Introduction

Implantable medical devices (IMDs) are a class of medical devices that can be introduced into the human body to interchange a lost body part, support an injured body part, or modify a significant body function. These devices are extensively used in the field of medicine, both

DOI: https://doi.org/10.1016/B978-0-12-820728-4.00005-8
© 2020 Elsevier Inc.
All rights reserved.

for diagnosis and treatment of numerous diseases. These IMDs act by networking with physiological processes such as heartbeat and facilitate sensing and local stimulation, data recording, and even drug delivery. These devices help to monitor blood pressure, blood glucose, and electrocardiogram, which is very important in clinical interpretation and also used as a personalized medical approach to diagnosis and treatment [1]. They also have the additional advantage of eluding the need for long periods of monitoring in hospitals and thus time and cost-effective. Orthopedic rods, pins, and screws used to repair fractured bones, artificial hip joints used to replace hipbones worn by arthritis, cardiac pacemakers, coronary stents, and defibrillators used to restore an irregular heart rhythm and widen narrowed blood vessel, neural prosthetics used to replace an injured and lost nerve, and drug-eluting stents used for controlling drug release are some of the extensively used IMDs. There are two types of IMDs namely passive and active based on the provision of the electrical source. Both these IMDs are inserted surgically or medically inside the human body, but the difference is that electrical energy is coupled with active type and is used to monitor physiological or pathological signals and to induce therapeutic effects; whereas, a bare-metal coronary artery stent is powerless and passive. Cardiovascular diseases (CVDs) are the ailments of the heart and blood vessels and comprise coronary heart diseases such as angina, myocardial infarction, stroke, heart failure, cardiomyopathy, congenital heart disease, aortic aneurysm, rheumatic heart disease, and other medical conditions. The most usual and threatening among all CVDs are coronary artery diseases (CAD). Many drugs and surgical procedures are available today to treat atherosclerosis, angina, myocardial infarction, cardiac arrhythmias, ventricular tachycardia, valvular heart disease, congestive heart failure, and other CADs but none could totally eliminate the likelihoods of mortality completely. A number of implantable devices are available to treat many diseases and increase the longevity of life of humans; still, cardiovascular diseases are considered as one of the major reasons of death if not closely monitored and treated. Hence, diagnosis and treatment of cardiovascular diseases are the chief concerns to the field of medicine. Artificial heart, heart valve, cardioverter defibrillator, cardiac pacemakers, and coronary stents are some of the important cardiovascular implants that are used currently to treat many cardiovascular diseases but have many requests to be satisfied to manufacture such devices. Even though cardiovascular implant devices have been successfully used in cardiology, the major setback that is foreseen is to its toxicological aspects that limit its widespread usage, and this puts forward to the need for strict regulations and guidelines for manufacture and sale of these implants. This chapter will throw light on the presently available state of the art implantable cardiovascular devices, the recent advances made in producing smart cardiovascular implants, the potential challenges, toxicological effects, and the regulations.

5.2 Implanted medical devices in treatment of cardiovascular disease

According to the World Health Organization and the American Heart Association, CVDs are considered as the leading cause of death globally and a number of people die annually from CVDs rather than from any other diseases. It is estimated that 17.6 million people died from CVDs in 2016, accounting for 31% of all global deaths, and 85% of which are caused due to heart attack and it is also expected to reach 23.6 million by 2030 based on a study conducted in 2014 [2,3]. In 2016, 840,678 people died per year in the United States due to CVDs, which is nearly one of every three deaths. Hence, CVDs account for 14% of total health expenditures when compared to any other diseases, thus increasing the medical costs in the form of hospitalization, drugs, and surgical interventions. CAD also known as ischemic heart disease caused due to the build-up of plaque in the arteries of the heart is the most common CVD that attributes to 43.8% deaths in the United States. Next to CAD, deaths due to stroke account for 16.8%, heart failure 9%, high blood pressure 9.4%, diseases of the arteries 3.1%, and other CVDs 17.9%. The aging population, obesity, suboptimal control of risk factors, and not using prevention methods are considered as a future CVD burden. In particular, men and women of ages 55–64 are under special concern. Children and young adults are also significantly important age groups because, when compared to adults, though only as low as 600 cases per year are recorded among children, but have been strongly linked to a greater risk of getting a sudden cardiac arrest (SCA), accounting for one in five unexpected deaths among 1–13 years old children and one in three among 14–21 years old children. Even though CVDs have been seen affecting extreme ranges of ages and races of people, still a positive trend is being documented in the past century, by showing a decline in the age-adjusted mortality rate. This decline is due to the prevention of acute myocardial infarction as well as to better acute medical treatment. However, in this century, childhood obesity and type 2 diabetes are major public health challenges, which are likely to increase the morbidity and mortality from CVDs. The management of CVDs is very extensive, based on the clinical situation of the patient. The various treatment methodologies include the use of drugs, surgical interventions, the use of cardiovascular implant devices, and education on the need for secondary prevention by risk factor and lifestyle modification. Still, all the above treatment and prophylactic methodologies are with the disadvantage of requiring hospitalization and the concurrent medical costs for continuous health monitoring. Introducing an IMD such as a cardiovascular electronic device that can continuously monitor and transmit the data could be a significant pillar in the treatment of CVDs. Thus they help in managing being away from the hospital and in early detection and treatment of disease before the appearance of symptoms. Some of the major clinically used cardiovascular implants such as the cardiac pacemakers, coronary stents, vascular grafts, pulse generators, and automated external defibrillators are class III medical devices that are approved by Food and Drug Administration (FDA). A coronary stent is a widely used cardiovascular implantable medical device that plays a significant role in the treatment of CAD. The main purpose of using cardiovascular implants is to provide functional support, structural support, and localized drug delivery (Table 5.1). A cardiac pacemaker, cardioverter defibrillator, drug-eluting coronary stents, and vascular grafts provide functional support to the body by substituting for an abnormal vein or artery. Although a heart valve, its accessories, loop recorders, and heart monitors help with structural and mechanical support. These implants significantly improve not only the patient's longevity but also the quality of life. The pacing device used for cardiac resynchronization therapy is the top sold IMDs. These cardiovascular implants' material qualities should resemble the original vessel wall and tissue and this factor still remains a challenge, which warrants for research on producing biocompatible materials in the future. While using cardiovascular stents and grafts, a thorough investigation is also essential for choosing it. In recent days, use of nanotopography, an advanced technology which employs titanium and titanium dioxide are considered for safer and successful implant preparation.

Table 5.1 Major purpose of using cardiovascular implants.

To provide functional support
Pacing devices
Cardiac resynchronization therapy devices
Implantable cardioverter—defibrillators
Implantable cardiac pacemakers
Pacing accessories—pacing leads, pacing batteries
To provide functional support and localized drug delivery
Cardiac stents and related implants
Coronary stents
Drug-eluting stents
Bare-metal coronary stents
Stent-related implants
Synthetic grafts—vascular grafts
Vena cava filters
To provide structural and mechanical support
Structural cardiac implants
Heart valves and accessories
Tissue heart valves
Ventricular assist devices
Implantable heart monitors
Insertable loop recorders
Implantable hemodynamic monitors

5.3 Selection of cardiovascular implantable device properties to avoid its toxicological aspects

A cardiovascular device to be best employed clinically to treat various cardiovascular diseases without producing any major adverse effect to the host must satisfy the following criteria:

1. Nature of the cardiovascular biomaterial
2. Suitable mechanical properties
3. Anticorrosive and biocompatibility

The selection of cardiovascular biomaterial is of major concern in the production of an ideal implantable device. The nature of the biomaterial refines its biomedical applications. The physical and mechanical characteristics of a biomaterial such as strength and deformation, fatigue and creep, friction and wear resistance, flow resistance and pressure drop are other criteria of a suitable biomaterial that has to be considered. The major feature that is needed by any ideal implant biomaterial and the one that limits the widespread use of especially cardiovascular implants is biocompatibility. Hence, an ideal biomaterial should be the best in its physical nature, mechanical properties, corrosion resistant, and biocompatible.

As the cardiovascular implant is in direct or indirect contact with the blood and tissue, it has to be biocompatible irrespective of the contact duration. Failing to meet this results in cardiovascular implant-induced complications. Biocompatibility indicates to the ability of a biomaterial to perform its required function with respect to a medical treatment, without provoking any adverse local or systemic outcomes in the recipient or beneficiary of that therapy, but producing the most suitable favorable cellular or tissue response in that specific situation and enhancing the clinically significant functioning of that therapy [4]. Biocompatibility of an implantable medical device can be studied by using complex in vitro and in vivo experiments to test for any local and systemic effects of the material on cell cultures, tissue sections, and in the whole body [5]. In vitro cell-culture studies are done using direct contact, agar diffusion, and elution methods, and the amount of dead cells is the measure of the cytotoxicity and biocompatibility of the biomaterial tested. In vivo studies are carried out in animal models (sheep, pig, rat) for testing the tissue section compatibility, for example, of a prosthetic device and also to assess whether the device is performing according to expectations without causing harm to the patient. Testing for toxicity, carcinogenicity, sensitization, and irritation helps in determining if the leachable products of the medical device affect the tissues near or far from the implant site.

Metals and its alloy, polymers, and biological materials are the best-used biomaterial in cardiology (Table 5.2). Metals such as stainless steel, cobalt, chromium, and titanium and its alloys are used to make heart valves, endovascular stents, and stent-graft combinations [6]. The most important applications of all are cardiovascular stents like bare-metal stents,

Table 5.2 Biomaterials used as implantable cardiovascular devices.

Metals and alloys	Polymers	Biological materials
Stainless steel	Polyamides	Homograft valves
Cobalt and its alloy	Polyolefin	Porcine valves
Chromium and its alloy	Polyesters	Bovine valves
Titanium and its alloy	Polytetrafluoroethylene	
	Polyurethane	

drug-eluting stents, and bioresorbable stents. Stainless steel is considered the gold standard in stent technology, which provides mechanical strength to the diseased arteries, and is also anticorrosive and made to provide mechanical strength to the heart valves. Cobalt and its alloy are the other biomaterials that can be employed for making coronary stents, pacing leads, stylets, and catheters. Recently, a combination of metals consisting of cobalt–chromium–tungsten–nickel (CoCrWNi) alloy has been used for producing heart valves [7]. Titanium and its alloy have been used in the medical field since the 1970s because of its lightweight, excellent tensile strength, and corrosion resistance and hence have ideal cardiovascular applications. Self-expanding shape-memory stents made of nickel–titanium (nitinol) alloy is a suitable biomaterial. However, titanium use is limited by its complication of stent-induced thrombosis requiring simultaneous antiplatelet therapy. The best remedy is the drug-eluting stents, where polymer-free stents or metallic stent with a polymer carrier to hold and release the drugs are used. Polymers have been considered as widely used cardiovascular biomaterials, which are both nonbiodegradable and biodegradable. Additionally, polymers are more biocompatible than metals and their alloy, and hence find its application as vascular grafts to stents, prosthetic heart valves, catheters, heart assist devices, and hemodialyzer. Some of the widely used nonbiodegradable polymers include ultra-high molecular weight polyethylene, polymethylmethacrylate, polyetheretherketone, and polyethylene terephthalate (PET). Polyamides are also known as nylon, the first thermoplastic used in cardiovascular implants to make transparent tubings. Polyolefins are used for producing blood bags and polypropylenes for heart valve structures. PET is also called as polyesters and popularly known as Dacron used for producing implantable sutures, surgical mesh, vascular grafts, sewing cuffs for heart valves, and components for percutaneous access devices. PET grafts are coated with collagen or albumin for reducing blood loss and better biocompatibility. Even though these nonbiodegradable polymers have wide applications in the medical field, its usage is minimized due to disadvantages and toxicities, and hence biodegradable polymers that are always beneficial over other materials replace them. The benefits include aiding in the temporospatial clearance of the material from the body and helping the neighboring tissue to independently refurbish its function over time. Synthetic biodegradable polymers such as polyesters (polyhydroxyalkanoate, PHA), polyorthoesters, polyanhydrides, polycarbonates, polyamides, polyurethanes, collagens, polysaccharides (hyaluronic acids), and some polyesters (e.g., PHA) offer the ability to control surface as well as mechanical properties and degradation kinetics. Resorbable polymers widely used in trauma surgery overcome the disadvantages of metal implants such as stress protection, potential for corrosion, wear, and debris formation as well as the necessity of implant removal. Among all bioresorbable polymers, polyhydroxy acids such as poly(L-lactide), poly(glycolide), and/or copolymers based on L-lactide, L/DL-lactide, DL-lactide, glycolide, trimethylene carbonate, and caprolactone top the list as implant material because of good biocompatibility and are nontoxic. Polymers made from glycolic acid and lactic acids have numerous uses in the medical industry. Poly(dioxanone), poly(trimethylene carbonate) copolymers, and polycaprolactone (PCL) homopolymers and copolymers are some of the others approved for use as medical devices. Polyanhydrides, polyorthoesters, and many more materials are still under research. Collagen with ideal characteristics of an implant material has been used for the closure of grafts and extraction sites. In cardiology, tissue-based collagen devices play a very important role as an implant material for heart valves and in vascular prostheses [8]. Polyether-based polyurethane elastomers are currently used in a variety of blood and tissue-contacting devices like a pacemaker lead, valve structures, and ventricular assisting device. Segmented polyurethanes have been used even for tissue engineering of vascular grafts and heart valves. (Table 5.3). Drug-coated implants help in

Table 5.3 Polymers and their biomedical applications.

Poly(tetrafluoroethylene)	Vascular graft, vascular prostheses
Polypropylene	Heart valve structures
Poly(ethylene terephthalate)	Vascular grafts and prosthesis, shunt, sutures
Polyamides (nylons)	Hemodialysis membrane
Poly(ether urethane) (e.g., pellethane)	Percutaneous leads, catheters, tubings, intraaortic balloons
Poly(ether urethane urea) (e.g., biomer)	Artificial heart components, heart valve
Low- and high-density polyethylene	Tubing
Polysulfones	Artificial heart components, heart valve
Polyvinylchloride	Tubing, blood bags
Poly(2-hydroxyethyl methacrylate)	Catheter coating
Polyesters	Vascular prostheses, drug delivery systems like drug-eluting stents, sutures
Hydrogels	Drug-delivery systems

localized drug delivery, and it is used to treat many diseases from cardiovascular to diabetes. By coating with drugs, the performance and duration of the implants are increased, which ensures in providing a better quality of life in patients. Drug-eluting stents are one of the trending and extensively used drug-coated implant materials, which have created a unique place in the pharma and medical industry. This drug-coated implant acts as a semipermeable compartment holding the drug while allowing passage of desired molecules in a controlled method. Various immunosuppressive drugs (sirolimus, everolimus, tacrolimus, ABT-578), antiproliferative drugs (paclitaxel, actinomycin, angiopeptin, etc.), antimigratory drugs (batimastat), and gene therapeutic reagents (antisense and siRNA, vascular endothelial growth factor, endothelial nitric oxide synthase (eNOS) and related genes) have been combined with stents and investigated for their local release and antirestenotic effects. FDA's approval of Cordis' CYPHERTM sirolimus-eluting stent (2003) opened the gate for adapting new technology combining both device and pharmaceutical designs [9]. Amazon Pax (MINVASYS) using Amazonia CroCo (L605) cobalt—chromium (Co—Cr) stent with antiproliferative drug Paclitaxel and abluminal coating as the carrier of the drug, and BioFreedom (Biosensors Inc.), Optima (CID S.r.I.), VESTA sync (MIV Therapeutics), and YUKON choice (Translumina) are made of stainless steel and combined with Tacrolimus, Sirolimus, and Probucol are some of the useful drug-eluting stents [10]. Cypher, Taxus, and Endeavour are the further improved drug-eluting stents that use bioresorbable polymers like polyethylene vinyl acetate and polybutyl methacrylate as a carrier matrix for the drugs that can be applied in prolonged stent requirement. Phosphorylcholine, polylactic acid, D-lactic polylactic acid, and polylactic-co-glycolic acid are some of the other widely used polymers widely used in cardiovascular devices. Limitations due to polymer nature result in vessel irritation, endothelial dysfunction, vessel hypersensitivity, and chronic inflammation in stent-implanted site that has been considered.

Biological tissues like humans (allograft) and xenografts can overcome the limitations of metals and polymers and proves to be a better alternative in cardiology. Homograft or allograft valves, porcine valves, and bovine pericardial valves are some of the currently available commercial bioprosthetic values [11]. Homografts are intact human valves obtained from donors and cryopreserved as entire aortic or pulmonary roots, in which are then modifications are made and the size adjusted according to the recipient. Xenografts are tissues from bovine, porcine, and equine. Pericardium isolated from porcine and bovine is used for producing bioprosthetic valves. However, they have the limitation of valve calcification and degradation, which can be overcome by coating with chemical agents, and hence have better biocompatibility and reduced immunogenicity.

Thus by adding a protective surface film, using a suitable alloy, selecting clean varieties of steel, advanced production methods, and surface treatment by ion beams we can produce an ideal implant material that is also corrosion resistant. Many of the causes of corrosion could be avoided by improvements in materials selection, implant design, quality control, materials handling, and education [12].

5.4 Implantable cardiovascular devices and their toxicity

5.4.1 Implantable blood pressure monitors in endovascular repair

Endovascular aneurysm repair (EVAR), in 1999, was the first FDA-approved implantable cardiovascular device that was used to treat the abdominal aortic aneurysm, an age-related ballooning of the main aorta that thins and ruptures leading to fatal consequences. EVAR is a stent-graft synthetic vascular mesh replacement that helps to prevent the aneurysm sac from systemic pressure. However, the toxicological effect that prevents its widespread use is the complication of endoleak, marked by high pressure within the aneurysm sac, and the challenge in diagnosing such endoleaks by conservative imaging techniques. Angiographies catheters are hence used to measure sac pressure again, with restrictions of keeping it inside the body for long periods of time, thus preventing long-term surveillance (Fig. 5.1).

EndoSure sensor (CardioMEMS) is a passive IMD, which is used within the aneurysm sac. It is surrounded by a wire basket and has an LC tank (inductive—capacitive), with a fixed inductive component and the capacitive component consists of flexible plates whose separation varies with blood pressure. As a result of the change in capacitance, the resonant frequency changes which is then transduced into real-time pressure measurements [13,14]. It also finds its application for monitoring and management of heart failure and reducing the rate of hospitalization. CardioMEMS HF system is a wireless pulmonary artery sensor used to reduce heart failure

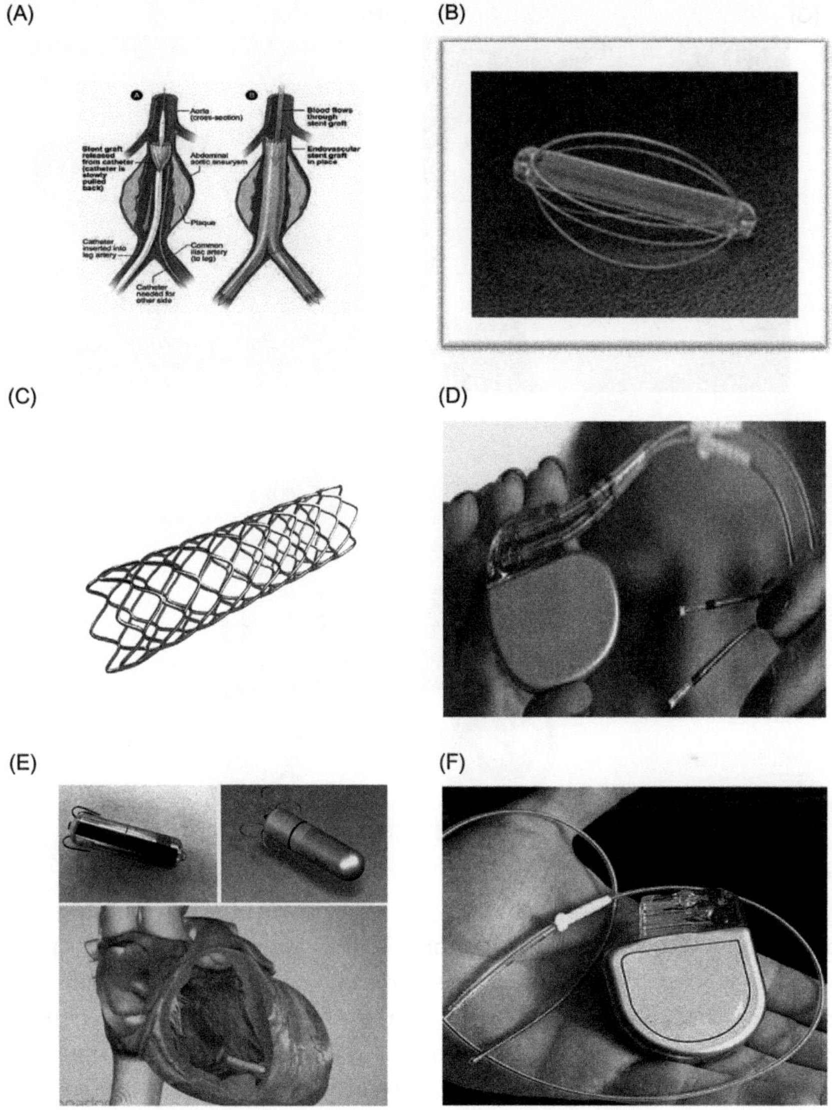

Figure 5.1 Cardiovascular implants. (A) Endovascular aneurysm repair (EVAR); (B) EndoSure sensor (CardioMEMS); (C) coronary stent; (D) permanent pacemaker; (E) leadless pacemaker (CRT); (F) cardioverter defibrillator; (G) subcutaneous ICD; (H) implantable loop recorders; (I) left ventricular assist device (LVAD).

hospitalization. The CHAMPION trial is a randomized, multicentered clinical trial called wireless pulmonary artery hemodynamic monitoring in chronic heart failure to test the effectiveness of the CardioMEMS heart failure system studied in 550 patients with NYHA functional class III heart

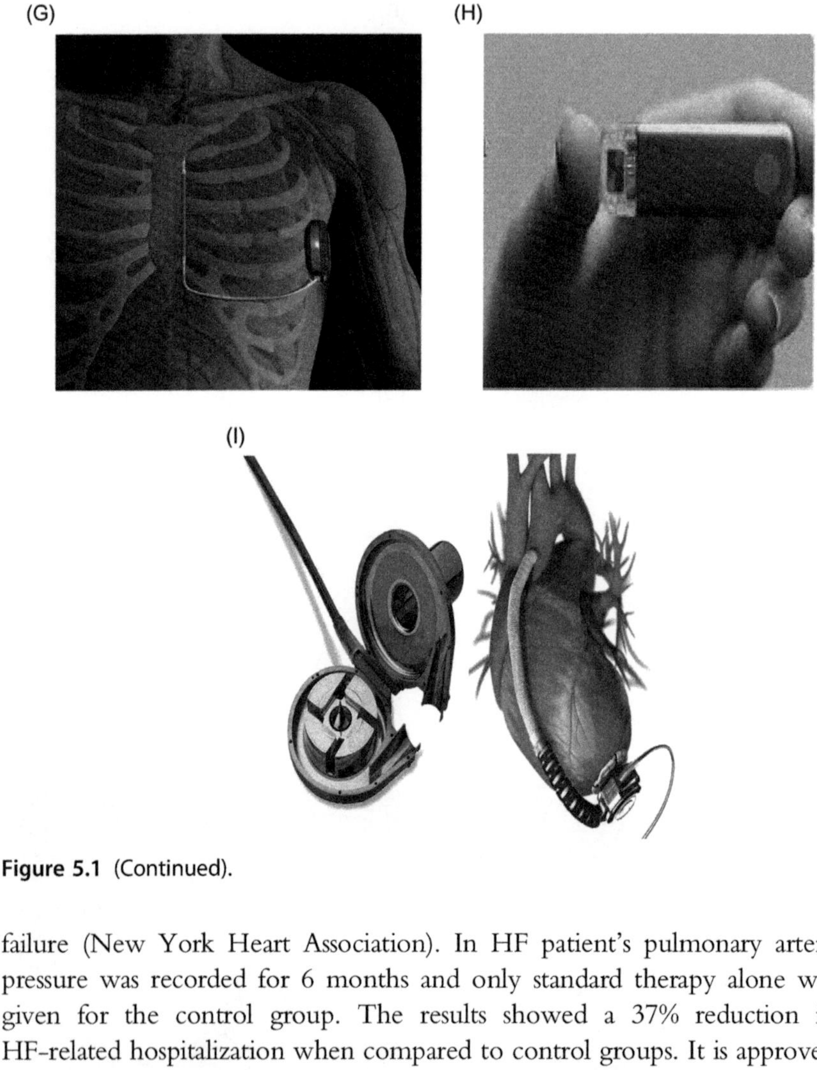

Figure 5.1 (Continued).

failure (New York Heart Association). In HF patient's pulmonary artery pressure was recorded for 6 months and only standard therapy alone was given for the control group. The results showed a 37% reduction in HF-related hospitalization when compared to control groups. It is approved by the US FDA and endorsed by European HF guidelines. It is used currently in older patients with major health issues and high baseline artery pressure with a successful reduction in pressure and rate of hospitalization [15]. The postmarket surveillance system, Manufacturer and User Facility Data Experience (MAUDE) database, records CardioMEMS HF system-related adverse effects within the first 3 years of FDA approval [16]. The toxicological effects included pulmonary artery injury or hemoptysis, infection, bleeding, and pulmonary embolism, which were lesser than other permanent implants that are employed in the treatment of heart failure.

ImPressure device is an IMD that is used for monitoring chronic heart failure (CHF) at home using pulmonary artery pressure by implantable device responding to ultrasonic signal (PAPIRUS II) study [17]. This device has two components: one implantable and the other an external unit. Implantable unit is composed of a pressure sensor, a piezoelectric transducer, a control chip, and a battery. In the external unit, ultrasonic energy is used to transmit a signal to the implant, stimulating its battery. Then the sensor measures full pressure waveforms for 10 seconds and the chip conducts the data to external units. ImPressure device is fixed to the outside of the endograft by hand sewing. Signal transmission in both Endosure and ImPressure is analog, but telemetric pressure sensor (TPS) uses digital signal transmission instead of analog to exclude surrounding interferences. The TPS is a passive, capsule-shaped IMD comprising a capacitor, receiver coil, and Zener diodes with the digital data processing unit. However, these devices possess the disadvantage of being highly costly for routine home use.

5.4.2 Coronary stents

Coronary stents such as metal bare stents are introduced in the 1980s. They are designed to provide mechanical support to the coronary arteries, which recoil after balloon angioplasty. Thus it assists in improving blood and oxygen perfusion to the heart. The major toxicity of using these bare-metal stents is that it removes the endothelial layer of blood vessels and induces an inflammatory response causing vascular smooth muscle cell proliferation and clot formation that once again blocks the blood vessel. Recently, FDA-approved drug-eluting stents with polymer timed-release coatings of cytotoxins such as sirolimus and paclitaxel are developed. These drug-eluting stents also pose the adverse effect of causing thrombosis and in-stent restenosis (ISR) that can be diagnosed by repeated angiography, with the drawback of low precision in clinical assessment. Another limitation includes the impossibility to clinically locate how the stent is working in the vessel. Studies have been conducted to find a reliable method to diagnose ISR, which can be done by inserting a pressure sensor in the stent, which helps in detecting the increase in pressure within the stent. Usually, coronary stents have mesh-like tube design. Brox et al. [18] designed a passive coronary stent that is a continuous helical coil that is integrated with a capacitive blood pressure sensor. This is an LC tank where the stent is the inductor and the senor the capacitor are inductively coupled to an external coil and the phase dip is measured. Schachtele [19] modified this method by integrating two pressure-sensitive transponders at either end of the stent. The delay between the resonances of the two transponders is used to calculate the local pulse wave velocity. Active coronary stent with electronic components was developed after research conducted by Son et al. [20]. These smart stents are bioresorbable and provide mechanical support, and it also possesses diagnostic and therapeutic potentials. The stent is incorporated with a blood flow sensor, a temperature sensor, and a nanoparticle shell containing antiproliferative drugs that are released photothermally.

5.4.3 Permanent pacemakers

A permanent pacemaker is a small device, which is implanted under the skin of the chest wall, beneath the collarbone under local anesthesia and sedation. It generates electrical impulses to keep the heart beating at a normal rate. A cardiac pacemaker is the most predominantly used cardiovascular implant effective in managing heart rhythm disorders like bradycardia, where the heart beats too slowly or an arrhythmia when it beats irregularly. A conventional pacemaker system consists of a small computer, a pulse generator, and a battery connected to a number of transvenous leads that are implanted prepectoral in the subcutaneous tissue. A dual-chamber pacemaker has an atrial lead implanted in the right atrium appendage and a ventricular lead at the right ventricle apex or septum. Usually, the implants are placed on the right side of the heart for those patients who had an earlier explantation from the left side of the heart. This procedure takes an hour and requires just a night's stay in the hospital. After 2 weeks of implantation, a review is done where a wand is used to transmit the information regarding battery life, condition of the lead, and about any occurrence of arrhythmias that are recorded in the device's generator to the computer. Later on, a periodic 6 months review can be made through telephone or Internet, thus reducing hospital visits and costs. However, the use of cardiac pacemakers may produce major health hazards leading to both mortality and morbidity in implanted patients due to the complications related to future lead extractions. Long-term use results in the lead-induced risks such as fracture, moderate-to-severe tricuspid regurgitation, venous obstruction, and infection resulting in bacteremia and endocarditis.

5.4.4 Leadless pacemakers

With a motive to overcome the lead-associated toxicity, a leadless pacemaker, a small independent device that is percutaneously implanted in the right ventricle of the heart via a large-bore femoral venous sheath capable of sensing and pacing the endocardium, is employed. The clinical advantage of using a leadless pacemaker is the absence of transvenous leads that have well-established issues related to lead toxicity. Another chief feature of a leadless pacemaker is that it can be used only for a single chamber cardiac pacing and has the advantage of having a greater battery life than traditional devices. Nanostim is the first leadless pacemaker successfully implanted on humans. Leadless II trial proved the efficacy, safety, and battery life of Nanostim. Micra transcatheter pacing system is yet another device showing a successful implantation rate of 99% and the safety endpoint was 96% including cardiac perforation and vascular injury [21].

5.4.5 Cardiac resynchronization therapy

A biventricular pacemaker, also called a resynchronization device, is like a conventional pacemaker but has a third lead that sends impulses to the heart to resynchronize the contractions of the ventricle. Cardiac resynchronization therapy (CRT) is the ultimate treatment for left ventricular systolic dysfunction and asynchronous left ventricular contraction. In both these medical conditions, CRT improves the patient's quality of life and reduces heart failure associated with hospitalizations and death [22]. In CRT, a transvenous lead is placed into a vein on the surface of the left ventricle via the coronary sinus that drains into the right atrium. This conventional treatment method resulted in various adverse events such as lead failure in 21% of patients within 10 years of implantation, infection, tricuspid valve insufficiency, and central vein obstruction [23]. This procedure takes 2 hours and requires just a night's stay in the hospital and a review after 2 weeks like a permanent pacemaker.

5.4.6 Leadless cardiac resynchronization therapy

Recently, in leadless cardiac resynchronization therapy, a self-contained, multicomponent designed device consisting of a pacing electrode and pulse generator is being used successfully. In leadless CRT, the energy is transferred wirelessly from the transmitter to the receiver unit via ultrasound-mediated energy transfer or electromagnetic induction. WiCS-LV, wireless chronic stimulation-left ventricle system, utilizes the acoustic energy that is coimplanted with a CRT device, implantable cardioverter-defibrillator (ICD) device, or pacemaker that allows biventricular pacing.

WiCS-LV detects the right ventricular pacing signal from the CRT device, and the pulse generator then generates ultrasonic energy that is received by the receiver unit implanted in the left ventricle, converts this ultrasonic energy into an electrical pulse allowing a synchronous right and left ventricular pacing. The energy transfer to the receiver unit is achieved using beamforming and using electromagnetic induction [24]. The subcutaneous transmitter unit is a coil that sends an alternating magnetic field. This transmitter unit induces a voltage in the receiver unit comprising a coil with ferrite core, bridge rectifier, and high impedance lead tip. One limitation is that the energy transfer efficiency is affected by the movement of the receiver unit due to the beating of the heart.

5.5 Implantable cardioverter-defibrillator

ICD is a small battery-powered device that is implanted under the skin in the chest or abdomen to treat most dangerous ventricular arrhythmias, both ventricular tachycardia and ventricular fibrillation, which leads to sudden cardiac arrest if the condition is not treated quickly [25,26]. ICD is considered as the most efficient treatment methods that notably improve the survival of the patients. It usually acts by either stopping the abnormal heartbeat by sending small, painless electrical pulses to the heart or by producing large energy that shocks the heart back to a normal rhythm. It stores information regarding when and how many electrical shocks are delivered to the heart, whether it corrected the arrhythmia and the status of the device's battery. An ICD consists of a pulse generator, one or two leads, electrodes, and a battery lasting for 5–10 years. It is usually implanted in the left side of the heart, and it can be single chamber or dual chamber and can be also be used to provide CRT. Many ICDs are combined with built-in pacemakers, which send electrical impulses to the heart when it is beating too slowly and help to beat at a normal rate. CRT-P is a device where a pacemaker is incorporated into cardiac resynchronization therapy; whereas, in CRT-D, a defibrillator is associated. A cohort study regarding safety and risk of CRT-P and CRT-D showed that both these methods were linked with periprocedural complications, but CRT-D was especially producing greater risk of long-term toxic effects importantly infection [27].

5.5.1 Subcutaneous implantable cardioverter-defibrillator

The best and latest alternative to traditional ICD is the subcutaneous ICD that provides the highest protection against SCA without touching the heart and the vasculatures. S-ICD is a sophisticated technology that uses a subcutaneous electrode and analyses the heart rhythm rather than single beats. Registry data show comparatively lower major toxicity rates for S-ICD implantation [28]. It eliminates the potential for vascular injury and hence reduces the chances of systemic infections. It is also not useful for patients who need permanent pacing. Combining an S-ICD with a leadless cardiac pacemaker is still understudies.

5.5.2 Implantable loop recorders

Implantable loop recorders (ILR) is a wireless small cardiac monitoring device that is implanted under the skin subcutaneously on the anterior chest wall under local anesthesia, which provides a temporal correlation between cardiac rhythm and intermittent symptoms such as syncope or palpitation. During experiencing syncope or palpitation the handheld recorder has to be placed over the device to record the heart's electrical activity. The recorded information can then be transmitted through a remote monitoring system to find the reason for the symptoms. It has a battery life of up to 3 years and records continuously the heart rhythms. LINQ and Confirm RX™ are the two newer generation ILRs, which are considerably smaller in size than conventional devices. These newest ILRs are extremely small and are loaded into a small plastic applicator and are implanted under the skin to the left of the breastbone. ILR can also be deployed for atrial fibrillation that causes a rapid and irregular heartbeat, and for stroke [29]. In a loop study carried out by Diederichsen et al. [30], LINQ was implanted in 1420 patients: 753 (53%) were done in the outpatient room and 667 (47%) in the electrophysiology lab and were being asked to follow up for 499 days to report for any adverse reactions. The results showed that 9 patients (0.63%) experienced adverse effects with device explantation, 15 (1.13%) found adverse reactions without device explantation. The rate of infection was seen in 12 patients (1.6%) when done in the procedure room, and it was lesser than 1 (0.1%) when it was carried out in electrophysiology lab, confirming that both methods possess only very low toxicological effects.

5.5.3 Left ventricular assist device

Left ventricular assist device (LVAD) is a battery-operated mechanical pump-type device that is surgically implanted to maintain the pumping action of the heart that cannot function on its own. It is also known as "bridge transplant" as it is useful in patients who are waiting for a donor for heart transplantation, where it reduces further heart weakening during this time. However, recently, it is even the long-term therapy as well as destination therapy in end-stage heart failure patients where transplantation is ruled out. LVAD has a tube that pulls blood from the left ventricle into a pump, and this pump then sends the blood into the aorta. This pump is placed in the upper part of the abdomen, and another tube attached to the pump is brought out of the abdominal wall to the outside of the body and attached to the pump's battery and control systems. These devices are used for weeks to months and help in providing an acceptable quality of life before heart transplantation (Tables 5.4 and 5.5; Fig. 5.1). However, they pose a high risk of infection, thrombus formation, and blood trauma complications. The first-generation LVADs (HeartMate 1) have textured blood-contacting surfaces that reduce thrombotic complications. A landmark first-generation LVAD study, REMATCH, showed a significant 46% decrease in death and a 1-year increase in the survival rate of 52% as compared to 25% of any medical therapy alone. The second-generation devices (HeartMate II) were small in size, more efficacious and durable with fewer adverse effects by decreasing prothrombotic sites. The blood-contacting surface was coated with titanium lining, which is an antithrombotic measure. HeartMate II BTT trial is another landmark study for LVAD that showed a 75% survival rate at 6 months and a 68% survival rate at 1 year, improved quality of life, and functional capacity [31].

Table 5.4 FDA-approved cardiovascular implantable medical devices for structural and mechanical support.

Implant	Polymer	Use
SAPIEN transcatheter Heart valve	Cow tissue with polyster	Heart valve
Trifecta valve	Bovine pericardial tissue-polyester-covered titanium stent	Trifecta valve-stented pericardial valve
Mitroflow aortic pericardial Heart valve	Bovine pericardium-polyester-covered polymer stent	Prosthetic aortic valves

Table 5.5 FDA-approved implantable medical devices for localized drug delivery and functional support.

Implant	Polymer/drug	Use
PROMUS element plus	Everolimus-eluting platinum chromium stent	Coronary stent
OVATION Abdominal stent graft system	Graft is a plastic tube with polymer filled ring and metallic stent	Abdominal aortic aneurysms
LeGoo	Poloxamer	Temporary plugging of blood vessel
Propel	Mometasone furoate (steroid)	Sinus surgery
ION	Paclitaxel-eluting Coronary stent system	Coronary stent system
Attain StarFix	Surgically implanted insulated wire	Bioventricular pacemaker Cardioverter-defibrillator
Endologix power link system	Endovascular graft with ePTFE	Abdominal aortic aneurysms

5.6 Latest innovative technologies in implantable cardiovascular devices

5.6.1 HeartWare ventricular assist device pump

HeartWare ventricular assist device (HVAD) is a leading implantable ventricular assist device. European CE 2009, Australian Therapeutic Goods Administration (TGA), and US FDA approved it in 2011 and 2012. Moreover, 11,000 patients with end-stage heart failure have successfully used it. It holds the advantage of being small and could be implanted with minimally invasive procedures. The major highlight of this device that makes it at the top is because of the integrated inflow cannula that eliminates the requirement for a separate pocket to hold the pump. There is also no contact between the rotor and the housing, thus no issue of hemolysis (Fig. 5.2).

5.6.2 HeartMate 3

HeartMate 3 is an LVAD, which received the Cardiostim—EHRA European Innovation Award. These implants are used by more than

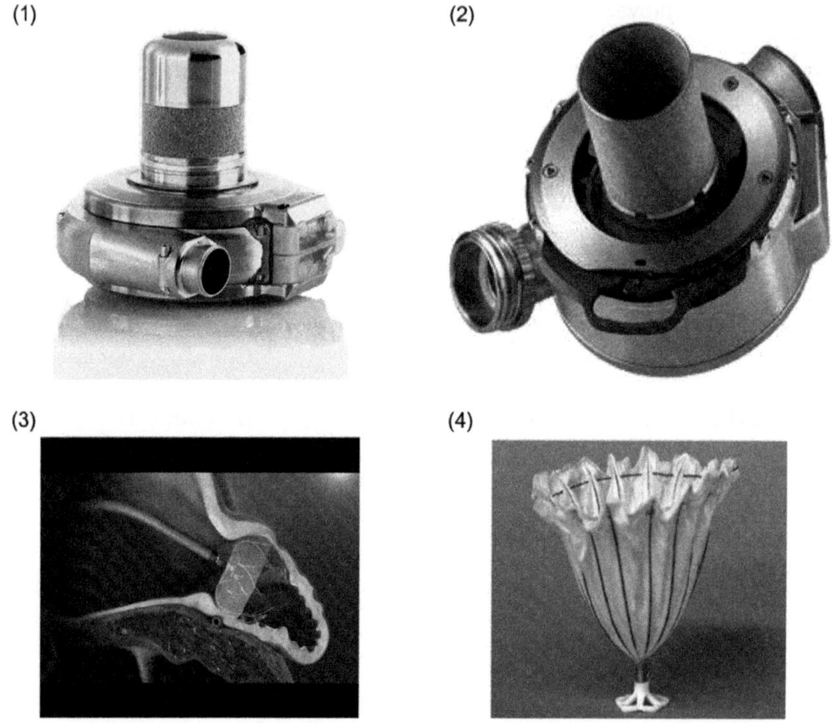

Figure 5.2 Latest innovations in cardiovascular implants. (1) HeartWare ventricular assist device; (2) HeartMate (LVAD); (3) Watchman left atrial appendage to occlude; (4) Parachute implant.

50,000 to a million advanced-stage heart failure patients in the United States. HeartMate 3 pumps up to 10 L of blood per minute. It was approved by CE in 2015 after successful clinical trials. It is the first commercially approved fully magnetically levitated LVAD.

5.6.3 Cardialen

This device restores the heart's natural rhythm in atrial fibrillation patients. It is a small-sized pacemaker that is surgically implanted with minimum invasiveness. The cardialen is used to continuously monitor the heartbeat and if it detects an atrial fibrillation, it emits low energy, electrical impulses that are hardly felt by the patients. The major advantage is low cost, and it can be switched on and off based on the patient's convenience.

5.6.4 Watchman

Watchman left atrial appendage occluder is used for atrial fibrillation patients who are under the risk of stroke, where an anticoagulant such as warfarin when used predisposes the risk of hemorrhages. This implant helps in stopping the use of anticoagulants in these patients. The device closes off the left atrial appendage in a transcatheter procedure and is usually suggested in patients whose condition is not primarily related to heart valves. This popular device has been approved for sale in Europe since 2005, and FDA clearance since 2015. Today, it is commercially available and implanted in 70 nations in more than 10,000 patients.

5.6.5 Parachute implant

Parachute implant is a transcatheter parachute structural heart implant from Cardio Kinetix Inc., which helps to compensate for the remodeling by separating the portion of the left ventricle that is damaged from the functional one. This then restores normal ventricular volume and improves the patient's heart's ability to pump blood effectively. Thus it helps to prevent left ventricular remodeling and worsening of heart failure. The size of this implant can be personalized according to the patient requirement through a computed tomography (CT) scan.

Even though these new technologies are trending in the implant field, the long-term impact will be based on clinical trial data, which are still understudies.

5.7 Tissue-engineered implants in cardiovascular diseases management

An emerging technology that could save the people from cardiovascular diseases and the implant-induced complication is the field of tissue engineering where a molecular, gene, or cell therapies can help in the development of a biological pacemaker that could be implanted efficiently, successfully, and safely. With the help of tissue engineering, ideal prostheses such as a myocardial valve and vascular device that is vital, growing, adaptive, autologous, and functionally optimally performing can be manufactured. Tissue engineering is a promising field for replacement in cardiovascular surgical procedures that offer better surgical outcomes and quality of life. It uses a biodegradable polymer scaffold (polyglycolic acid, PGA), hydrogels, and decellularized tissue composed of natural ECM proteins such as collagen, fibrin, and elastin that provide a structure for cells or tissues to grow. Embryonic stem cells, skeletal myoblasts, and induced pluripotent stem cells are generally used for cardiac tissue engineering. An ideal tissue-engineered cardiovascular implant should be biocompatible, functional, withstand high pressure, and highly vascular to produce a myocardium patch. Tissue engineering heart values require complex molds and cellularized with myofibroblasts to obtain a functional valve. The limitation of tissue-engineered valves is due to the calcification of tissue [32]. Currently, cardiovascular implants in tissue engineering follow three approaches:

1. Cell seeding of biodegradable valve matrices
2. Cell seeding of decellularized allograft or xenograft valves
3. Promote repopulation and adaptive remodeling of decellularized allograft valves.

Bypass vascular grafts have been tissue engineered using cellularized smooth muscle cells used in coronary bypass surgery to treat atherosclerosis. Tissue-engineered cardiac patches find use in the treatment of acute myocardial infarction, which helps in augmenting contractile function by promoting revascularization of ischemic tissue. Cell-based cardiac pumps are hollow structures tissue engineered with myocytes on cell surface and endothelial cells in the lumen, which helps to generate intramural pressure when stimulated electrically, and contracts in synchronization with the normal heart. It is most useful in treating chronic heart failure. Some of the toxicological effects that lead to vascular graft failure included thrombosis, intimal hyperplasia, atherosclerosis, or infection, which may be due to mismatch of graft, original vessel, diameter of the vessel, and damage due to procedure; specifically, atherosclerosis is the major cause for failure. The main application of tissue engineering technology is to overcome the above adverse effects and produce effective cardiovascular implants.

5.8 Smart cardiovascular implants and technologies that overcome its toxicological aspects

Conventional cardiovascular coronary stents are passive IMDs that act without requiring an electrical source. However, the recent novel breakthrough is the production of an active coronary stent, which is linked with electrical energy such that it monitors physiological or pathological signals and also stimulates therapeutic effects. Even the use of drug-eluting coronary stent induces intimal hyperplasia (IH) or restenosis that can be monitored using active IMDs. By providing a battery supply that will give a consistent, uninterrupted source of electrical energy, we can make smart implants. In the late 1950s, zinc or mercury oxide batteries were used for manufacturing cardiac pacemakers, but stopped due to their host toxicity, further in 1980s it was replaced with lithium or iodine batteries for use with pulse generators [33]. High-tech cardiac pacemakers are available nowadays by integrating memory to it to help record and transmit the heart's electrical activity. Lithium batteries with hybrid cathodes generate higher power density, but still with the limitation of life of these batteries and their replacement by another surgical procedure. Microelectronics has been yet another development in the field of IMDs, which help in producing implants of millimeter scale by minimizing the battery size that is a major challenge for the researchers. To overcome this challenge, the new innovation is wireless powering, where an electrical coil receives energy from another coil (transmitter) that is kept outside the body [34]. Research conducted at Stanford University by Ada Poon and his group came out with high-performance wireless powering systems that can be incorporated into miniature coronary stents. Excess energy in the form of gravitational, chemical, thermal, and electromagnetic energy produced in the human body can also be converted into electrical energy through human energy harvesting systems when fabricated using ultra low power circuits. Tashiro et al. [35] have found that using variable-capacitance-type electrostatic generators to power a cardiac pacemaker without a battery could create 36 μW power for 2 hours. We still need ample of research to produce a stent, which can produce more energy and consume less energy. A smart stent has a biosensor, a wireless module, and a mini computer [36]. This wireless module can monitor the condition of the patient continuously and changes according to the required treatment strategy at a particular time. The stent communicates with a remote server via a receiver Medical Implant Communication Service, which then interacts through a wired network with the server thus saving the long-term data. WLAN (wireless local area network), WPAN (wireless personal area network), and LR-WPAN (low rate wireless personal area network) are used for on the body communication services, and WBAN (wireless body area network) is useful for communications inside the body. E2R MedRadio is a WBAN that consumes less energy because it has a reliable communication system [37].

New smart devices include an electronic wrist ring or patch that can be worn by a patient and acts as a wearable device. Through microfabrication techniques, integrated circuits have been modified to create sensors for biomedical devices. Microelectromechanical systems (MEMS) produce very small implants, which have a mechanical part, and an integrated circuit that helps in the detection of physical forces is used to monitor health, and sense and treat diseases with very less invasive procedures [38]. Recent advancement in MEMS in cardiac resynchronization therapy is the use of a miniaturized sensor for heart sound that fits into the pacemaker. These sensors are attached to the tip of the leads in direct contact with the heart wall. As they are in direct contact with the organs, the need for biocompatible implant materials is of foremost concern. Silicon and glass are some of the best biocompatible material. The sensors are connected to an application-specific integrated circuit (ASIC) that transmits the signal to the external world. These sensors and ASIC are arranged vertically on printed circuit boards and form a system on package. Tsai et al. [39] made a micromachined capacitive sensor with a readout circuit on a single chip. The only disadvantage is that silicon is less flexible and brittle and hence is replaced by stretchable interconnects such as polyurethane. While producing implants, not only the size and nature of the material but also the shape of the implant material counts for its smartness. Smart implants of helical or serpentine wavy shapes at the milli- and microscale are recently developed. Sekitani et al. [40] produced stretchable material using uniformly dispersed single-walled carbon nanotubes. Nanocomposite-based inks for printing using either dispersed carbon or a metal-based filler material is an innovative printing technique that offers alternatives to soft lithography. Micra is a new and smallest pacemaker approved by the FDA in April 2016, which is implanted directly into the patient's heart via a vein in the leg and hence possesses an advantage of being less invasive eliminating the possible medical complications. Multifunctional shape memory polymers are finding its wide application as a smart implant biomaterial.

5.9 Cardiovascular implant-induced toxicity and management methods

At present, although there is a voluminous growth in cardiovascular implant technology, production, and wide application of high-tech cardiovascular implants in various cardiovascular diseases, still there are many toxicological effects that limit the utmost usefulness of these implants. Infection, inflammation, pain, rejection, coagulation, allergic response, superficial thrombosis, embolization, and organ injury are considered as among some of the major adverse effects of cardiovascular implants. These toxicological effects are also the major challenges in the use of many cardiovascular implants that have to be overcome. Infection is a serious toxic effect leading to morbidity and mortality. Management of infection is a major challenge in implant technology. Cardiac permanent pacemakers (PPM) induced endocarditis has been reported even since the 1970s [41,42]. Most of these infections are pocket infection, and frank permanent pacemaker endocarditis accounts for 10% of PPM infections [43]. Prepectoral ICD induced infection rate is as low as 7% when compared to the conventional ICD. It is reported that among Medicare beneficiaries the rate of cardiac device infections (PPMs, ICDs, Valves and Ventricular Assist Devices) increased 124%, from 0.94 to 2.11 per 1000 beneficiaries from 1990 to 1999 [44]. Data from the Truven MarkestScan database about Medicare and US healthcare claims studied in 72,701 patients with TV-PPM show 15%–16% complications in 3 years representing a significant economic burden to both the patient and the healthcare system. It was also found that the infection rate was higher in patients using ICDs than PPMs. It is shocking to observe that there is an increased risk of hospitalization deaths due to implant use. Implanted patients when predisposed to other complications such as diabetes mellitus, kidney dysfunction, fever, and oral anticoagulant and long-term corticosteroid users are at greater risk for infections [45–47]. In a cohort study from Olmsted Country, Minnesota, 55% out of 22 cardiovascular device-implanted patients with subsequent *Staphylococcus aureus* bacteremia developed infections [48]. There was also the risk of mortality during device replacement after pocket infection. Kapa et al. [49] reported a 1.4% complication risk at the Mayo clinic. Perioperative antimicrobial prophylaxis, use of the pectoral transvenous device, and a well-experienced physician while doing implantation can prevent the rate of these infections. Identifying and understanding the pathogenesis of these infections may better help in the management of these challenges. Oral antibiotic therapy against staphylococci with oral vancomycin as empirical therapy or with cefazolin or nafcillin and percutaneous lead extraction can help in treating the infection. However, lead extraction might also introduce to risks of tamponade, hemothorax, pulmonary embolism, lead migration, and death even when done by an experienced physician. Antimicrobial therapy is given usually for 7–10 days for pocket infection and if with inflammation, 10–14 days treatment is advisable. In bloodstream infection, parenteral antibiotics for 4 weeks is preferred.

The conventional cardiac pacemakers cause thrombosis, lead failure, pneumothorax, and tricuspid regurgitation, and these toxic effects can be overcome by using a leadless transvenous pacing device (Table 5.6). Most of the conventionally used coronary stents pose serious adverse effects such as from a common thrombosis to restenosis. In active IMDs, the electronic components added to the stent are a major challenge. These electronic modules have to resist stent crimping procedures, stent expansion, and all chemical and biological reactions that happen in the blood vessel of the patient during its stay in the body. A smart stent developed by Chen et al. overcomes the above procedures [50]. Their stent included a pressure sensor that is incorporated using laser microwelding. They also added Parylene C and gold coatings to warrant biocompatibility and X-ray opacity. This stent was found to be positive in diagnosing the blood pressure when studied in a swine model. Cardiovascular implants show blood and soft tissue interaction with biomaterials; currently, there are numerous FDA-approved cardiovascular implants that are commercially available and used by millions of patients, but none is found to completely treat the cardiovascular disease. There is always a problem of the implant surface and tissue interaction that can be overcome by surface modification and by supplementation of material surfaces with a specific peptide that will cause an inflammatory response but induces functional endothelialization.

Table 5.6 Cardiovascular implant-induced toxicity.

Implants	Toxicological effects
Heart valve prostheses	Thrombosis, embolism, paravalcular leak, anticoagulation-related hemorrhage, infective endocarditis, extrinsic dysfunction, incomplete valve closure, cloth wear, hemolytic anemia, component fracture, tissue valves, cusp tearing, cusp calcification
Vascular grafts	Thrombosis, embolism, infection, perigraft erosion, perigraft seroma, false aneurysm, disintegration/degradation
Cardiac assist/replacement devices	Thrombosis, embolism, endocarditis, extraluminal infection, Component fracture, hemolysis, calcification
Vascular stents	Thrombosis, proliferative restenosis, strut-related inflammation, foreign-body reaction, incomplete expansion, overexpansion, infection, malposition

Toxicological challenges while using an implantable cardiovascular device can be overcome by FDA approval or clearance for sale, premarket review, postmarket review, tracking, monitoring efficacy, and patient safety.

5.10 Marketing strategies and regulations to prevent cardiovascular implant-induced toxicity

The growing prevalence of cardiovascular diseases has led to high demand for the use of cardiovascular implants across the globe irrespective of the developed or developing nations. Moreover, this has given way for the recent advancement in the medical field, thus providing diagnosis and treatment of various diseases, which were once considered fatal. One such advance is in the production of smart cardiovascular stents, which top the sales of implant market with a good profit, as well as providing quality of life and cost-effective treatment for the heart patients. Cardiac pacemakers are lifesaving, and worldwide millions of people are using these implants. The global market for cardiovascular implants in the United States in 2018 was $ 19.8 billion, and it is estimated to reach the US $ 27.1 billion by 2024. While these implants possess the best therapeutic effects, eventually they also pose a serious risk due to toxicity, which limits their use. To overcome these limitations, the United States has framed strict regulations for the medical device industry. The device manufacturers have to pass through stringent product approval procedures, clinical trials, pay user fees, and conduct periodic audits/inspections to market a cardiovascular implant. There are abundant cardiovascular implant manufacturers in the United States, but only a few of them produce all the major devices. Surprisingly, only three manufacturers produce cardiac defibrillators and four drug-eluting coronary artery stents with anticoagulant drugs. Recently, a tissue-engineered cardiovascular implant alone has accounted for $6.9 billion in global markets. The regulations help to streamline the manufacturing and sale of quality implants. The FDA has regulatory frameworks that have to be cleared for approval and market of the cardiovascular implant. Such regulatory frameworks are based on the complexity and amount of risk it poses to patients; the higher the risk, the greater is the strict regulatory needs. Although the manufacturers are following strict FDA rules globally, still certain factors act as limitations such as lack of price transparency, lack of knowledge about various implants its quality, performance, and lack of control over buying decisions restricted by both manufacturer and physician. These limitations can be overcome through appointing technology assessment committees that can collect data regarding the quality, performance, and patient outcomes and assess the effectiveness of these hospital-implanted devices. Besides these committees, the Agency for Healthcare Research and Quality, in the US Department of Health and Human Services, collects research data based on reviews and published works. Additionally, device registry data provide information on safety, effectiveness, and performance of the implantable devices, and a unique device identifier, given for high-risk implants, helps in studying the patient safety [51].

5.11 Conclusion

Despite recent advances in the medical field, there is an alarming percentage of mortality rate due to many diseases especially cardiovascular diseases. As cardiovascular implants have been extensively deployed clinically, it accounts for the major contribution to the treatment of cardiovascular diseases. With more scientific innovations, there is also a parallel increase in the number of complicated diseases, which requires hospitalization, time, and money. Even though many diseases have emerged, the life expectancy of individuals has increased, which is indirectly due to the development of more sophisticated and advanced implantable medical devices with diagnostic and therapeutic effects. Smart-advanced cardiovascular implants produced abiding to strict regulatory frameworks have become the golden standards in both cardiovascular patients and healthcare professionals.

References

[1] Bussooa A, Neale S, Mercer JR. Future of smart cardiovascular implants. Sensors 2018;18:1–11.
[2] Smith SC, Collins A, Ferrari R, Holmes DR, Logstrup S, McGhie DV, et al. Our time: a call to save preventable death from cardiovascular disease (heart disease and stroke). J Am Coll Cardiol 2012;60:2343–8.
[3] World Health Organization, World Heart Federation, World Stroke Organization. Global atlas on cardiovascular disease prevention and control: policies, strategies, and interventions, August 7; 2012.
[4] Williams DF. On the mechanisms of biocompatibility. Biomaterials 2008;29:2941–53.

[5] Onuki Y, Bhardwaj U, Papadimitrakopoulos F, Burgess DJ. A review of the biocompatibility of implantable devices: current challenges to overcome foreign body response. J Diabetes Sci Technol 2008;2:1003–15.
[6] Hermawan H, Ramdan D, Djuansjah RP. Metals for biomedical applications. In: Reza Fazel, editor. Biomedical engineering – from theory to applications, vol. 29; 2011. p. 441–30.
[7] BomBac D, Brojan M, FajFar P, Kosel F, Turk R. Review of materials in medical applications. RMZ-Mater Geoenviron 2007;54(4):471–99.
[8] Ramshaw JAM, Werkmeister JA, Glattauer V. Collagen-based biomaterials. Biotechnol Genet Eng Rev 1995;13:335–82.
[9] Wu P, Grainger DW. Drug/device combinations for local drug therapies and infection prophylaxis. Biomaterials 2006;27:2450–67.
[10] Abizaid A, Costa JR. New drug-eluting stents an overview on biodegradable and polymer-free next-generation stent systems. Circ Cardiovasc Interv 2010;3 (4):384–93.
[11] Carpentier A. From valvularxenograft to valvularbioprosthesis. Med Instrum 1977;11 (2):98–101.
[12] Kamachimudali U, Sridhar TM, Raj B. Corrosion of bio implants. In: Sadhana, editor. Academy proceedings in engineering sciences. Indian Academy of Sciences; 2003. p. 601–37.
[13] Maisel WH. Medicine and public issues medical device regulation: an introduction for the practicing physician. Ann Intern Med 2004;140:296–302.
[14] Springer F, Gunther RW, Schmitz-Rode T. Aneurysm sac pressure measurement with minimally invasive implantable pressure sensors: an alternative to current surveillance regimens after EVAR? Cardiovasc Intervent Radiol 2008;31:460–7.
[15] Abraham WT, Adamson PB, Bourge RC, Aaron MF, Costanzo MR, Stevenson LW, et al. Wireless pulmonary artery haemodynamic monitoring in chronic heart failure: a randomized controlled trial. Lancet 2011;377:658–66.
[16] Vaduganathan M, DeFilippis EM, Fonarow GC, Butler J, Mehra MR. Post marketing adverse events related to the CardioMEMS HF system. JAMA Cardiol 2017;2 (11):1277–9.
[17] Ohki T, Ouriel K, Silveira PG, Katzen B, White R, Criado F, et al. Initial results of wireless pressure sensing for endovascular aneurysm repair: the APEX Trial-Acute pressure measurement to confirm aneurysm sac exclusion. J Vasc Surg 2007;45:236–42.
[18] Brox D, Chen X, Mirrabbasi S, Takahata K. Wireless telemetry of stainless steel based smart antenna stent using a transient resonance method. IEEE Antennas Wirel Propag Lett 2013;394:164–71.
[19] Schachtele J. A bifrequent passive sensor system for measurement of the pulse wave velocity in a stent. In: Proceedings of the 2016 38th annual international conference of the IEEE engineering in medicine and biology society (EMBC), Orlando, FL, August 16–20; 2016. p. 1926–9.
[20] Son D, Lee J, Lee DJ, Ghaffari R, Yun S, Kim SJ, et al. Bioresorbable electronic stent integrated with therapeutic nanoparticles for endovascular diseases. ACS Nano 2015;9:5937–46.
[21] Bernard ML. Pacing without wires: leadless cardiac pacing. Ochsner J 2016;16 (3):238–42.
[22] McAlister FA, Ezekowitz J, Hooton N, Vandermeer B, Spooner C, Dryden DM, et al. Cardiac resynchronization therapy for patients with left ventricular systolic dysfunction: a systematic review. JAMA 2007;297:2502–14.
[23] Miller MA, Neuzil P, Dukkipati SR, Reddy VY. Leadless cardiac pacemakers back to the future. J Am Coll Cardiol 2015;66:1179–89.

[24] Wieneke H, Rickers S, Velleuer J, Bruck G, Bai Z, Kocks C, et al. Leadless pacing using induction technology: impact of pulse shape and geometric factors on pacing efficiency. Europace 2013;15:453–9.
[25] Connolly SJ, Gent M, Roberts RS, Dorian P, Roy D, Sheldon RS, et al. Canadian implantable defibrillator study (CIDS): a randomized trial of the implantable cardioverter defibrillator against amiodarone. Circulation 2000;101:1297–302.
[26] Moss AJ, Zareba W, Hall WJ, Klein H, Wilber DJ, Cannom DS, et al. Prophylactic implantation of a defibrillator in patients with myocardial infarction and reduced ejection fraction. N Engl J Med 2002;346:877–83.
[27] Barra S, Providencia R, Boveda S, Duehmke R, Narayanan K, Chow AW. Device complications with addition of defibrillation to cardiac resynchronization therapy for primary prevention. Heart 2018;104(18):1529–35.
[28] Burke MC, Gold MR, Knight BP, Barr CS, Theuns DA, Boersma LV, et al. Safety and efficacy of the totally subcutaneous implantable defibrillator: 2-year results from a pooled analysis of the IDE study and EFFORTLESS registry. J Am Coll Cardiol 2015;65:1605–15.
[29] Wiles BM, Illingworth CA, Paisey JR, Roberts PR, Harden SP. Keeping up appearances: the radiographic evolution of cardiovascular implantable electronic devices. Br J Radiol 2017;91:1–6.
[30] Diederichsen SZ, Haugan KJ, Hojberg S, Holst AG, Kober L, Pedersen KB, et al. Complications after implantation of a new-generation insertable cardiac monitor: results from the LOOP study. Int J Cardiol 2017;15:229–34.
[31] Rodriguez LE, Suarez EE, Loebe M, Bruckner BA. Ventricular assist devices (VAD) therapy: new technology, new hope? Methodist Debakey Cardiovasc J 2013;9 (1):32–7.
[32] Klopsch C, Steinhoff G. Tissue-engineered devices in cardiovascular surgery. Eur Surg Res 2012;49:44–52.
[33] Chen K, Merritt DR, Howard WG, Schmidt CL, Skarstad PM. Hybrid cathode lithium batteries for implantable medical applications. J Power Sources 2006;162:837–40.
[34] Ho JS, Kim S, Poon ASY. Midfield wireless powering for implantable systems. Proc IEEE 2013;101:1369–78.
[35] Tashiro R, Kabei N, Katayama K, Tsuboi E, Tsuchiya K. Development of an electrostatic generator for a cardiac pacemaker that harnesses the ventricular wall motion. J Artif Org 2002;5:239–45.
[36] Zheng G, Shankaran R, Orgun MA, Qiao L, Saleem K. Ideas and challenges for securing wireless implantable medical devices: a review. IEEE Sens J 2017;17:562–76.
[37] Hsu JM, Chiang TC, Yu YC, Teng WG, Hou TW. A new energy efficient and reliable medradio scheme based on cooperative communication for implanted medical devices. Int J Distrib Sens Netw 2015;2015:1–11.
[38] Deterre M. MEMS integration for smart medical devices: opportunities and challenges. In: Proceedings of the 2012 symposium on design, test, integration and packaging of MEMS/MOEMS, Cannes, France; April 25–27 2012. p. 253–7.
[39] Tsai TH, Tsai HC, Wu TK. A CMOS micromachined capacitive tactile sensor with integrated readout circuits and compensation of process variations. IEEE Trans Biomed Circuits Syst 2014;8:608–16.
[40] Sekitani T, Noguchi Y, Hata K, Fukushima T, Aida T, Someya T. A rubberlike stretchable active matrix using elastic conductors. Science 2008;321:1468–72.
[41] Schwartz IS, Pervez N. Bacterial endocarditis associated with a permanent transvenous cardiac pacemaker. JAMA 1971;218:736–7.

[42] Corman LC, Levison ME. Sustained bacteremia and transvenous cardiac pacemakers. JAMA 1975;233:264–6.
[43] Arber N, Pras E, Copperman Y, Schapiro JM, Meiner V, Lossos IS, et al. Pacemaker endocarditis: report of 44 cases and review of the literature. Med (Baltim) 1994;73:299–305.
[44] Cabell CH, Heidenreich PA, Chu VH, Moore CM, Stryjewski ME, Corey GR. Increasing rates of cardiac device infections among medicare beneficiaries: 1990–1999. Am Heart J 2004;147:582–6.
[45] Bloom H, Heeke B, Leon A, Mera F, Delurgio D, Beshai J, et al. Renal insufficiency and the risk of infection from pacemaker or defibrillator surgery. Pacing Clin Electrophysiol 2006;29:142–5.
[46] Lekkerkerker JC, Nieuwkoop C, Trines SA, Bom JG, Bernards A, Velde ET, et al. Risk factors and time delay associated with cardiac device infections: leiden device registry. Heart 2009;95:715–20.
[47] Sohail MR, Uslan DZ, Khan AH, Friedman PA, Hayes DL, Wilson WR, et al. Risk factor analysis of permanent pacemaker infection. Clin Infect Dis 2007;45:166–73.
[48] Uslan DZ, Sohail MR, Sauver JL, Friedman PA, Hayes DL, Stoner SM, et al. Permanent pacemaker and implantable cardioverter-defibrillator infection: a population-based study. Arch Intern Med 2007;167:669–75.
[49] Kapa S, Hyberger L, Rea RF, Hayes DL. Complication risk with pulse generator change: implications when reacting to a device advisory or recall. Pacing Clin Electrophysiol 2007;30:730–3.
[50] Chen X, Assadsangabi B, Hsiang Y, Takahata K. Enabling angioplasty-ready 'smart' stents to detect in-stent restenosis and occlusion. Adv Sci 2018;5(5):1–10.
[51] Keith D, Lind JD. Understanding the market for implantable medical devices. AARP Insights 2017;129:1–15.

CHAPTER SIX

Breasts and birth control

Krishna Gautam[1,3], Shreya Dwivedi[1], Dhirendra Singh[2] and Sadasivam Anbumani[1,3,*]

[1]Ecotoxicology Laboratory, Regulatory Toxicology Group, CSIR-Indian Institute of Toxicology Research, Lucknow, India

[2]Pathology Laboratory, Regulatory Toxicology Group, CSIR-Indian Institute of Toxicology Research, Lucknow, India

[3]Academy of Scientific and Innovative Research (AcSIR), CSIR-Indian Institute of Toxicology Research, Lucknow, India

*Corresponding author

Abstract

In this chapter, we discussed the two widely used medical implants and their role, application, and effectiveness among women. An implant is an artificial implement or a device that is used in the medical field to restore the natural appearance of body structure or to correct any sort of deformities. The evacuation of the implant is basically depending on the durability and the type of implant. Since the 19th century, breasts implant has been done to bring back the semblance of breasts, lost due to mastectomy or to ameliorate innate defects or reconstruction of breasts distorted by accident or disease (breasts cancer) and to correct the impairment of chest wall. Birth control implant is the hormonal-based contraceptive to prevent the unintended and unplanned pregnancy. Unplanned and unintended pregnancies are the most common health issue at the global level and imposing the socioeconomic burden to the society and the family. Therefore the prevention of these kinds of pregnancies is always an essential part of the practice of medicine. The regulation and the classification of the medical implants are necessary, to ensure the effectiveness and the safety of the patient.

Keywords: Birth control implants; breasts implants; anaplastic large cell lymphoma

6.1 Introduction

An implant is an artificial implement or a device that is used in the medical field to restore the natural appearance of body structure or to correct any sort of deformities. Implants can be inserted or placed either on the surface of the body or inside the body. They can be implanted for lifelong or can be evacuated when not required. The evacuation of the

Toxicological Aspects of Medical Device Implants.
DOI: https://doi.org/10.1016/B978-0-12-820728-4.00006-X

© 2020 Elsevier Inc.
All rights reserved.

implant is basically depending on the durability and the type of implant. Medical implants are made up of a variety of organic and inorganic materials that are biofunctional, biocompatible, corrosive resistance, bioadhesive, and easily processable [1]. Among these properties, biofunctionality and biocompatibility are two of the utmost important regulatory characteristic features of the human body. Some of the materials that are used in the manufacturing of implants are silicone, silicate, polyethylene, polyurethane foam, titanium, prolactic acid metals, ceramics, plastic, skin, human tissues, and others. Magnesium used in implant manufacture is highly acceptable as they are easily absorbable and compatible. Food and drug administration (FDA) classified and grouped different types of materials used in implant into three classes, that is, class I (subjected to lowest risk and used for general control), class II (require extensive and exclusive control involving appropriate scrutiny and obligatory performance standards), and class III (comprises both class I and II properties along with review) [2]. However, implants involve varied risks and complications such as failure and rupture of the implant, soreness, and puffiness around the implanted area, site burnishing, and infection. Breasts implant, contraceptive implant, artificial hip, and pacemaker implantation are responsible for major health injuries and may require further surgeries to correct the defect and sometimes it may result in the death of the patient (Fig. 6.1). Between 2015 and 2018, around 62,000 cases of adverse effects were

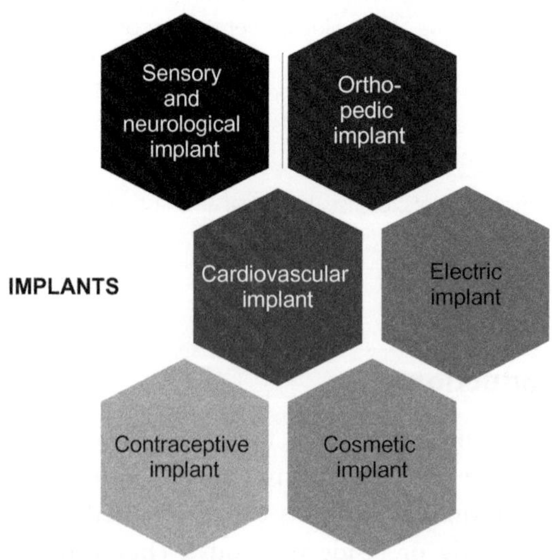

Figure 6.1 Types of various implants used in the medical field.

reported alone in the United Kingdom, out of which 1004 resulted in the death of the patients [3]. Capsular contracture, breasts implant rupture, and breasts implant–associated anaplastic large cell lymphoma (BIA-ALCL) are some of the severe complications that result after breasts implantation surgeries. BIA-ALCL first reported in 1997 that a rare T-cell lymphoma may arise either in situ or infiltrative disease [4]. In this chapter, authors have discussed two types of implants, that is, breasts implant and birth control implants, their types, mode of action, adverse effect, and the effectiveness with acceptability in women.

6.2 Breasts implant

The breasts implant is a surgical process that is done by placing the implants behind breasts tissues and is intended to modify the form, size, and surface contour of a person's breasts. Since the 19th century, breasts implant has been done to bring back the semblance of breasts lost due to mastectomy or to ameliorate innate defects or reconstruction of breasts distorted by accident or disease (breasts cancer) and to correct the impairment of chest wall. In 1895, Czerny corrected a breasts defect through transplanting a tissue, lipoma (fatty lump) from the pelvis of a patient [5]. This was considered to be the first cosmetic surgery of breasts by autonomous reconstruction. There are various ways for breasts augmentation. On the position of the implant, it can be subglandular or retroglandular (implant will be placed deep to the glandular muscle) and subpectoral or retropectoral (implant will be placed deep to the pectoralis major muscle) [6]. In 1962 Cronin and Frank Gerow, American plastic surgeons, introduced the first-generation silicone gel-filled breasts implant created by Dow Corning Corporation [7]. However, due to poor quality and less viscosity of the shell, there are more cases of capsular contracture and implant rupture and this problem resulted in the development of second-generation silicone gel-based breasts implant in the 1970s. After that to further improve the quality of implants, the third-generation implant was developed but in 1992 due to restriction pose by the FDA to the use of third-generation implants in the United States, fourth and fifth-generation silicone gel-based implant came into existence [6]. In the United Kingdom, cosmetic breasts augmentation is one of the most frequently performed breasts implant surgery [8,9]. According to a study, each year in the United Kingdom around 55,000 women were diagnosed with breasts cancer and 40% of them necessitate breasts augmentation as foremost operative treatment [8]. Breasts implants are categorized in different types based on the filler material used in the implant, that is, saline breasts implant, silicone breasts implant, structured breasts implant, composite breasts implant (discontinued), gummy bear breasts implant, smooth breasts implant, textured breasts implant, and round breasts implant. Out of these implants, saline and silicone breasts implants are most recommended. According to the analyzed data, out of 100,000 patients, 80,000 patients underwent silicone gel-based breasts implant and 20,000 patients received saline-based breasts implants in the year 2007–2010 (Fig. 6.2) [10].

In 1964, a saline breasts implant was put forward as a prosthetic implement that can be used in the pharmaceutical sector. Saline solution is used as filler material in saline breasts implants. Laboratories Arion company in France manufactured this saline solution for the very first time. Saline breasts implant became more recommended as it is the physically less invasive surgical technique and can be performed through smaller and shorter incisions comparative to the usual surgical incisions [11]. It gives more satisfactory results than other implants and is considered a safer implant than the other. In the case of implant rupture, the saline solution can be safely absorbed or ejected by the body. In silicone breasts implants, silicone gel is used as a filler material that is prefilled in a silicone shell that

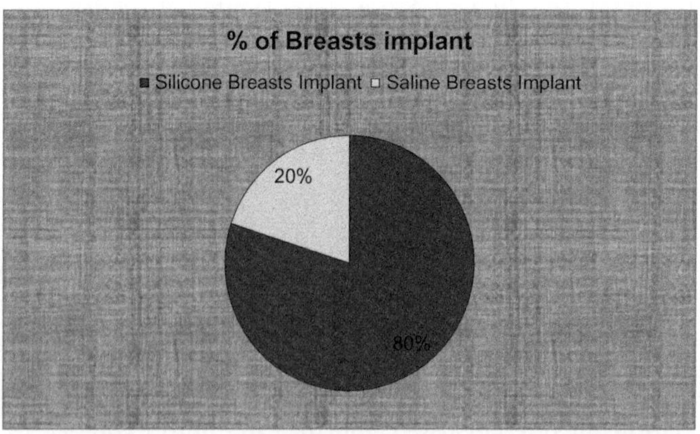

Figure 6.2 Percentage of silicone and saline breasts implant received by patients in the year 2007–2010.

is inserted through longer incisions than a saline breasts implant. The texture of the gel is more or less similar to the natural tissues of the breasts. In the case of breasts implant rupture, the gel may persist within the implant shell or may break out into the implant pocket but it will not disrupt.

Silicone implant incompatibility syndrome (SIIS) is a clinical syndrome that arises from silicone implants with consecutive symptoms such as arthralgias, myalgias, cognitive impairment, sleep disturbance, and chronic fatigue [12]. In 2011, Schoenfeld reported that SIIS is a subtype of autoimmune syndrome induced by adjuvants (ASIA). Around 4497 cases of ASIA have been reported; among them, 305 cases are of severe ASIA along with 11 deaths [13]. Instead of the above-mentioned complications due to breasts augmentation surgeries, it is one of the most frequently performed cosmetic surgeries. In 2011, around 320,000 individuals under the age of 18 years underwent breasts augmentation surgery [14]. The US Food and Drug Administration recommended a minimum age limit for women looking forward to breasts implants as it involves certain risks and medical complications [14]. There is a different age range for silicone and saline breasts implant; silicone gel-filled breasts implants are accepted for the women of 22 years old or above and saline-filled breasts implants are accepted for the users of 18 years old or above. FDA has approved a structured breasts implant as a third category of breasts implants [15]. Structured breasts implant has been considered to be safer as the rate of implant rupture and capsular contracture is much lesser than saline and silicone breasts implant. One of the reasons behind this is that structured breasts implants are of dual lumen saline-filled implants [16]. Composite breasts implants are terminated due to associated health risks and complications. The filler materials that are practiced in this implant are silastic rubber, soy oil, polypropylene string, ground rubber, and Teflon-silicone prostheses. In gummy bear breasts implants, silicone gel is used as a filler material but the viscosity of the gel inside the implant is richer than the usual silicone gel implant. These are sometimes also referred to as form-stable implants as they maintain their shape even when the implants get ruptured. Breasts augmentation poses various health risks and complications that include breasts implant rupture, breasts pain, infection, capsular contraction, being unable to breastfeed or producing less milk than before, nerve damage to the nipples, and many more. Surgical treatments are more or less suspected to cause infection at the surgical site, and overuse of prosthetic materials increases the probability to cause infection.

Infection is one of the major risks associated with breasts implants. Based on a study, 2.9% of women are diagnosed to be affected by infection after breasts implant surgery [17]. ALCL is a rare form of breasts implant malignancy identified by the FDA and considered to be associated with chronic inflammation.

The FDA has reported that cosmetic augmentation of the breasts may be linked with the atypical form of cancer called ALCL, believed to be related to chronic microbial inflammation [18]. According to a medical report, the FDA has come across a sum of 359 cases of BIA-ALCL, along with 2.5% deaths [19].

6.2.1 Breasts implant technique

Breasts augmentation is a surgical process by which an implant is placed within the breasts tissues to get better the shape and enhance the size of the breasts. There are mainly five surgical techniques for the placement of breasts implants, that is, subglandular, subfascial, subpectoral, submuscular, and pectoral or subcutaneous (Table 6.1).

6.2.2 Breasts implant rupture

Breasts augmentation involves various types of risks: breasts implant rupture or leakage is one of those. Silicone gel breasts implant rupture can be of two types: extracapsular and intracapsular; there cannot be extracapsular rupture without intracapsular rupture. As a usual natural reaction to any foreign implant, the human body creates a fibrous capsule scar. In an intracapsular rupture, the ruptured implant will remain within the fibrous capsule or an implant pocket whereas there is the exudation of silicone gel outside the fibrous capsule in extracapsular rupture. Saline breasts implant rupture results in the leakage of the saline solution, and the implant quickly gets compressed; thus, it can be removed readily.

Table 6.1 Various techniques of breasts implant and their description.

Techniques	Description
Subglandular	The implant is placed in the retromammary space (the space between the breasts tissues and the chest muscles)
Submuscular	The implant is placed beneath the chest muscles
Subfascial	The implant is kept inside the fascia of pectoralis major muscle
Subpectoral	The implant is placed under pectoralis major muscle
Pectoral	The implant is placed above the pectoralis major muscle

Some of the most frequent causes of implant rupture are secondary to the normal aging of the implant as all prostheses' walls will rupture eventually. Literature and personal experience allow physicians to estimate this time frame from 25 to 35 years. All ruptures occurring within 20 years are premature. These early ruptures have different causes that include incompetent valves, manufacturing defects, and underfilling that lead to folds thus provoking a premature weakness in the wall. Most traumas do not because prosthesis ruptures except, possibly, in the case of blunt trauma. Nonpenetrating traumas were encountered in closed capsulotomy of old silicone prostheses, but these are seen less today [20–23].

6.2.3 Breasts implant complications

Breasts augmentation is a surgical procedure that involves severe risks and complication with at least 1% of breasts implant patients showing adverse results after implantation. Complication of breast implant involves atrophy of breasts tissues that involves shrinking and thinning of breasts skin, formation of hematoma and seroma that may cause swelling, contusion, and pain near the surgical site, swelling of lymph nodes or lymphedema, necrosis (skin near the implant become dead) that can be caused by infection, deformation of chest wall, and capsular contracture (Fig. 6.3) [24]. Sometimes the skin around the implant breaks down and the implant becomes visible or there will be chances of palpability. Asymmetry of breasts, redness around implant, deflation, infection, inflammation, displacement of implant, and loss of sensation around the breasts are some of

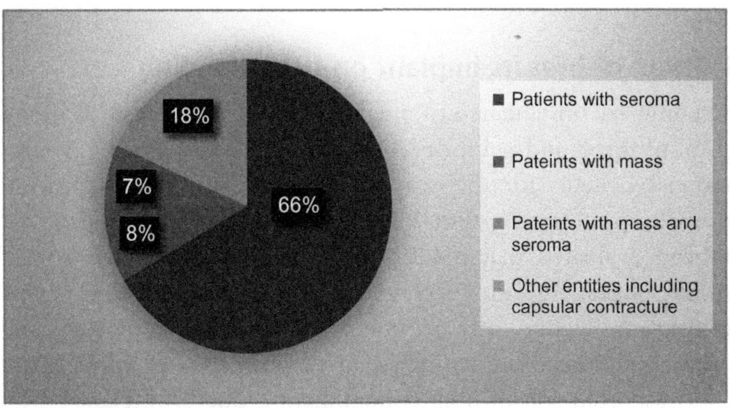

Figure 6.3 Percentage of different complications in patients.

the most probable complications after breasts implant. BIA-ALCL is a kind of non-Hodgkin's lymphoma, cancer of the immune system, and is found to be associated with breasts implant by FDA in 2011.

6.2.4 Breasts implant–associated anaplastic large cell lymphoma

ALCL is an atypical type of cancer that attributes to non-Hodgkin's lymphoma (2%–3%) and T-cell lymphomas (12%) and considered as an abnormal growth of lymphocytes that is linked with the breasts implant [25]. However, apart from its connection with the breasts implant, it has also been diagnosed in patients of age 55–60 years, more frequently in males at stages III–IV, a high International Prognostic Index score, with B-symptoms, and an aggressive course [25]. During the previous decade, more than 300 instances of anaplastic large cell lymphoma (ALCL) related with breasts implants, with nine deaths, have been accounted for the US FDA, with the greater part happening in patients after breasts reconstruction for cancer [24]. On the basis of a number of published cases all over the world, women with breasts implant pose 18.2–67.7 times higher risk to be diagnosed with ALCL. BIA-ALCL can be diagnosed through standard diagnostic procedures prescribed by varied federal and medical organizations such as the National Comprehensive Cancer Network (NCCN, USA), the Institute National du Cancer (Inca, France), and the Netherlands Association for Plastic and Reconstructive Surgery (NVPC, Netherlands) [26]. After a year of breasts implantation, if there is the formation of seroma that is not due to any trauma or infection then it should be treated as apprehensive BIA-ALCL [18].

6.2.5 Effect of breasts implant on breastfeeding

Breastfeeding has instantaneous and long-term gastrointestinal, immunological, nutritional, and neurodevelopmental well-being to the infants and psychosocial benefits for the women [27]. Breastfeeding appears to be exceptionally protective against some early day's complications in infants. It has been evaluated that millions of women all over the world have undergone breasts implant surgery that can be either saline or silicone breasts implant. Hence, this became an issue of concern regarding the health of the children who are breastfed on women with implants as there will be a suspected risk of milk contamination due to implant rupture or leakage as silicone gel and saline solution are used as a filler material in breasts implant, which can be harmful. According to a published report, silicone from the breasts implant from mother to child can be transferred through breasts milk during breastfeeding and may cause childhood "rheumatoid symptoms" or "scleroderma-like" abnormal esophageal motility [28,29]. Women with breasts implants were significantly less likely to breastfeed than women without implants [30]. The breasts implant may also destruct the nerves and ducts of the breasts during the surgery that imposes difficulties in functional breastfeeding.

6.2.6 Capsular contracture

Capsular contracture is an immunological response of the body to foreign material such as an implant. It can also be understood as the formation of a clot around the implant can be painful. Capsular contracture may also follow by bacterial infection or seroma (accumulation of fluid after surgery) and hematoma (accumulation of blood outside the blood vessels). There are four grades of capsular contracture based on the baker's scale (Fig. 6.4).

Capsular contracture of grades III and IV appears to be more severe and may require further surgery. However, there may be a reoccurrence of capsular contracture after surgery. Capsular contraction is one of the most severe complications that lead to compaction, distortion, or displacement of the implant. It is reported that there are 15%–45% cases of capsular contracture and around 92% of cases are reported with the occurrence of capsular contracture within a year of postbreast implantation [20].

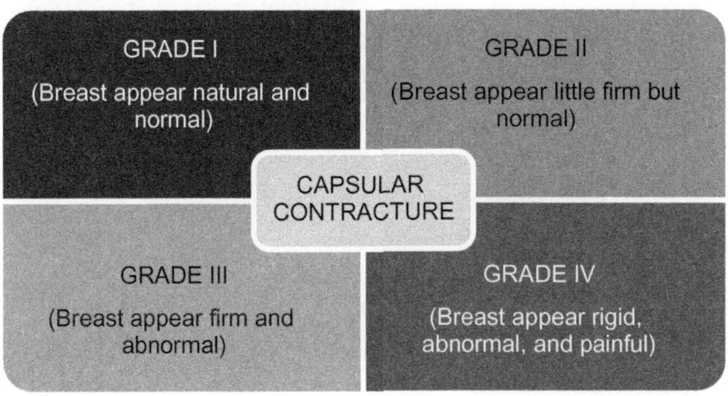

Figure 6.4 Grades of capsular contracture on the basis of morphology.

6.3 Birth control implant

Birth control implant (BCI) is the hormonal-based contraceptive to prevent the unintended and unplanned pregnancy. BCI is a thin rod-shaped small tube-like, having size same as a matchstick and implanted by doctors under the dermal or subdermal region of skin [31], where they release the hormone in a particular concentration depending upon the type of implant. Both the insertion and the removal technique are very important in the case of subdermal BCI and required trained and professional personals. Unplanned and unintended pregnancies are the most common health issues at the global level, imposing the socioeconomic burden to the society and the family. These pregnancies are more likely to end in abortion, while infants born are more likely to face health problems. Health-related risks like physical and mental issues have been accounted for in the offspring of women who have unintended pregnancies [32]. However, major reproductive health-related issues are also associated with these unwanted pregnancies worldwide [33]. Therefore the prevention of these kinds of pregnancies is always an essential part of the practice of medicine. Currently, four types of subdermal, namely Norplant, Implanon NXT/Nexplanon, Sino-implant, and Jadelle are commercially available (Fig. 6.5).

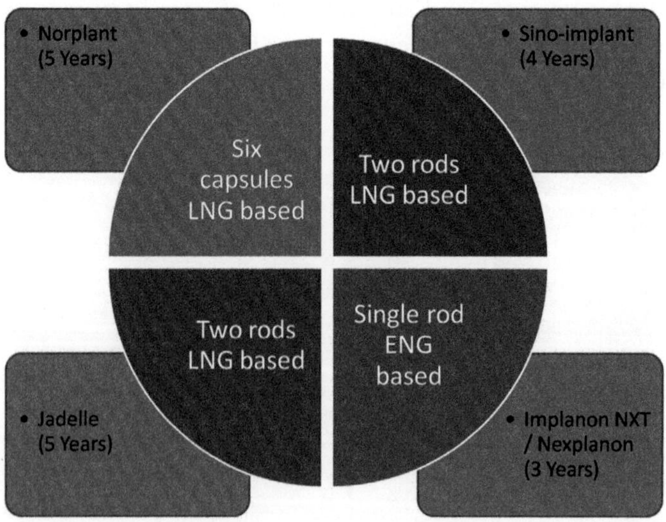

Figure 6.5 Types of subdermal implants on the basis of duration of use and hormone.

6.3.1 The implant as long-acting reversible contraceptives

As of now various methods such as contraceptive pills (known as the first line of prevention), intrauterine devices (IUD), contraceptive patch, contraceptive implants, depot medroxyprogesterone acetate injection, and monthly vaginal ring are taken care by healthcare facilities to prevent the unplanned conception [34]. These methods are known as long-acting reversible contraceptives. American Congress of Obstetrician and Gynecologists (ACOG) is the first who recommended the LARCs as the most effective and appropriate method for birth control. The women's selections of contraception methods to prevent unplanned pregnancy depend on the lifestyle, affordability, convenience, product efficacy, and accessibility. The medical assessment, patient medical history, menstrual cycle, and adherence are also part of the choice of contraception method [35]. Apart from that, the provider education is also essential for promoting the appropriate LARCs method. In the United States, majorly, two types of BCI are available: IUD and etonogestrel subdermal implants [36]. The IUDs are T-shaped thin devices implanted inside and left the side of the uterus and a medical practitioner places the birth control implant (Nexplanon) under the skin of the upper arm. They prevent the unintended pregnancies for 3–10 years, and the Food and Drug Administration approves the duration of use for the various IUDs and the subdermal implants. Nowadays, the FDA approved one copper and four levonorgestrel, and one progestin hormone-based contraceptive implant is available in the market. ACOG has reported that the success rate of IUD and birth control implant in the first year of typical use is the same as the range of sterilization methods to prevent unplanned pregnancy [37].

6.3.2 Subdermal BCI: mode of action and side effects

The subdermal BCI has certain features that make them an appropriate method for contraception. This method of birth control is most appropriate and effective against the aforementioned preexisting methods of contraception. The yearly unsuccessful rate of the subdermal implant is 0.05% [38]. The etonogestrel implants come in the category of a subdermal implant having rod-shaped and releases etonogestrel that is a synthetic biologically active metabolite of progestin desogestrel [38]. In 2006, this type of subdermal implant was approved by the FDA. The etonogestrel implants showed long-lasting effects and estrogen-free, and there is no need to implant inside the uterus, which makes them safe irrespective of the conditions during delivery [39–41]. Recently, the US selective way of recommendations for birth control makes use of the implants in the immediate postpartum period [40,42]. The currently available subdermal implant is a single rod-shaped implant having diameter 2 mm and the length 4 cm, made up of ethylene-vinyl acetate core embedded with progestin active metabolite, etonogestrel [38]. A layer of ethylene-vinyl acetate covers the inner core of the implant and regulates the releasing concentration of the hormone. The total concentration of hormone progestin is 68 mg, which is released gradually in starting at the rate of 60–70 mg/day and by the first year the rate of flow is decreased to 35–45 mg/day and similarly, at the end of 3 years, the rate is decreased to the level of 30–40 mg/day, respectively. Three birth control subdermal implants are currently in use and made up of flexible nonbiodegradable rods [43,44]. The single rod implants are Implanon having a total of 68 mg of etonogestrel [44]. Implanon NXT/Nexplanon is a radiopaque having 15 mg barium sulfate, and this is bioequivalent to the nonradiopaque Implanon. These implants are provided for the single-use, a preloaded disposable applicator that accesses the proper implanting beneath the skin [45]. Apart from the single rod, two-rod birth control implants are also available such as Sino-implant (II) and Jadelle containing 70 and 150 mg of levonorgestrel in each rod, respectively [43,46]. These two-rod BCIs are provided with the onetime use of disposable trocar [47]. In 2008, the Norplant, the first-generation implant, which consisted of a set of six silicon capsules, with a total concentration of 216 mg levonorgestrel, was discontinued globally [48]. Concerning the mode of action, BCI is the progestin reservoirs that release the hormone into the serum that goes finally to the targeted organ or part of the body of women and shows the immediate effect to induce the process of contraception. These changes associated with these implants also provide some therapeutic benefits to some extent in women [49]. These implants mainly affect the ovulation process or ovarian function in women through the continuous release of progestin in deficient concentration and also thickens the cervical mucus [43,44]. In many studies, the vaginal ultrasound monitoring is used to evaluate the effect of levonorgestrel-based birth control implants on follicular growth as well as endocrine profiling [50–53]. The first condition that was observed in these studies during the follicular growth was the rupturing, followed by the elevated level of progesterone at the end. The second one was the development of luteinized unruptured follicles with increasing concentration of progesterone, and the last observation was the development of persistent unruptured follicles that are functionally active till 21 days and continue to produce the estradiol while the level of progesterone remains declined. It has been reported that the birth control implants tend to alter the physiological and functional parameters of the reproductive system both in the hypothalamus and genital tract, and the pharmacological action of these implants includes alteration of endometrial structure, tubal motility, and their function [54]. Reduced forearm bone density has been reported in the case of levonorgestrel and etonogestrel implant users [55]. Previously, the bleeding pattern associated with Implanon (subdermal implant) has been analyzed via reference period analysis. In this study, the pattern showed (33.6%) infrequent, (22.2%) amenorrhea, (6.7%) frequent, and (17.7%) prolonged bleeding [56]. Apart from the developed countries, the side effects of BCI also reported in developing countries like India. In 2011, Bhatia et al. reported the same or little high percentage of menstrual disorder due to which women discontinue the use of implant, that is, polymenorrhagia (22.5%), irregular bleeding (27%), prolonged spotting (23%), and amenorrhea 48 (24%) (Fig. 6.6) [57]. A case had been reported in which due to persistent vaginal bleeding, a 27-year-old woman go for the removal of birth control implant. The implant had been located at the left upper arm for over 5 years. During the removal process, the area had been measured (6 × 4 cm) where fat atrophy appeared [58]. During the insertion of BCI, various types of complications or side effects have been seen on the skin such as

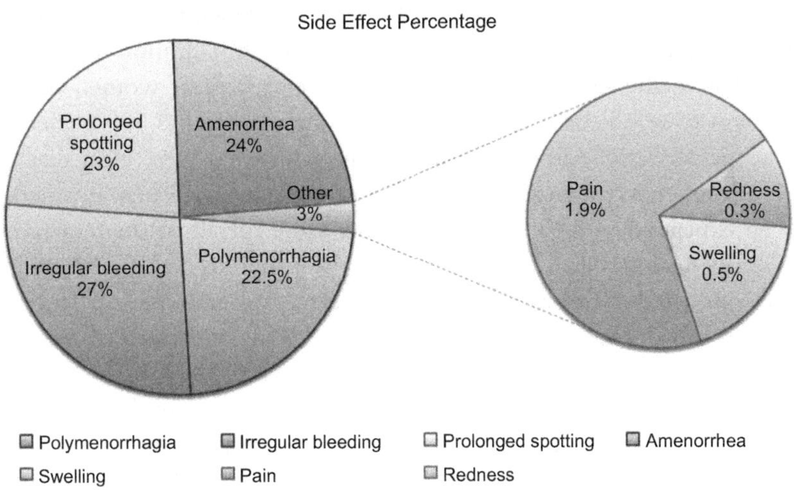

Figure 6.6 Reported percentage adverse effect of Implanon in healthy women.

tenderness, irritation, pain, and redness at the early stage. Similar kind of adverse effects against all trails of Implanon has been reported in 0.5% swelling, 1.9% pain, and 0.3% in redness cases (Fig. 6.6) [59]. Similarly, the adverse effect such as weight gain, headache, acne, viral infection, stomach pain, breasts pain, vaginitis, mood swings, depression, nausea, dizziness, pain at the site of insertion, ectopic pregnancy, and neuropathy, and follicular cysts has been reported after using the Nexplanon BCI [60]. In a study, it was reported that Norplant makes blood vessels fragile after interacting with Cytokeratin, beginning them to leak into the endometrial cavity [61]. Among all of them, the headache is the most frequent side effect among the patients using progestin-based subdermal implants [60]. In most of the studies, the weight gain has been recorded with all types of BCI, and the average weight gain was found approx. 0.4–1.5 kg/year [62–66]. This continuous weight gain and related factors subsequently make the insertion and the removal technique more difficult and lead to the removal procedure more technically challenging [67]. However, in thin or underweight women, the chances of the deep insertion of subdermal implants with the scant subcutaneous tissue are more [68]. Therefore it was reported that the chance of neurovascular injury is greater in underweight thin women and it has been noticed for all five structures of neurovascular bundles and musculocutaneous nerves [69–71].

6.3.3 Effectiveness of BCI

The effectiveness of any birth control implants is depending on the working action and the consistency of use by the user. In common terms, processes that totally inhibit the ovulation in every cycle of women or stop the sperm to reach the egg in the meantime are termed as 100% effective and work perfectly. After reviewing the literature, it is very clear that the high effectiveness and the efficacy of birth control implants are neither can be explained in a simple way nor the same for all of them, and not necessarily constantly active throughout their life. In 1991, a study has been conducted to assess the in vivo release rate and the efficiency of progestin-based 3-keto-desogestrel subdermal BCI. In this study, the process of ovulation was inhibited in women having the level of 3-keto-desogestrel >0.28 nmol/La and decreased progesterone level. It was reported that BCI 3 keta desogestrel was released at a rate of 0.01 mg/day thereby maintaing the plasma concentration of 0.28 nmol/L [72]. However, ovulation is rarely seen in the third year of use [73]; however, still, the implants remain the most efficient and appropriate method for preventing unintended pregnancies by inhibiting the sperm penetration of the cervical mucus and the thinning of endometrium. Similarly, sometimes the typical use (inconsistent and incorrect) and perfect use (consistent and correct) show how the effective method can be used for birth control implant. The percentage of women encountering unplanned pregnancy during the first year of perfect and typical use of the different preventive measures is shown (US data) in Fig. 6.7 [74]. Several studies have reported the effective percentage of various implants and contraceptives in successful cases (Fig. 6.8).

6.3.4 Return to fertility

As per the aforementioned, the BCI is effective for a time being period. If women want to discontinue this contraceptive method, they can easily return to ovulation within 3 weeks of implant removal and there is a need to take any additional prevention or care. It was reported that after removing the Implanon, the level of etonogestrel drops down to the detection limit, that is, (20 pg/mL) within a week's time [75]. A 4 year pilot study demonstrated that 6 women out of 29 got conceived within three months after removing the Implanon as BCI [76]. Similarly, in a comparative study of Norplant and Norplant II, it was revealed that out of 10 Norplant and 11 Norplant II users, 9 and 6 had conceived within a year after removal, respectively [77]. Recently, in 2011, a study was conducted in which 74 implant removals were done, out of which 50 implant users take another contraceptive. However, out of 24 remaining cases, 29.16% conceived within 3 months, 62.50% within 6 months, 66.66% within 9 months, and 95.8% within a year [57].

However, if we compare the implants with other contraceptive methods, there is no difference found except injectable contraceptives. Therefore users can be suggested that there is no problem in come again of fertility after removing birth control implant.

6.3.5 Acceptability among users

Previously, it was seen that the continuation rate in ENG implant users for 2 years is 50%–75% [78–81]. Similarly, in the United States, project reports showed that, among the users of another contraceptive method, 79% were satisfied with implants and 83% continued this contraceptive method for 1 year [82]. Suddenly, the continuation rate fell down to 69%

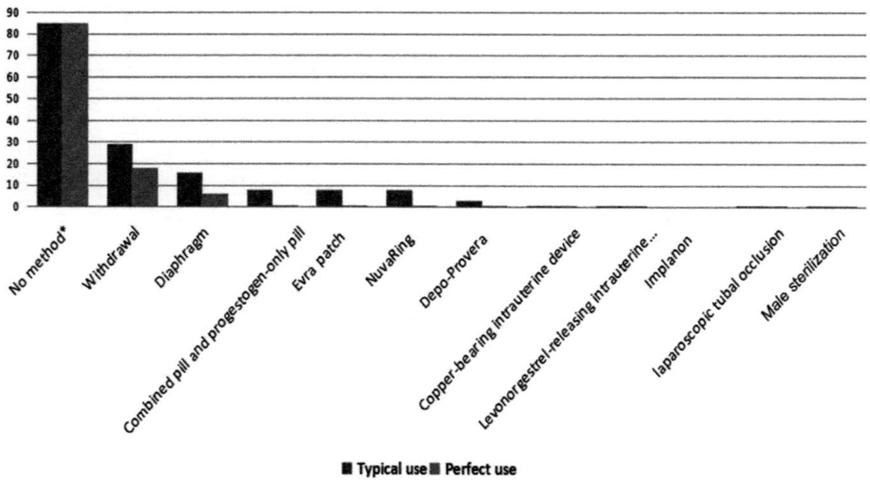

Figure 6.7 Total percentage of women experiencing unplanned pregnancies using various contraceptive methods.

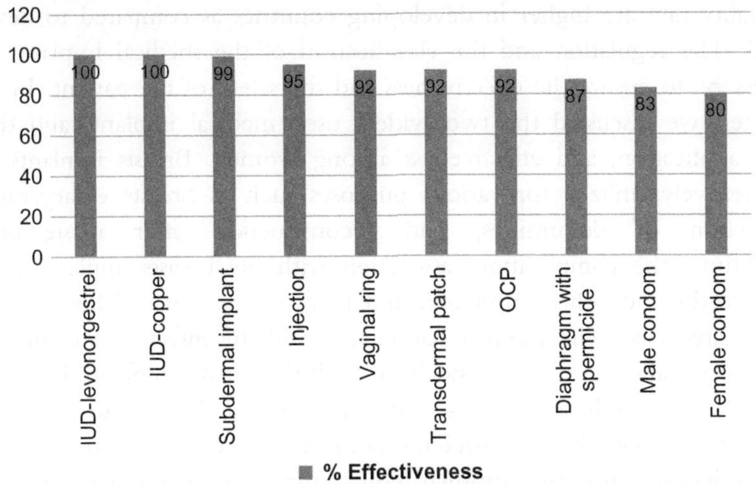

Figure 6.8 Effective percentage of various contraceptive methods in successful cases.

after 2 years [83]. Among implant users in four European countries, successful and satisfactory rate with this contraceptive technique was 66% in those deciding on inserts initially, and the continuation rate was 86% per year [84]; after 2 years in this examination, satisfaction was somewhat higher, at 70%, and continuation was 83% [85]. In 3 years of study in Australia, initially, 85% of women continued the method for a year, 70% of users for 2 years, and 53% of women used this method for 3 years [86]. In the last three reported studies, the birth control implant came firmly following the intrauterine framework concerning both continuation and satisfaction. This ought to be centered around how much higher continuation rates with implants are differentiated and joined hormonal contraception; they are in like manner fundamentally higher than the rates for injectables.

6.4 Conclusion

The worldwide economy is progressively interconnected although there is a very big difference between the developed and the developing countries. This is seen in all parts of life, perhaps no place more prominent than in medical care, where malnutrition, communicable diseases, and mortality rate are higher in developing countries as compared to developed. The regulation and the classification of the medical implants are necessary, to ensure the effectiveness and the safety of the patient. In this chapter, we discussed the two widely used medical implants and their role, application, and effectiveness among women. Breasts implants are progressively utilized for various purposes such as breasts enlargement, correction of deformities, and reconstruction after mastectomy. Sometimes the complications associated with the breasts implants cause noteworthy morbidity, mortality, and increase the time of hospital stay and related cost. The capsular contracture and the infection are the two common challenges that are associated with the breasts implant. The utilization of breasts implants keeps on expanding, and the load related to implant-associated health problems because of breasts rupture, bacterial contamination, necrosis, capsular contracture, and nerve damage, and related deferred recuperation, severe pain, and loss of capacity will keep on expanding. With new approaches, the quality of implant during manufacturing has been improved; for this reason, the minimum cases of capsule formation have been reported. Submuscular placement of cohesive gel implants has limited the risk associated with capsule formation. Nevertheless, the attention is still on advancing autologous and implant-based reconstructive surgical methods. Settling on the proper implant size, based on the individual plans for surgery, has turned out to be altogether simpler after the advancement of better than ever materials; the parameters are gone into calculations, and the signs and complexities are examined in forthcoming investigations.

Apart from this, women also used contraceptive implants to prevent unwanted pregnancy. Retrospective studies showed the effectiveness of birth control implants for the benefit of both mother and child by reducing the risk of mortality, morbidity, and improving the socioeconomic status of families. However, the cases of the poor health of the infant and the rate of mortality and morbidity of mother and child are very high in developing countries as compared to the developed countries. The rate of fertility is regulated by the use of modern contraceptive implants. Time-to-time examination of the cases of unplanned pregnancy is required so that the researcher, stakeholders, and policymakers may provide the new approaches toward helping the women to achieve reproductive goals. This shows the need for effective contraceptive services and the impact of policies and the programs on unplanned pregnancies and their final outputs. These estimates can furthermore be used to observe the variations in how women determine effective contraceptive services provided after pregnancy help women who want to hold-up or prevent subsequent pregnancies, select the contraceptive procedure that is effective, safe, convenient, and best meet their short-term and long-term family planning needs.

Conflict of interest

The authors declare that they have no conflict of interest.

References

[1] Li J, Stachowski M, Zhang Z. Application of responsive polymers in implantable medical devices and biosensors. In Switchable and responsive surfaces and materials for biomedical applications. 2015. pp. 259–298.
[2] Van Eck CF, Chen AF, Klatt BA, D'Antonio J, Fu F. The classification of implants: class I, II, III. J Long Term Eff Med Implants 2009;19(3).
[3] Support the guardian. Revealed: faulty medical implants harm patients around the world. Available at: <https://www.theguardian.com/society/2018/nov/25/>.
[4] DePaola NE, Coggins H. Breast implant-associated anaplastic large cell lymphoma: what we know. J Adv Pract Oncol 2019;10(1):54.
[5] Yang N, Muradali D. The augmented breast: a pictorial review of the abnormal and unusual. Am J Roentgenol 2011;196(4) W451-60.
[6] Maxwell GP, Gabriel A. The evolution of breast implants. Clin Plast Surg 2009;36 (1):1–3.
[7] Peters W, Fornasier V. Complications from injectable materials used for breast augmentation. Can J Plast Surg 2009;17(3):89–96.
[8] Potter S, MacKenzie M, Blazeby JM. Does the addition of mesh improve outcomes in implant-based breast reconstruction after mastectomy for breast cancer? Bmj 2018;362:k2607.
[9] Parthasarathy M, Orrell J, Mortimer C, Ball L. Chemotherapy-resistant breast implant-associated anaplastic large cell lymphoma. Case Rep 2013;2013 bcr2013201950.
[10] Coroneos CJ, Selber JC, Offodile AC, Butler CE, Clemens MW. US FDA breast implant postapproval studies: long-term outcomes in 99,993 patients. Ann Surg 2019;269(1):30–6.
[11] Gilbert AH. Inventor. Retromammary prosthesis. United States patent US 3,416,160, December 17; 1968.
[12] Fuzzard SK, Teixeira R, Zinn R. A review of the literature on the management of silicone implant incompatibility syndrome. Aesthetic Plast Surg 2019;1–5.
[13] Jara LJ, García-Collinot G, Medina G, del Pilar Cruz-Dominguez M, Vera-Lastra O, Carranza-Muleiro RA, et al. Severe manifestations of autoimmune syndrome induced by adjuvants (Shoenfeld's syndrome). Immunol Res 2017;65(1):8–16.
[14] Jordan SW, Corcoran J. Considerations in breast augmentation in the adolescent patient. Seminars in plastic surgery, vol. 27. Thieme Medical Publishers; 2013. p. 067–71.

[15] Nichter LS, Hardesty RA, Anigian GM. Ideal implant structured breast implants: core study results at 6 years. Plast Reconstr Surg 2018;142(1):66.
[16] Brandon HJ, Nichter LS, Back DD. New evaluation procedure for multi-dimensional mechanical strains and tangent moduli of breast implants: ideal implant® structured breast implant compared to silicone gel implants. Bioengineering 2019;6 (2):43.
[17] Rubino C, Brongo S, Pagliara D, Cuomo R, Abbinante G, Campitiello N, et al. Infections in breast implants: a review with a focus on developing countries. J Infect Dev Countries 2014;8(09):1089−95.
[18] Mukhtar RA, Holland M, Sieber DA, Wen KW, Rugo HS, Kadin ME, et al. Synchronous breast implant−associated anaplastic large cell lymphoma and invasive carcinoma: genomic profiling and management implications. Plast Reconstr Surg−Global Open 2019;7(4):e2188.
[19] Berlin E, Singh K, Mills C, Shapira I, Bakst RL, Chadha M. Breast implant-associated anaplastic large cell lymphoma: case report and review of the literature. Case Rep Hematol 2018;2018.
[20] Prasad K, Zhou R, Zhou R, Schuessler D, Ostrikov KK, Bazaka K. Cosmetic reconstruction in breast cancer patients: opportunities for nanocomposite materials. Acta Biomater 2018;.
[21] Magill LJ, Tanska A, Keshtgar M, Mosahebi A, Jell G. Mechanical and surface chemical analysis of retrieved breast implants from a single centre. J Mech Behav Biomed Mater 2019;91:24−31.
[22] Bachour Y, Heinze ZC, Dormaar TS, van Selms WG, Ritt MJ, Niessen FB. Poly implant prothèse silicone breast implants: implant dynamics and capsular contracture. Eur J Plast Surg 2018;41(5):563−70.
[23] Syal S, Mwansa V, Chhabra L. Unexpected silicone breast implant rupture after implantation of insertable loop recorder. Methodist DeBakey Cardiovasc J 2018;14 (2):e4.
[24] Leberfinger AN, Behar BJ, Williams NC, Rakszawski KL, Potochny JD, Mackay DR, et al. Breast implant−associated anaplastic large cell lymphoma: a systematic review. JAMA Surg 2017;152(12):1161−8.
[25] Kaartinen I, Sunela K, Alanko J, Hukkinen K, Karjalainen-Lindsberg ML, Svarvar C. Breast implant-associated anaplastic large cell lymphoma−from diagnosis to treatment. Eur J Surg Oncol (EJSO) 2017;43(8):1385−92.
[26] Barbé E, de Boer M, de Jong D. A practical cytological approach to the diagnosis of breast-implant associated anaplastic large cell lymphoma. Cytopathology 2019;30 (4):363−9.
[27] Gartner LM, Morton J, Lawrence RA, Naylor AJ, O'Hare D, Schanler RJ, et al. Breastfeeding and the use of human milk. Pediatrics 2005;115(2):496−506.
[28] Teuber SS, Gershwin E. Autoantibodies and clinical rheumatic complaints in two children of women with silicone gel breast implants. Int Arch Allergy Immunol 1994;103(1):105−8.
[29] Levine JJ, Ilowite NT. Scleroderma like esophageal disease in children breast-fed by mothers with silicone breast implants. JAMA 1994;271(3):213−16.
[30] Schiff M, Algert CS, Ampt A, Sywak MS, Roberts CL. The impact of cosmetic breast implants on breastfeeding: a systematic review and meta-analysis. Int Breastfeed J 2014;9(1):17.
[31] Iftikhar T, Ara J, Arshad H, Sultana N. Evaluation of levonorgestrel subdermal implant as long term reversible contraceptive. J Rawalpindi Med Coll 2018;22:164−7.
[32] Kost K, Lindberg L. Pregnancy intentions, maternal behaviors, and infant health: investigating relationships with new measures and propensity score analysis. Demography 2015;52(1):83−111.

[33] Yazdkhasti M, Pourreza A, Pirak A, Abdi F. Unintended pregnancy and its adverse social and economic consequences on health system: a narrative review article. Iran J Public Health 2015;44(1):12.
[34] Roe AH, Bartz D. Society of family planning clinical recommendations: contraception after surgical abortion. Contraception 2018 Sep 6.
[35] Colquitt CW, Martin TS. Contraceptive methods: a review of nonbarrier and barrier products. J Pharm Pract 2017;30(1):130−5.
[36] Baron M, Potter B, Schrager S. A review of long-acting reversible contraception methods and barriers to their use. WMJ 2018;117(4):156−9.
[37] Weber TL, Briggs A, Hanson JD. Exploring the uptake of long-acting reversible contraception in south dakota women and the importance of provider education. South Dak Med J South Dak State Med Assoc 2017;70(11):493.
[38] Meckstroth KR, Darney PD. Implant contraception. Sem Reprod Med 2001;19 (04):339−54.
[39] Tocce K, Sheeder J, Python J, Teal SB. Long acting reversible contraception in postpartum adolescents: early initiation of etonogestrel implant is superior to IUDs in the outpatient setting. J Pediatr Adolesc Gynecol 2012;25(1):59−63.
[40] Centers for Disease Control and Prevention (CDC). US medical eligibility criteria for contraceptive use, 2010. MMWR. Recommendations and reports: morbidity and mortality weekly report. Recommendations and reports, vol. 59, no. RR-1; 2010. p. 1.
[41] American College of Obstetricians and Gynecologists. Adolescents and long-acting reversible contraception: implants and intrauterine devices. Committee opinion no. 539. Obstet Gynecol 2012;120(983):8.
[42] American College of Obstetricians and Gynecologists. Long-acting reversible contraception: implants and intrauterine devices. practice bulletin no. 121. Obstet Gynecol 2011;118(1):184−96.
[43] Sivin I, Nash H, Waldman S. Jadelle levonorgestrel rod implants: a summary of scientific data and lessons learned from programmatic experience. New York: Population Council; 2002.
[44] Darney P, Patel A, Rosen K, Shapiro LS, Kaunitz AM. Safety and efficacy of a single-rod etonogestrel implant (Implanon): results from 11 international clinical trials. Fertil Steril 2009;91(5):1646−53.
[45] Mansour D, Mommers E, Teede H, Sollie-Eriksen B, Graesslin O, Ahrendt HJ, et al. Clinician satisfaction and insertion characteristics of a new applicator to insert radiopaque implanon: an open-label, noncontrolled, multicenter trial. Contraception 2010;82(3):243−9.
[46] Steiner MJ, Lopez LM, Grimes DA, Cheng L, Shelton J, Trussell J, et al. Sino-implant (II)—a levonorgestrel-releasing two-rod implant: systematic review of the randomized controlled trials. Contraception 2010;81(3):197−201.
[47] Steiner MJ, Boler T, Obhai G, Hubacher D. Assessment of a disposable trocar for insertion of contraceptive implants. Contraception 2010;81(2):140−2.
[48] Jacobstein R, Polis CB. Progestin-only contraception: injectables and implants. Best Pract Res Clin Obstet Gynaecol 2014;28(6):795−806.
[49] Bahamondes L, Valeria Bahamondes M, Shulman LP. Non-contraceptive benefits of hormonal and intrauterine reversible contraceptive methods. Hum Reprod Update 2015;21(5):640−51.
[50] Olsson SE, Bakos O, Lindgren PG, Odlind V, Wide L. Ovarian function during use of subdermal implants releasing low doses of levonorgestrel. Br J Family Plan 1990;16(3):88−93.
[51] Shoupe D, Horenstein J, Mishell Jr DR, Lacarra M, Medearis A. Characteristics of ovarian follicular development in norplant users. Fertil Steril 1991;55(4):766−70.

[52] Shaaban MM, Segal S, Salem HT, Ghaneimah SA, Khalifa EA, Ahmed AG. Sonographic assessment of ovarian and endometrial changes during long-*term* norplant use and their correlation with hormonal levels. Fertil Steril 1993;59 (5):998–1002.

[53] Alvarez F, Brache V, Faundes A, Tejada AS, Thevenin F. Ultrasonographic and endocrine evaluation of ovarian function among norplant® implants users with regular menses. Contraception. 1996;54(5):275–9.

[54] Goldstuck ND, Le HP. Delivery of progestins via the subdermal versus the intrauterine route: comparison of the pharmacology and clinical outcomes. Expert Opin Drug Deliv 2018;15(7):717–27.

[55] Monteiro-Dantas C, Espejo-Arce X, Lui-Filho JF, Fernandes AM, Monteiro I, Bahamondes L. A three-year longitudinal evaluation of the forearm bone density of users of etonogestrel-and levonorgestrel-releasing contraceptive implants. Reprod Health 2007;4(1):11.

[56] Mansour D, Korver T, Marintcheva-Petrova M, Fraser IS. The effects of Implanon® on menstrual bleeding patterns. Eur J Contracept Reprod Health Care 2008;13(sup1):13–28.

[57] Bhatia P, Nangia S, Aggarwal S, Tewari C. Implanon: subdermal single rod contraceptive implant. J Obstet Gynecol India 2011;61(4):422.

[58] Chadha-Gupta A, Moss A. Fat atrophy at the site of a subdermal contraceptive implant. J Family Plan Reprod Health Care 2007;33(2):123.

[59] Mascarenhas L. Insertion and removal of Implanon®. Contraception. 1998;58 (6):79S–83S.

[60] Brache V, Faundes A, Alvarez F, Cochon L. Nonmenstrual adverse events during use of implantable contraceptives for women: data from clinical trials. Contraception. 2002;65(1):63–74.

[61] Wonodirekso S, Au CL, Hadisaputrat W, Affandi B, Rogers PA. Cytokeratins 8, 18 and 19 in endometrial epithelial cells during the normal menstrual cycle and in women receiving Norplant®. Contraception. 1993;48(5):481–93.

[62] Coutinho EM. One year contraception with a single subdermal implant containing nomegestrol acetate (Uniplant). Contraception. 1993;47(1):97–105.

[63] Zenger E, Shuhua Q, Huimin F. Introduction of Norplant® implants in four counties of rural China: a two-year evaluation. Contraception. 1995;52(6):349–55.

[64] Coutinho EM, De Souza JC, Athayde C, Barbosa IC, Alvarez F, Brache V, et al. Multicenter clinical trial on the efficacy and acceptability of a single contraceptive implant of nomegestrol acetate, Uniplant. Contraception. 1996;53(2):121–5.

[65] Sivin I, Mishell Jr DR, Darney P, Wan L, Christ M. Levonorgestrel capsule implants in the United States: a 5-year study. Obstet Gynecol 1998;92(3):337–44.

[66] Barbosa I, Coutinho E, Athayde C, Ladipo O, Olsson SE, Ulmsten U. The effects of nomegestrol acetate subdermal implant (Uniplant) on carbohydrate metabolism, serum lipoproteins and on hepatic function in women. Contraception 1995;52 (2):111–14.

[67] Navani M, Robinson C. Clinical challenge with Implanon removal: a case report. J Fam Plann Reprod Health Care 2005;31(2):161–2.

[68] Mansour D, Walling M, Glenn D, Egarter C, Graesslin O, Herbst J, et al. Removal of non-palpable etonogestrel implants. BMJ Sex Reprod Health 2008;34(2):89.

[69] Hueston WJ, Locke KT. Norplant neuropathy: peripheral neurologic symptoms associated with subdermal contraceptive implants. J Family Pract 1995;40(2):184–7.

[70] Rowlands S. Legal aspects of contraceptive implants. BMJ Sex Reprod Health 2010;36(4):243–8.

[71] Brown M, Britton J. Neuropathy associated with etonogestrel implant insertion. Contraception 2012;86(5):591–3.

[72] Diaz S, Pavez M, Moo-Young AJ, Bardin CW, Croxatto HB. Clinical trial with 3-keto-desogestrel subdermal implants. Contraception 1991;44(4):393–408.
[73] Croxatto HB. Mechanisms that explain the contraceptive action of progestin implants for women. Contraception 2002;65(1):21–7.
[74] Trussell J. Contraceptive failure in the United States. Contraception 2004;70 (2):89–96.
[75] Huber J. Pharmacokinetics of Implanon®: an integrated analysis. Contraception 1998;58(6):85S–90S.
[76] Kiriwat O, Patanayindee A, Koetsawang S, Korver T, CoelinghBennink HJ. A 4-year pilot study on the efficacy and safety of Implanon®, a single-rod hormonal contraceptive implant in healthy women in Thailand. Eur J Contracept Reprod Health Care 1998;3(2):85–91.
[77] Singh K, Viegas OA, Ratnam SS. Norplant contraceptive implants—a comparison of capsules versus rods in Singapore. Singapore Med J 1990;31(6):568–72.
[78] Lakha F, Glasier AF. Continuation rates of Implanon® in the UK: data from an observational study in a clinical setting. Contraception 2006;74(4):287–9.
[79] Arribas-Mir L, Rueda-Lozano D, Agrela-Cardona M, Cedeño-Benavides T, Olvera-Porcel C, Bueno-Cavanillas A. Insertion and 3-year follow-up experience of 372 etonogestrel subdermal contraceptive implants by family physicians in Granada, Spain. Contraception 2009;80(5):457–62.
[80] Harvey C, Seib C, Lucke J. Continuation rates and reasons for removal among Implanon® users accessing two family planning clinics in Queensland, Australia. Contraception 2009;80(6):527–32.
[81] Teunissen AM, Grimm B, Roumen FJ. Continuation rates of the subdermal contraceptive Implanon® and associated influencing factors. Eur J Contracept Reprod Health Care 2014;19(1):15–21.
[82] Peipert JF, Zhao Q, Allsworth JE, Petrosky E, Madden T, Eisenberg D, et al. Continuation and satisfaction of reversible contraception. Obstet Gynecol 2011;117 (5):1105.
[83] O'Neil ME, Peipert JF, Zhao Q, Madden T, Secura G. Twenty-four–month continuation of reversible contraception. Obstet Gynecol 2013;122(5):1083.
[84] Short M, Dallay D, Omokanye S, Hanisch JU, Inki P. Acceptability of the levonorgestrel releasing-intrauterine system and etonogestrel implant: one-year results of an observational study. Eur J Contracept Reprod Health Care 2012;17(1):79–88.
[85] Short M, Dallay D, Omokanye S, Stauch K, Inki P. Acceptability of long-acting, progestin-only contraception in Europe: a two-year prospective, non-interventional study. Eur J Contracept Reprod Health Care 2014;19(1):29–38.
[86] Weisberg E, Bateson D, McGeechan K, Mohapatra L. A three-year comparative study of continuation rates, bleeding patterns and satisfaction in Australian women using a subdermal contraceptive implant or progestogen releasing-intrauterine system. Eur J Contracept Reprod Health Care 2014;19(1):5–14.

CHAPTER SEVEN

Gastroenterology

Somnath Pandey[1,*] and Shobana Navaneeethabalakrishnan[2]
[1]Radiation Oncology, Massachusetts General Hospital, Harvard Medical School, Boston, MA, United States
[2]Department of Endocrinology, Dr. ALM Postgraduate Institute of Basic Medical Sciences, University of Madras, Chennai, India
*Corresponding author

Abstract

The gastrointestinal tract (GIT) allows the absorption of processed food and checks the entry of risky luminal toxicants and pathogens. The inability to do so leads to innumerable diseases. Implants provide unimpeded access to the remote and complex environment in the GIT, thereby allowing fast and accurate disease detection and management. Gastroesophageal reflux disease, gastroparesis, and short-bowel syndrome are just a few examples where implants have made a huge difference in the quality of life of a patient. The success of such implants is contingent upon not only its own physicochemical properties but also on the physical location where the implant is positioned inside the body that can pose serious challenges. Herein, we gain an insight into the numerous aspects of implants used in GIT. Industries designing and manufacturing GIT implants are on the rise and so is the ever-increasing need for cognizance relating to the biological risks and adverse events associated with such implants.

Keywords: Gastroesophageal reflux disease; gastrointestinal tract; adjustable gastric band; LINX; gastric electrical stimulation

7.1 Introduction

The gastrointestinal tract (GIT) is an anatomically intricate continuous hollow organ that orchestrates a variety of functions to facilitate the transport and digestion of complex food, absorption of nutritive elements, and expulsion of waste products. The GIT involves esophageal, gastrointestinal, and colonic sensory together with motor functions. The interstitial cells of Cajal or ICC (pacemaker cells in the GIT) help to initiate and coordinate the motility in the GIT by giving rise to a bioelectric activity known as "slow waves" [1]. In addition to ICC, smooth muscle cells and the enteric nervous system play an important role in regulating gut

Toxicological Aspects of Medical Device Implants.
DOI: https://doi.org/10.1016/B978-0-12-820728-4.00007-1
© 2020 Elsevier Inc.
All rights reserved.

motility, and any aberrant changes in the normal functioning of these cells result in dysmotility and GI disorders [2].

Disturbances in the GIT affect a large number of people worldwide [3] not only undermining their quality of life but also resulting in substantial healthcare costs. A number of GIT disorders are known to date [4]. Gastrointestinal neuromuscular disorders are marked by inadequate functionality of the intestinal muscle layer involving any part of GIT. Such disorders manifest in form of and are not limited to dyspepsia, dysphagia, transit blockade, gastroparesis, or obstruction of the GIT that is responsible for 40% of the GIT disorders in patients seeking care gastroenterology clinics [5] and gastroesophageal reflux disease (GERD). Given that about 20% of the population in western society is affected by GERD, it is imperative to understand this condition.

GERD occurs when the sphincter muscle that connects the esophagus to the stomach weakens (Fig. 7.1). This muscle is called the lower

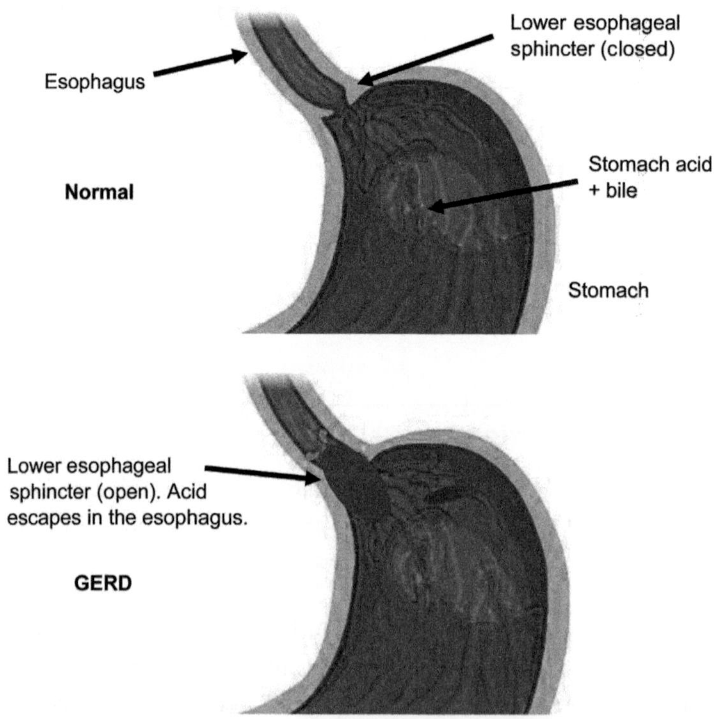

Figure 7.1 Gastroesophageal reflux disease (GERD) is caused due to the weakening of the lower esophageal sphincter (LES) muscle. *Created in Biorender.com.*

esophageal sphincter (LES) muscle. A normally functioning LES allows food to pass through into the stomach and prevents the back passage of the food and stomach acid into the esophagus. Once the LES weakens, the stomach acid bile flows back into the esophagus, leading to symptoms such as acid reflux and heartburn. In the United States alone, GERD is known to affect one in every five adults.

It is, therefore, of paramount importance to design suitable interventions and establish therapeutic strategies to ameliorate conditions such as GERD and other GIT-related disorders. The past decades have seen major advances toward the development of gastrointestinal implants. A number of different medical devices that have successfully made a significant impact in improving the quality of life of such patients have been designed. Herein, we will review the frequently utilized devices in GIT disorders and later study various adverse events associated with them.

7.2 Commonly used implants in gastrointestinal tract disorders

7.2.1 LINX reflux management system

The LINX reflux management system was approved by the United States Food and Drug Administration (FDA) in 2012 for GERD patients. The LINX device is shaped in the form of a ring, featuring a series of rare-earth metal beads with magnetic cores covered in titanium alloy, linked by wires that are surgically implanted through a minimally invasive procedure, around the LES of GERD patients (Fig. 7.2).

The magnetic force associated with the LINX device overcomes the increased gastric pressure linked with GERD, thereby reinforcing the obstruction of the LES to the aberrant opening known to be associated with the disease. This way the contents of the stomach are prevented from entering into the esophagus.

During the process of swallowing of food bolus, the magnetic beads separate temporarily and the LINX band expands, thereby allowing the food bolus to pass through into the stomach. This event is followed by band closure that keeps food, acid, and bile inside the stomach where they belong. The LINX band similarly expands during the events of belching and vomiting. The LINX procedure is completely reversible and the device can be removed at any time.

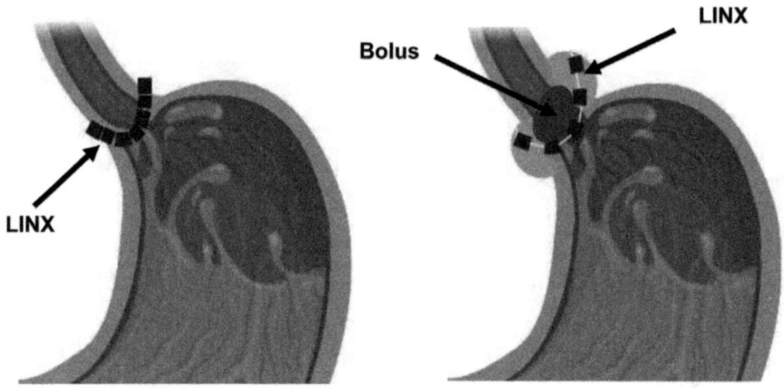

Figure 7.2 The LINX device is surgically placed around the LES of GERD patients where it prevents the flow of stomach acid and bile into the esophagus while allowing the passage of food bolus from the esophagus into the stomach. *Created in Biorender.com.*

7.2.2 Adjustable gastric band

An adjustable gastric band, also known as a lap band or an A-band, is an inflatable silicone-based device that is placed around the upper part of the stomach to create a small pouch (Fig. 7.3). This limits the amount of food that can be consumed at one time, thereby offering an apparent sense of satiety through the release of neuroendocrine peptide YY (PYY), while there is no change in the way food is absorbed. In 2011, the FDA approved A-bands to patients with a body mass index between 35 and 40 and a weight-related condition, like hypertension and diabetes. Patients with this band achieve uninterrupted weight loss by choosing healthy diet options, and limiting the amount and volume of food intake. Establishing the A-band in a patient is minimally invasive and completely reversible. This is normally performed using laparoscopic surgery resulting in smaller scars, shorter hospital stays, faster recovery, and less pain than open surgical procedures.

Such bands are entirely made of biodegradable materials, so they can be left in the patient's body without causing any sort of damage. The A-band is used to treat obesity, GERD, metabolic syndrome amongst other disorders.

7.2.3 Gastric electrical stimulation

Gastric electrical stimulation (GES) has been used for treating gastroparesis for more than 10 years [6–9]. While GES has been approved only based

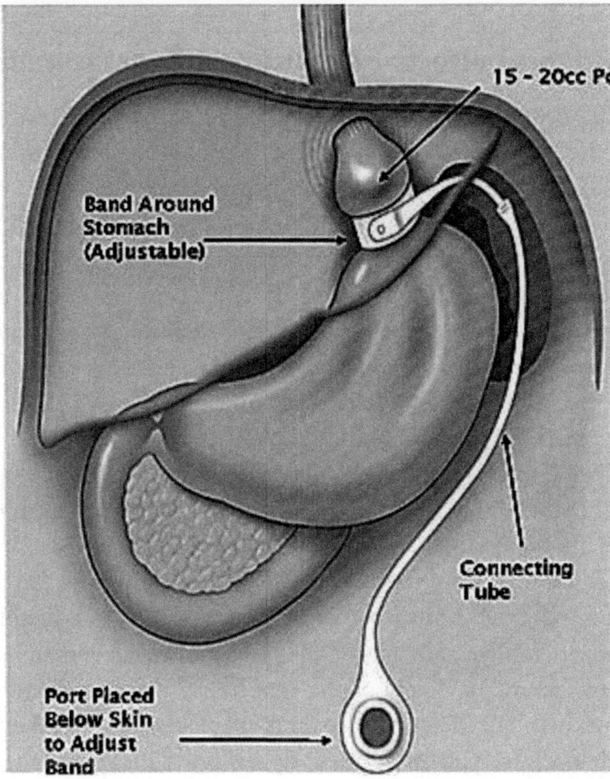

Figure 7.3 The A-band is used to divide the stomach into two sections: A smaller pouch (which has a capacity equivalent to a tablespoon volume) and a large stomach compartment. A tube is used to connect the A-band with a port located on the abdominal muscles of the patient. Depending on the weight loss goals, a surgeon injects saline using a needle through the port that causes the band to tighten, thereby restricting food intake. Conversely, when the saline is removed, the A-band expands to allow food intake. *Taken with permission from internet source: https://misnorthcounty.com/bariatric-surgery/gastric-band-lap-band/.*

on the humanitarian device exemption rule rather than as effective therapy by the Federal Drug Administration [10], it has become the most accepted and used treatment option for patients with otherwise refractory symptoms of gastroparesis. GES, also referred to as implantable gastric stimulation, involves the usage of a pacemaker-like device that provides electrical stimulation to the stomach surface, thereby breaking the motility cycle or inducing the enteric nervous system. GES is also used for treating obese patients who suffer from diabetes. Currently, there are a number of such devices in the market such as Diamond, Maestro, and Transend.

7.3 Adverse effects of gastric electrical stimulator

Several studies have attested to the relatively low probability of detrimental effects of pocket infection, lead perforation, and bowel obstruction caused because of implantations. Such complications, however, require surgical interventions [9,11]. These risks are highly significant as only one of the controlled trials showed a marginal benefit with decreased vomiting frequency during the period of active stimulation compared to the sham phase [12–16]. A recent study used a voluntary reporting system of FDA, where the authors examined the type and frequency of adverse events of the implant [17]. The Manufacturer and User Device Experience (MAUDE) databank of FDA is a repository of voluntarily reported adverse events involving medical devices. It has been used to determine the type and relative frequency of approved and marketed devices used in the United States [18–20]. Bielefeldt in 2017 [17] conducted an electronic search of MAUDE databank using the keyword "Enterra" for the time period between January 2001 and October 2015 and summarized information about the year of device implantation, the type of adverse event, and year of the report and the outcomes of operative interventions. The deleterious events were broadly classified as perioperative, device, or patient-related. Specifically these included device components (generator, battery, leads), nature of complaints or patient experiences (lack/loss of efficacy, pain with specific emphasis on experiences of shocks or jolts), events leading to surgical interventions (generator movement, pocket revision, battery exchange, generator or lead exchange, device explant, lead perforation, pocket infection, pocket erosion, small bowel obstruction), and events that interfered with normal device function (electromagnetic interference, inability to communicate with or program the device, logistic difficulties with system support services). A total of 1587 entries were retrieved using "Enterra" as a search term in the MAUDE databank [17]. Of these, 36 reports indicated cases involving initial implantation and were put under perioperative complications. Three deaths were documented: one due to cardiac arrest and two due to septic complications that resulted in multiple organ failure. Several cases reported stroke, after myocardial infarction, which was further complicated by pulmonary embolism. About seven reports outlined bleeding, complicating the initial surgery. During the procedure itself, lead damage had occurred 10 times, with eight reports related to the connection between leads and generator, and accidental gastric perforation [17,21]. Operations were successfully conducted indeed with none of these problems leading to clinically manifest adverse outcomes for the patients.

Pain was the second-most concern in patients, exhibiting most frequently as a shock, occasionally also associated with muscle contractions. Reports also recorded discomfort at the generator site additionally to intermittent shocks or jolts [17]. A few reports included data about actions been taken that included changes in stimulation intensity, assessment for possible lead fracture or generator dysfunction, which often led to surgical intervention. Sometimes rare events ranged from syncopal episodes, seizure, sensory abnormalities [8], worsening reflux symptoms, psychiatric emergencies to increased urinary tract infections, attributable to the implantation or the presence of the device [17].

Forty-five reports listed shifting or flipping of the generator within its pocket (Fig. 7.4), associated with discomfort, finally requiring surgical intervention [17,22]. Lead perforation into the stomach and erosion of the generator through the skin also added to the increased plausibility for surgical corrections. A patient's death was recorded owing to sepsis in the sequel to lead-induced colonic perforation. Intestinal obstruction due to stimulator leads was reported in 20 patients, who had required

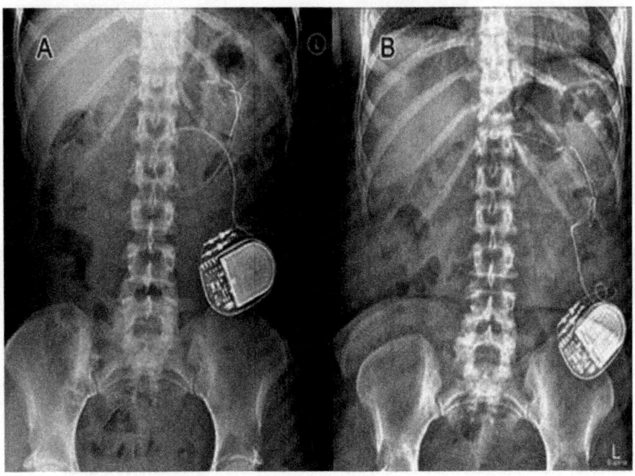

Figure 7.4 Abdominal X-ray depicts gastric stimulator (A) in correct position after 1 year of implantation and (B) displaced stimulator after 5 years. *Taken with permission from Tetangco EGP, Harrell S, Abboud R, Rao SSC, Hilton LR, Sharma A. Goo due to gastric stimulator electrode migration: add this to your DDX of gastroparesis exacerbation. Program no. P1269. ACG annual scientific meeting abstracts. Philadelphia, PA: American College of Gastroenterology; 2018.*

surgery, and besides these nine cases of incisional hernia formation, it was linked to stimulator insertion [17,23]. Some patients were diagnosed with esophagitis, and there was a displacement of gastric stimulator lead (Fig. 7.5) [22].

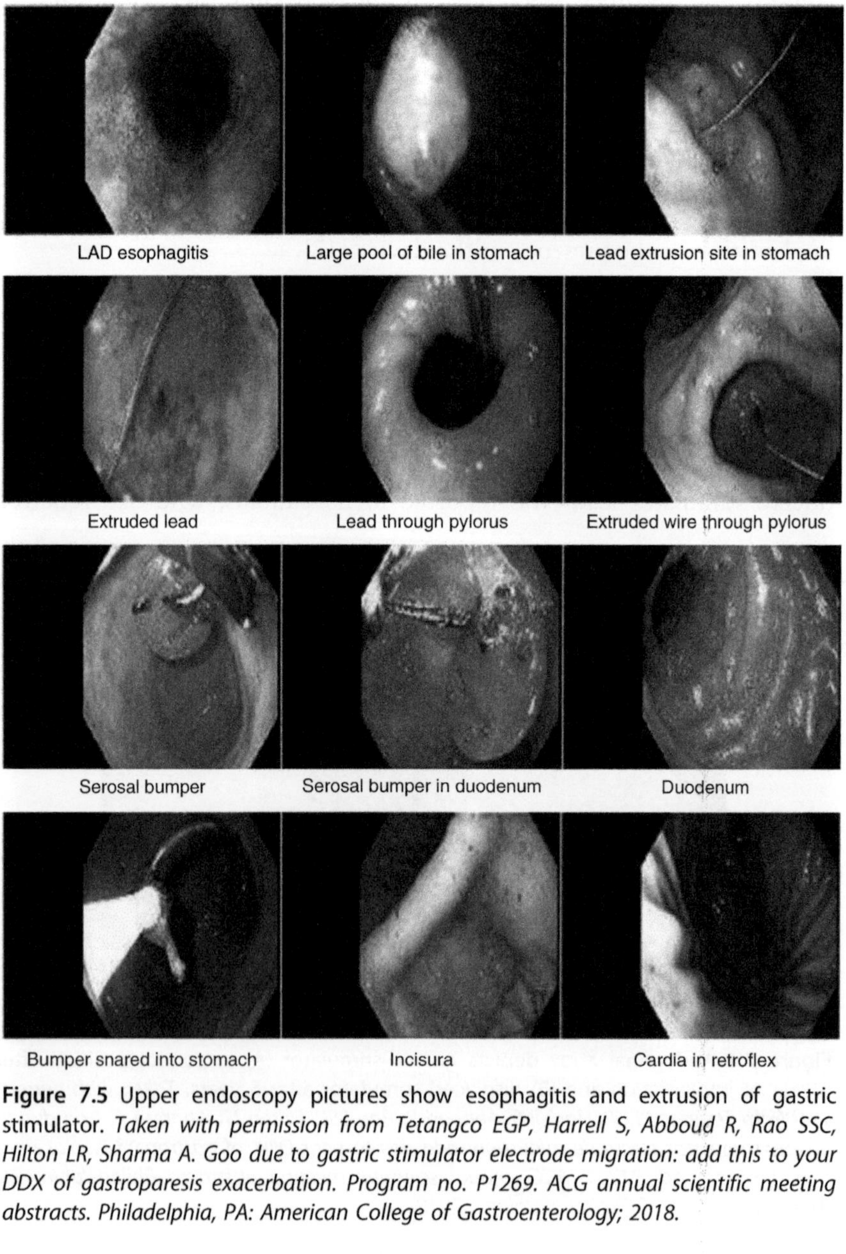

Figure 7.5 Upper endoscopy pictures show esophagitis and extrusion of gastric stimulator. *Taken with permission from Tetangco EGP, Harrell S, Abboud R, Rao SSC, Hilton LR, Sharma A. Goo due to gastric stimulator electrode migration: add this to your DDX of gastroparesis exacerbation. Program no. P1269. ACG annual scientific meeting abstracts. Philadelphia, PA: American College of Gastroenterology; 2018.*

Hematomas are known to be caused because of inadequate hemostasis as a result of injury to the blood vessel by the gastric electric stimulator implantation [13,14,23]. Further, coiling of the small intestine around the GES has previously been shown to result in the obstruction of the small intestine [23].

Device-related complications in human patients are highlighted by Bielefeldt et al. [17]. Generator malfunction or battery depletion was the major drawback in the implant, prompting device explant or replacement [17]. Surprisingly, battery depletion was too early than what was originally expected as based on 47 complaint cases. Electromagnetic interference was also observed in 27 reports, leading to the alteration of stimulator function and required reprogramming. There were also cases showing faulty or expired device components during surgery but did not cause any major harm. It was described in five reports that device programming was complicated or incorrect. Three reports indicated interactions with other programmable and implanted devices. Additionally, two patients experienced severe pain during transcutaneous electrical nerve stimulation for coexisting medical problems. With these results focusing on the side effects of GES, the number of reports about repeated operations clearly indicates a risk associated that should not be underestimated [17].

7.4 Adverse effects of magnetic sphincter augmentation

The LINX [magnetic sphincter augmentation (MSA)] reflux management system was designed for the treatment of GERD [24]. However, the most common complication of a LINX device was dysphagia observed in 43% of the patients in a study conducted by Bonavina et al. [25]. This knowledge was further supported by another pivotal study that involved 100 patients who underwent laparoscopic insertion of the LINX device and 68% of patients had dysphagia immediately after the operation [24]. The second-most common side effect was painful esophageal spasm [26]. The most threatening complication of MSA is device migration and erosion into the esophagus [27,28]. In a study of 3283 patients who underwent MSA, 0.15% had device erosion along with dysphagia or odynophagia, and was removed endoscopically or laparoscopically without any complication. In a few cases, patients subsequently underwent an uncomplicated laparoscopic fundoplication [29]. Two cases with penetration of the device into the esophagus were reported accompanied by progressive and severe dysphagia after the MSA [29,30]. These possible outcomes may help in educating the patients before surgery.

7.5 Adverse effects of endoscopic duodenal–jejunal bypass liner

Duodenal–jejunal bypass liner (DJBL), also known as an Endobarrier, is an implantable medical device consisting of a self-broadening ring equipped with barbs endoscopically anchored in the duodenal bulb and a 60 cm impervious Teflon-liner coating the proximal jejunal mucosal resorption area that prevents the interaction of food with hormones and enzymes in the proximal intestine. The DJBL is an endoscopic approach extensively used for treating obesity and type 2 diabetes mellitus [31,32]. However, its use was stopped by the FDA in the United States because of the development of liver abscesses [33]. According to the German DJBL registry analysis, adverse events, particularly gastrointestinal symptoms (abdominal pain, nausea, vomiting, diarrhea, constipation, and flatulence), were observed in patients. One patient was found with severe dehydration along with acidosis due to diarrhea and vomiting. Other serious adverse events included dislocation/migration, GI bleeding, sleeve obstruction, duodenal ulcer with perforation, biliary obstruction without cholecystitis or cholangitis, and esophageal lesion without perforation [32]. During the explantation visit, patients manifested with mucosal bleeding, gastritis, intestinal erosions, and liver abscess [34].

A retrospective study, highlighting the safety and effectiveness of the DJBL [35], reported that 84 out of the 114 patients experienced at least one adverse event. Major adverse events included epigastric pain (43%) and nausea and vomiting (15%). The DJBL caused 16 patients to experience a severe adverse event and 4 patients to experience a life-threatening adverse event. The life-threatening events included gastrointestinal hemorrhages and liver abscesses. The overall severe-to-life-threatening adverse event rate was found to be 18%. Out of the total 114 patients, 112 underwent endoscopic removal of the device. Complications observed included mucosal tears of the esophagus, gastroesophageal junction, soft palate, fundus, and pylorus. There was difficulty in the removal of one arm of the DJBL device that prolapsed through the pylorus in one of the patients. Among 112 patients explanted, 11 were reported to have distal migration of the device [35].

These reports were supported by another study in which three patients experienced an adverse event during the DJBL implantation procedure [36]. After delivering the sleeve in a patient, during the procedure, the anchor unfolded incompletely. During the DJBL explantation procedure, two patients experienced the damage to their esophagus. Seven patients were diagnosed with GI bleeding after implantation; among those, two patients complained of hematemesis and melena, 3 and 6 weeks after implantation of the DJBL, respectively. There were no reports of lowered hemoglobin or hematocrit or any signs of hypovolemia observed in both the cases. One patient was reported to elicit slight erosions of the duodenal mucosa and in another patient three longitudinal ulcers with two blood clots were found below the anchor. After 40 weeks of implantation, one patient complained of fatigue and dizziness and was later detected with ulcerations. The DJBL implantation caused mild pancreatitis in two patients. The first patient experienced severe abdominal pain and vomiting. Migration of DJBL was observed via CT scan (Fig. 7.6A). Esophagogastroduodenoscopy (EGD) confirmed CT scan results (Fig. 7.6B–D). The second patient presented with 3 days of abdominal pain and like patient one, the EGD showed migration of DJBL past the major duodenal papilla. After the DJBL retrieval, both patients recovered quickly. Further, after 12 months of implantation, EGD showed perforation of one of the barbs of the anchor through the duodenal wall into the stomach in one patient during the explantation process (Fig. 7.7) [36].

7.6 Adverse effects of bile duct endoprosthesis

Duodenal perforation was reported in a 66-year-old woman following bile duct endoprosthesis placement [37]. The patient manifested abdominal pain and jaundice and was diagnosed with hepatic metastases

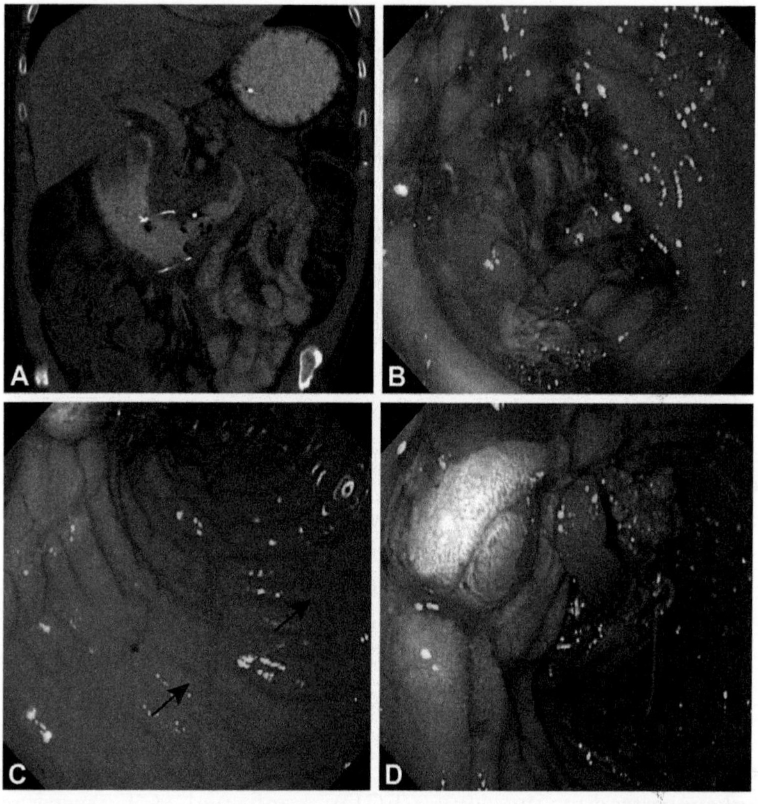

Figure 7.6 Movement of duodenal–jejunal bypass liner and associated adverse events. (A) A CT scan picture showing the migration of the DJBL, (B) EGD confirms passing of DJBL across the swollen major duodenal papilla, (C) ulcerations of duodenal mucosa was observed due to migration of DJBL, and (D) blockage of papilla due to the presence of residual food at the entrance of the DJBL. *Taken with permission from Betzel B, Koehestanie P, Aarts EO, Dogan K, Homan J, Janssen IM et al. Safety experience with the duodenal–jejunal bypass liner: an endoscopic treatment for diabetes and obesity. Gastrointest Endosc 2015;82(5):845–52.*

having distension of bile duct, indicating a primary malignancy of the pancreas or bile ducts. A 15-cm long endoprosthesis was inserted to fix the outflow of bile from the left hepatic system. Endoscopic retrograde cholangiopancreatography confirmed the penetration of endoprosthesis into the duodenal wall [37]. This might be attributed to the high pressure by the malignant process on the endoprosthesis that pushed it toward the duodenal wall, after which it penetrated the wall. Later, the endoprosthesis was removed and the perforation was sealed with endoclips [37].

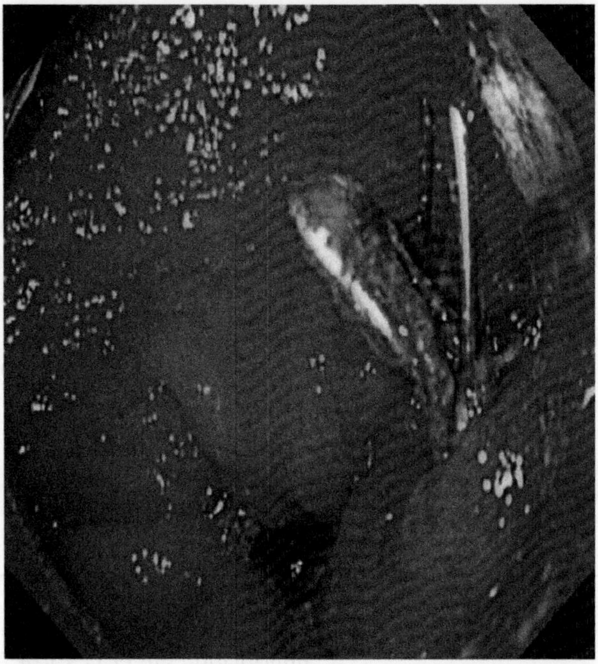

Figure 7.7 EGD shows the perforation of a barb of the anchor of the DJBL through the duodenal wall, adjacent to the pylorus, into the stomach. *Taken with permission from Betzel B, Koehestanie P, Aarts EO, Dogan K, Homan J, Janssen IM et al. Safety experience with the duodenal–jejunal bypass liner: an endoscopic treatment for diabetes and obesity. Gastrointest Endosc 2015;82(5):845–52.*

7.7 Adverse effects of long nasointestinal tubes

Long nasointestinal tubes have been extensively used in treating acute bowel obstruction and intestinal plication with great results [38–40]. A clinical study was conducted with a total of 88 patients (59 males and 29 females) who were treated with long nasointestinal tubes for acute bowel obstruction [41]. About 95.4% of the patients experienced nasopharynx discomfort and pain; 44.3% had electrolyte disorders and 3.4% were diagnosed with aspiration pneumonia. There were also cases in which sustained catheter-related accidents were recorded including tube obstruction (15.9%), unexpected catheter shedding (5.6%), anterior balloon rupture (1.1%), and dislodgement of the guide (2.3%). There were no cases with intestinal hemorrhage, perforation, and necrosis [41].

7.8 Conclusion

The previously discussed implants are used for treating various gastrointestinal tract related ailments. Although they provide a minimally invasive and promising treatment approach, unintended adverse effects may emerge. As the side effects of the implant are unavoidable, proper precautionary measures have to be carried out to avoid severe and life-threatening outcomes. Thus the secret of successful and favorable results of the implants depends on the proper preoperative assessment and appropriate patient selection. A summary of the adverse effects associated with implants is mentioned in Table 7.1.

Table 7.1 Adverse effects of implants.

Serial number	Implant	Side effects
1.	Gastric electrical stimulator	Vomiting, bowel obstruction [9,11], pocket infection, lead perforation, hematoma at implantation site [9,11,13,14,23], displacement of gastric stimulator lead and esophagitis [22], septic complications which resulted in multiple organ failure, stroke, myocardial infarction, pulmonary embolism [17], gastric perforation [21], pain during muscle contractions and intermittent shocks or jolts in the generator site [9,11,17,23], syncopal episodes, seizure, sensory abnormalities [8]
2.	Magnetic sphincter augmentation	Dysphagia [25], painful esophageal spasm [26], device migration and erosion [27,28], penetration of the device into the esophagus [29,30]
3.	Distraction enterogenesis	Multiple surgeries to exploit and safely remove the device [42]
4.	Endoscopic duodenal–jejunal bypass liner	Liver abscesses [33], abdominal pain, nausea, vomiting, diarrhea, constipation, and flatulence, severe dehydration along with acidosis, device dislocation/migration, GI bleeding, sleeve obstruction, duodenal ulcer with perforation, biliary obstruction

(*Continued*)

Table 7.1 (Continued)

Serial number	Implant	Side effects
		without cholecystitis or cholangitis, and esophageal lesion [32], mucosal bleeding, gastritis, intestinal erosions [34], mucosal tears of the esophagus, gastroesophageal junction, soft palate, fundus and pylorus, epigastric pain, gastrointestinal hemorrhages [35], hematemesis, melena, erosion of the duodenal mucosa, and perforation of the device into the stomach [36]
5.	Bile duct endoprosthesis	Penetration into the duodenal wall [37]
6.	Long nasointestinal tubes	Nasopharynx discomfort and pain, electrolyte disorders, aspiration pneumonia [41], tube obstruction, unexpected catheter shedding, anterior balloon rupture, and dislodgement of the guide [41]

References

[1] Huizinga JD, Lammers WJ. Gut peristalsis is governed by a multitude of cooperating mechanisms. Am J Physiol Gastrointest Liver Physiol 2009;296(1):G1−8.

[2] Lo YK, et al. A wireless implant for gastrointestinal motility disorders. Micromachines (Basel) 2018;9(1).

[3] Yamazaki S, et al. Homeostasis of thymus-derived Foxp3 + regulatory T cells is controlled by ultraviolet B exposure in the skin. J Immunol 2014;193(11):5488−97.

[4] Dumic I, et al. Gastrointestinal tract disorders in older age. Can J Gastroenterol Hepatol 2019;2019 6757524.

[5] Halder SL, et al. Natural history of functional gastrointestinal disorders: a 12-year longitudinal population-based study. Gastroenterology 2007;133(3):799−807.

[6] Abell TL, Van Cutsem E, Abrahamsson H, Huizinga JD, Konturek JW, Galmiche JP, et al. Gastric electrical stimulation in intractable symptomatic gastroparesis. Digestion 2002;66(4):204−12.

[7] Cutts TF, Luo J, Starkebaum W, Rashed H, Abell TL. Is gastric electrical stimulation superior to standard pharmacologic therapy in improving GI symptoms, healthcare resources, and long-term health care benefits? Neurogastroenterol Motil 2005;17:35−43.

[8] Maranki JL, Lytes V, Meilahn JE, Harbison S, Friedenberg FK, Fisher RS, et al. Predictive factors for clinical improvement with enterra gastric electric stimulation treatment for refractory gastroparesis. Dig Dis Sci 2008;53(8):2072−8.

[9] McCallum RW, Lin Z, Forster J, Roeser K, Hou Q, Sarosiek I. Gastric electrical stimulation improves outcomes of patients with gastroparesis for up to 10 years. Clin Gastroenterol Hepatol 2011;9(4):314−19 e1.

[10] FDA. Humanitarian device exemption. <http://www.fda.gov/MedicalDevices/DeviceRegulationandGuidance/HowtoMarketYourDevice/PremarketSubmissions/HumanitarianDeviceExemption/default.htm/>; 2010.

[11] Anand C, Al-Juburi A, Familoni B, Rashed H, Cutts T, Abidi N, et al. Gastric electrical stimulation is safe and effective: a long-term study in patients with drug-refractory gastroparesis in three regional centers. Digestion 2007;75(2–3):83–9.
[12] Frokjaer JB, Ejskjaer N, Rask P, Andersen SD, Gregersen H, Drewes AM, et al. Central neuronal mechanisms of gastric electrical stimulation in diabetic gastroparesis. Scand J Gastroenterol 2008;43(9):1066–75.
[13] McCallum RW, Sarosiek I, Parkman HP, Snape W, Brody F, Wo J, et al. Gastric electrical stimulation with enterra therapy improves symptoms of idiopathic gastroparesis. Neurogastroenterol Motil 2013;25(10):815–e636.
[14] McCallum RW, Snape W, Brody F, Wo J, Parkman HP, Nowak T. Gastric electrical stimulation with enterra therapy improves symptoms from diabetic gastroparesis in a prospective study. Clin Gastroenterol Hepatol 2010;8(11):947–54.
[15] Abell T, McCallum R, Hocking M, Koch K, Abrahamsson H, Leblanc I, et al. Gastric electrical stimulation for medically refractory gastroparesis. Gastroenterology 2003;125(2):421–8.
[16] Abell TL, Johnson WD, Kedar A, Runnels JM, Thompson J, Weeks ES, et al. A double-masked, randomized, placebo-controlled trial of temporary endoscopic mucosal gastric electrical stimulation for gastroparesis. Gastrointest Endosc 2011;74 (3):496–503 e493.
[17] Bielefeldt K. Adverse events of gastric electrical stimulators recorded in the manufacturer and user device experience (maude) registry. Auton Neurosci 2017;202:40–4.
[18] Tremaine AM, Avram MM. FDA maude data on complications with lasers, light sources, and energy-based devices. Lasers Surg Med 2015;47(2):133–40.
[19] Overbey DM, Townsend NT, Chapman BC, Bennett DT, Foley LS, Rau AS, et al. Surgical energy-based device injuries and fatalities reported to the food and drug administration. J Am Coll Surg 2015;221(1):197–205 e191.
[20] Naumann RW, Brown J. Complications of electromechanical morcellation reported in the Manufacturer and User Facility Device Experience (MAUDE) database. J Minim Invasive Gynecol 2015;22(6):1018–21.
[21] Becker JC, Dietl KH, Konturek JW, Domschke W, Pohle T. Gastric wall perforation: a rare complication of gastric electrical stimulation. Gastrointest Endosc 2004;59 (4):584–6.
[22] Tetangco EGP, Harrell S, Abboud R, Rao SSC, Hilton LR, Sharma A. Goo due to gastric stimulator electrode migration: add this to your DDX of gastroparesis exacerbation. Program no. P1269. ACG annual scientific meeting abstracts. Philadelphia, PA: American College of Gastroenterology; 2018.
[23] Zoll B, Jehangir A, Malik Z, Edwards MA, Petrov RV, Parkman HP. Gastric electric stimulation for refractory gastroparesis. J Clin Outcomes Manag 2019;26(1):27–38.
[24] Ganz RA, Peters JH, Horgan S, Bemelman WA, Dunst CM, Edmundowicz SA, et al. Esophageal sphincter device for gastroesophageal reflux disease. N Engl J Med 2013;368(8):719–27.
[25] Bonavina L, Demeester T, Fockens P, Dunn D, Saino G, Bona D, et al. Laparoscopic sphincter augmentation device eliminates reflux symptoms and normalizes esophageal acid exposure: one- and 2-year results of a feasibility trial. Ann Surg 2010;252(5):857–62.
[26] Reynolds JL, Zehetner J, Bildzukewicz N, Katkhouda N, Dandekar G, Lipham JC. Magnetic sphincter augmentation with the LINX device for gastroesophageal reflux disease after U.S. Food and Drug Administration approval. Am Surg 2014;80 (10):1034–8.
[27] Lipham JC, Taiganides PA, Louie BE, Ganz RA, DeMeester TR. Safety analysis of first 1000 patients treated with magnetic sphincter augmentation for gastroesophageal reflux disease. Dis Esophagus 2015;28(4):305–11.

[28] Bielefeldt K. Adverse events after implantation of a magnetic sphincter augmentation device for gastroesophageal reflux. Clin Gastroenterol Hepatol 2016;14(10):1507–8.
[29] Salvador R, Costantini M, Capovilla G, Polese L, Merigliano S. Esophageal penetration of the magnetic sphincter augmentation device: history repeats itself. J Laparoendosc Adv Surg Tech A 2017;27(8):834–8.
[30] Zadeh J, Andreoni A, Treitl D, Ben-David K. Spotlight on the LINX reflux management system for the treatment of gastroesophageal reflux disease: evidence and research. Med Devices (Auckl) 2018;11:291–300.
[31] Endobarrier. The endobarrier® gastrointestinal liner with delivery system – instructions for use. Lexington: GI Dynamics; 2017.
[32] Sauer N, Aberle J, Lautenback A, Seufert J, Laubner K. Safety- and efficacy-outcomes of the duodenal–jejunal bypass liner (DJBL) registry in obese patients with type 2 diabetes. In: Paper presented at the 52nd annual meeting of the European association for the study of diabetes; September 12–16, 2016, Munich, Germany; 2016.
[33] K L. Final efficacy and safety results of U.S. ENDO Trial announced at Ada. Boston, MA: GI Dynamics; 2016.
[34] Riedel N, Laubner K, Lautenbach A, Schön G, Schlensak M, Stengel R, et al. Longitudinal evaluation of efficacy, safety and nutritional status during one-year treatment with the duodenal–jejunal bypass liner. Surg Obes Relat Dis 2018;14 (6):769–79.
[35] Forner PM, Ramacciotti T, Farey JE, Lord RV. Safety and effectiveness of an endoscopically placed duodenal–jejunal bypass device (endobarrier®): outcomes in 114 patients. Obes Surg 2017;27(12):3306–13.
[36] Betzel B, Koehestanie P, Aarts EO, Dogan K, Homan J, Janssen IM, et al. Safety experience with the duodenal–jejunal bypass liner: an endoscopic treatment for diabetes and obesity. Gastrointest Endosc 2015;82(5):845–52.
[37] Kusters PJ, Keulen ET, Peters FP. Duodenal perforation following bile duct endoprosthesis placemen. Endoscopy 2014;46:E646–7.
[38] Gowen GF. Long tube decompression is successful in 90% of patients with adhesive small bowel obstruction. Am J Surg 2002;185(6):512–15.
[39] Ishizuka M, Nagata H, Takagi K, Kubota K. Transnasal fine gastrointestinal fiberscope-guided long tube insertion for patients with small bowel obstruction. J Gastrointest Surg 2009;13(3):550–4.
[40] Guo SB, Duan ZJ. Decompression of the small bowel by endoscopic long-tube placement. World J Gastroenterol 2012;18(15):1822–6.
[41] Wang K, Yang G, Han C, Bi W, Zhang G. Clinical analysis of common complications induced by long nasointestinal tubes: a retrospective cohort study. Transl Surg 2018;3:28–33.
[42] Rouch JD, Dunn JC. New insights and interventions for short bowel syndrome. Curr Pediatr Rep 2017;5(1):1–5.

CHAPTER EIGHT

Obstetrics and gynecology

Mounika Gudeppu[1], Jesudas Balasubramanian[1], Pramila Bakthavachalam[1], Logesh Chokkalingam[2] and Prakash Srinivasan Timiri Shanmugam[2,*]

[1]HCL, Chennai, Tamil Nadu, India
[2]HCL America Inc., Sunnyvale, CA, United States
*Corresponding author

Abstract

There are many controversies resulting recently, surrounding the medical devices used for maintaining women's health and for contraception. There are many risks and complications occurring due to the approval of intrauterine devices or the other contraceptive devices without proper regulatory clearance. Hence, the special concern should be reserved during the classification of these OB/GYN devices; thus, stringent regulatory requirements can be imposed on them for its market approval. The high-risk devices must be categorized into class II and class III rather than class I; thus, they have to clear premarket approval requirements for their market clearance. However, postmarketing surveillance must also be conducted for continuous monitoring of the devices; if some risk befalls, the classification can be changed by the higher authority of regulatory bodies. This chapter mainly describes about various OB/GYN devices, their toxicity, applications, and market range. It provides a detailed description of the regulatory requirements of OB/GYN devices with biocompatibility approach.

Keywords: OB/GYN devices; regulatory requirements; toxicity; applications; biocompatibility

Highlights

- Provides a detailed overview of OB/GYN devices, types, and applications.
- Biocompatibility tests required for meeting the safety and efficacy requirements of OB/GYN devices were mentioned.
- Different kinds of toxicities resulted due to long-term usage and/or other causes were reported.

Toxicological Aspects of Medical Device Implants.
DOI: https://doi.org/10.1016/B978-0-12-820728-4.00008-3
© 2020 Elsevier Inc.
All rights reserved.

- The controversies in OB/GYN device classification were described.
- Stringent regulatory requirements were defined.
- Market range of OB/GYN devices was demarcated.

8.1 Introduction to medical devices used in obstetrics and gynecology

Obstetrics and gynecology are mainly encompassed with females and are considered as a medical specialty with two subspecialties of obstetrics that covers pregnancy, childbirth, and the postpartum period and gynecology that covers the health of the female reproductive system—vagina, uterus, ovaries, and breasts. The terms obstetrics and gynecology were generally abbreviated as *OB-GYN* or *OB/GYN* in American English and *obs* and *gynae* in British Language [1].

According to US-FDA, OB/GYN devices were classified into class III devices, that is, "designated life sustaining" and they possess greater potential risks to the patients. FDA was more concerned about approving certain "high-risk devices" and the organization was too hasty in approving the devices without any sufficient efficacy and safety data. FDA has framed stringent rules for trails for medical devices used in OB/GYN. In the case of controversial devices, a permanent sterilization method must be employed for women and a device must be used for the purpose of reducing postsurgical adhesions. Some devices like transvaginal mesh and power morcellators went through the short 510(k) approval process by using a predicting device that was already in the market. These devices have got approved by the 510(k) approval process without any rigorous premarket approval (PMA) process where new medical devices must undergo. The postmarketing surveillance data have reported that the usage of these devices led to serious adverse effects that resulted in severe health concerns. However, the power morcellators were withdrawn from the market, whereas transvaginal mesh was reclassified as PMA, a "high-risk" device. Along with the growing "innovations" in the medical devices field, the need for "burden of proof" related to the device's safety and efficacy is growing to reduce the adverse effects and complications of medical devices [2].

The obstetrics and gynecology devices panel (OGDP) monitors the safety and effectiveness of the marketed and investigational devices by reviewing and evaluating the data. It makes appropriate recommendations to the Commissioner of Food and Drugs [3].

Let us take an example of the OB/GYN device "Pressure Wedge" and consider its requirements to satisfy its intended purpose safely. The primary use of pressure wedge is to reduce cesarean delivery. It is used as a doctor's prescription by providing mechanical support into the perianal region of the mother externally during the labor and inducing the vaginal delivery process, thus reducing the cesarean delivery. Special controls must be maintained for these devices' usage, that is, the patient-contacting parts of the device should be biocompatible and do not cause any adverse effects. The other nonclinical parameters like the device sensitivity must be demonstrated and checked before use, as the device must be stable and should not break when subjected to the forces during labor. Sterility of the device should be validated as a part of performance data, which demonstrate the sterility and package integrity of the device over a certain period of labeled shelf life; the rate of skin/tissue trauma must be characterized based on clinical performance data. Regarding the accurate placement and use of the device, specific instructions should be maintained [3,4].

8.2 Biocompatibility of OB/GYN devices

Biocompatibility is the most primary and imperative concern for OB/GYN devices, as their nature and duration of the contact are more complex and long-term usage. The incidence of genotoxicity, carcinogenicity, and mutagenicity was high with OB/GYN devices. In addition, hypersensitivity and other miscellaneous toxicities were common. Hence, higher attention should be specified to these devices to ensure their safety and efficacy by analyzing their biocompatibility as well as hemocompatibility [4].

Some of the metals such as copper, nickel, and titanium were present in OB/GYN devices. Intrauterine contraceptive devices (IUD) fall under the category of OB/GYN devices containing metals, specifically copper, which was used for reversible contraception in approximately 5% of British women and 10% of Danish women. Some of the copper IUDs like Paragard 380A (from Duramed Pharmaceuticals) are without any contamination and had a composition of polyethylene, barium sulfate, and 99.9% pure copper wire. However, the most adverse effect found very often during their usage is dermatitis, due to its systemic allergic contact effect. This was confirmed by performing patch tests. It was suggested to remove the product that has resulted in the resolution of the symptoms [5–10]. Some of the permanent contraceptive devices such as the Essure device (Bayer Corp) and the Filshie clip (Cooper Surgical) containing metals like nickel and titanium reported with the incidence of hypersensitivity. The Essure devices induce permanent contraception by inducing fibrosis and tubal occlusions after their transvaginal implantation and expansion into fallopian tubes. The outer coils of permanent contraceptive devices were composed of Nitinol (55% titanium/45% nickel) and their inner coils were covered with SAE 316L stainless steel. The nickel releases slowly from the Nitinol and results in systemic allergic contact dermatitis [11]. Owing to the severe adverse effects cause of nickel release from the device, the users have submitted a registered complaint in the Manufacturer and User Facility Device Experience database. Hence, on September 24, 2015, FDA has reconvened OGDP and evaluated the effectiveness of safety [12]. After the discussion, the FDA has recommended the manufacturer to conduct postmarketing surveillance study to ensure the safety of the product. If any unavoidable risk occurred, on considering risk–benefit ratio proper labeling with a warning about the risk to be mentioned [13].

The regulations employed on OB/GYN devices are more stringent than the other devices and it involves the implantation of general and special controls after the device classification. Let us consider an example of fetal head elevator, which is a prescription device by possessing a mechanism that elevates the fetal head to facilitate delivery during a cesarean section [14]. FDA has classified the device as a class II by employing special controls along with the general controls by considering the components coming in patient contact. Initially, after classifying the device the probable risks have to be identified and then suitable mitigation measures can be taken against the risks. The possible risks, with their suitable mitigation measures, were as follows [15].

- The incidence of adverse tissue reaction—biocompatibility evaluation should be performed.
- Incidence of infection—sterilization, validation, shelf-life testing, and labeling need to be performed.

- Occurrence of fatal injury due to device failure—nonclinical performance testing, shelf-life testing, and labeling need to be performed.
- Incidence of maternal injury due to device failure—nonclinical performance testing, shelf-life testing, and labeling need to be performed.
- Any usage error—labeling.

In this case, both special and general controls were employed. The following are the identification and classification of the device, fetal head elevator, and special controls employed for its safety [15].

- *Identification*—the intended use of the device should be identified—in case of the fetal head elevator the intended purpose is to facilitate the delivery during cesarean section by elevating the fetal head.
- *Classification*—the device should be classified depending on its risk factors and suitable controls (general controls or special controls) should be implemented—the fetal head elevator was classified as a class II with the implementation of special controls.

The following special controls were employed for the fetal head elevator:

- The device components coming in patient contact should be identified and ensure their *biocompatibility*.
- The sterility of the patient-contacting device components should be ensured by *performance data.*
- The shelf life of the device based on sterility, package integrity, and device functionality was analyzed, and it should be supported by performance data.
- To ensure the performance of the device during anticipated conditions, *nonclinical performance data* should be observed, and the following performance characteristics must be tested:
    - Under relevant use conditions, reliability testing should be performed during device deployment and retrieval.
    - The maximum force applied on to fetal head was tested by using an anatomic model.
    - The elevator mechanism of the uniform application was tested on the fetal head.
- The *labeling* on the device must include the following:
    - If the user/patient has any genital infection, the device usage must be contraindicated.
    - During its proper placement and use of the device, specific instructions must be followed.
    - Shelf life should be maintained appropriately.

According to ISO 10993:1, the OB/GYN devices can be classified as following and respective studies should be conducted for ensuring their safety [16] (Table 8.1).

8.3 Regulatory requirements of the devices

The regulatory requirement of OB/GYN devices was very high, as the associated risks and complications are more compared to the other devices. It affects women's health to the highest extent and becomes life threatening. The probable causes of these adverse effects are as follows [23]:

- The manufacturers instead of performing the suitable tests, they compare the device with predicting device and assures its safety; the method of testing may vary when compared to the device of interest.
- The devices were monitored after entering into the market rather than monitoring the device effects in animals and patients before releasing into the market.
- The name of 510(k) was scrapped more descriptive, the "Safety and Performance Based Pathway."

Hence, as the associated risk and complications are more, US-FDA has increased the regulatory burden on the manufacturers to release their OB/GYN products into the market. However, if suitable laboratory data are available proving the device safety, then the regulatory burden can be reduced by reclassifying the class III devices into class I and class II categories. A similar incident has occurred in the case of "single-use female condoms" [24].

8.3.1 Reclassification of "single-use female condom" into "multiple-use condom" by US-FDA [25]

8.3.1.1 Description of the device and its regulation history

The single-use condom, a device that is mainly intended for females, is like a sheath that can be inserted into the vagina before the initiation of coitus. The device holds the flexible rings for holding the device in place during the sexual intercourse, and the device functions as a mechanical barrier that protects the user from sexually transmitted diseases (STDs) and aids in contraception. The female condoms are different from that of male condoms, as in the case of the male's complete penis was covered with a

Table 8.1 Represents the end points in biological risk assessment of OB/GYN devices.

Category	Nature of contact	Duration of contact	Recommended tests	Specific parts of ISO 10993 involved
Surface medical devices	Mucosal membrane	A—limited (≤24 h)	Cytotoxicity	ISO 10993:5 [17]
			Sensitization	ISO 10993:10 [18]
			Irritation/intracutaneous	ISO 10993:10
		B—Prolonged (> 24 h to 30 d)	Cytotoxicity	ISO 10993:5
			Sensitization	ISO 10993:10
			Irritation/intracutaneous	ISO 10993:10
			Acute systemic toxicity	ISO 10993:11 [19]
			Subacute toxicity	ISO 10993:11
			Implantation effects	ISO 10993:6 [20]
		C—Long-term (> 30 d)	Cytotoxicity	ISO 10993:5
			Sensitization	ISO 10993:10
			Irritation/intracutaneous	ISO 10993:10
			Acute systemic toxicity	ISO 10993:11
			Subacute toxicity	ISO 10993:11
			Subchronic toxicity	ISO 10993:11
			Chronic toxicity	ISO 10993:11
			Implantation effects	ISO 10993:6
			Genotoxicity	ISO 10993:3 [21]
	Breached or compromised surface	A—limited (≤24 h)	Cytotoxicity	ISO 10993:5
			Sensitization	ISO 10993:10
			Irritation/intracutaneous	ISO 10993:10
			Material-mediated pyrogenicity	ISO 10993:11
			Acute systemic toxicity	ISO 10993:11

(*Continued*)

Table 8.1 (Continued)

Category	Nature of contact	Duration of contact	Recommended tests	Specific parts of ISO 10993 involved
		B—Prolonged (>24 h to 30 d)	Cytotoxicity	ISO 10993:5
			Sensitization	ISO 10993:10
			Irritation/intracutaneous	ISO 10993:10
			Material-mediated	ISO 10993:11
			pyrogenicity	ISO 10993:11
			Acute systemic toxicity	ISO 10993:11
			Subacute toxicity	ISO 10993:6
			Implantation effects	
		C—Long term (>30 d)	Cytotoxicity	ISO 10993:5
			Sensitization	ISO 10993:10
			Irritation/intracutaneous	ISO 10993:10
			Material-mediated	ISO 10993:11
			pyrogenicity	ISO 10993:11
			Acute systemic toxicity	ISO 10993:11
			Subacute toxicity	ISO 10993:11
			Subchronic toxicity	ISO 10993:11
			Chronic toxicity	ISO 10993:6
			Implantation effects	ISO 10993:3
			Genotoxicity	ISO 10993:3
			Carcinogenicity	

(Continued)

Table 8.1 (Continued)

Category	Nature of contact	Duration of contact	Recommended tests	Specific parts of ISO 10993 involved
Implant medical device	Blood	A—limited (≤24 h)	Cytotoxicity	ISO 10993:5
			Sensitization	ISO 10993:10
			Irritation/intracutaneous	ISO 10993:10
			Material-mediated	ISO 10993:11
			pyrogenicity	ISO 10993:11
			Acute systemic toxicity	ISO 10993:6
			Implantation effects	ISO 10993:4 [22]
			Hemocompatibility	ISO 10993:3
			Genotoxicity	
		B—Prolonged (> 24 h to 30 d)	Cytotoxicity	ISO 10993:5
			Sensitization	ISO 10993:10
			Irritation/intracutaneous	ISO 10993:10
			Material-mediated	ISO 10993:11
			pyrogenicity	ISO 10993:11
			Acute systemic toxicity	ISO 10993:11
			Subacute toxicity	ISO 10993:6
			Implantation effects	ISO 10993:4
			Hemocompatibility	ISO 10993:3
			Genotoxicity	
		C—Long-term (> 30 d)	Cytotoxicity	ISO 10993:5
			Sensitization	ISO 10993:10
			Irritation/intracutaneous	ISO 10993:10
				ISO 10993:11

(Continued)

Table 8.1 (Continued)

Category	Nature of contact	Duration of contact	Recommended tests	Specific parts of ISO 10993 involved
			Material-mediated	ISO 10993:11
			pyrogenicity	ISO 10993:11
			Acute systemic toxicity	ISO 10993:11
			Subacute toxicity	ISO 10993:11
			Subchronic toxicity	ISO 10993:6
			Chronic toxicity	ISO 10993:4
			Implantation effects	ISO 10993:3
			Hemocompatibility	
			Genotoxicity	

Note: Before the above tests, physical and/or chemical information about the device was collected in common in spite of the difference in their categorization.

closely fitting membrane and was categorized into class II devices under §§ 884.5300 and 884.5310 (21 CFR 884.5300 and 884.5310). The first single-use female condom was received by FDA 510(k) on January 1989 for its approval by Wisconsin Pharmacal Company LLC (WPC) and was received. Initially, it was named as WPC-333 device and later it was renamed as Femsheild/reality female condom and regulated as a class III device under section 513(f)(1) of the FD&C Act. During this classification, FDA was unaware of the existence of a Gee Bee ring, a pouch-like device intended to line the vaginal wall for contraception and prophylaxis of STDs. In the provided WPC documentation to the 510(k), the information about the Gee Bee ring was provided; however, this cannot be compared with the real female condom as it is intended for single use, whereas Gee Bee ring was intended for reuse. Moreover, the Gee Bee ring was made of animal tissue. Once the FDA came to know about the existing evidence of Gee Bee ring, they verified its preamendment status and uses and presented them to an OGDP/classification panel on March 7, 1989. After a wide range of review, OGDP classified the device into class III, as there is no availability of laboratory test reports or clinical study data. The OGDP also confirmed that the device is different from a male condom and recommended the FDA to establish special controls for the device to substantiate the importance in preventing the impairment of human health. FDA accepted the recommendations of OGDP, in the Federal Register of June 10, 1999 (64 FR 31164) and proposed a rule for creating a new classification regulation (§ 884.5330 (21 CFR 884.5330) for classifying the female condom as class III and a finalized rule was released on May 18, 2000 (65 FR 31454). In all types of the female condom, the Gee Bee ring was regulated under § 884.5330 and by using the FDA product code OBY it was identified.

The Center for Devices and Radiological Health 2014–2015 has strategically prioritized the right balance between Premarket and Postmarket Data Collection, which was considered as a retrospective review of class III devices subject to PMA. On April 29, 2015, the FDA has given a notice in the Federal Register entitled "Retrospective Review of Premarket Approval Application Devices; Striking the Balance Between Premarket and Postmarket Data Collection," where FDA has considered reclassification of single-use female condoms from class III to class II and the MBU product was used for its identification. With respect to the notice, FDA received seven comments, where six comments were supported for reclassification of MBU and one comment was against to the reclassification and stated that the FDA has failed in gathering the information to determine the type of risks involved for female condoms of different design, materials, and manufacturing processes. By consideration of all negative and positive comments, FDA has decided to reclassify the female condoms from class III to class II [26].

8.3.1.2 Reclassification of the device

As there is sufficient information that exists for establishing the special controls, FDA has proposed to reclassify a single-use female condom from class III to class II. By framing the special controls and combining them with general controls, reasonable assurance of device safety and efficacy can be provided. The FDA has proposed to reclassify the postamendments from class III to class II (special controls), in accordance with the section 513(f)(3) of the FD&C Act and 21 CFR part 860, subpart C. FDA has gathered sufficient information of nonclinical and clinical data from submitted PMA applications [27]: P910064, P940033, and P080002, available to FDA under section 520(h)(4) of the FD&C Act; postmarket experience; and peer-reviewed literature for establishing special controls to mitigate the risks to the health of females using single-use female condoms. Special controls are required as the general controls are insufficient to provide reasonable assurance of the safety and effectiveness of the device. However, FDA proposed to rename the single-use female condom to multiple-use female condoms by consideration of preamendments of the class III device. The multiple-use female condom (a postamendment female condom—product code OBY) was cleaned at the conclusion of coitus and reused, whereas this is not possible with a single-use female condom (a preamendment female condom—product code MBU). There specified another revision of changing the term "diseases" to "infections," which is more appropriate in clinical terminology [28].

According to the section 520(h)(4) of the FD&C Act [29], postmarket experience and peer-reviewed literature, and the recommendations provided to the OGDP by FDA, the following are the risks associated with the health of users:

- Pregnancy—slippage, breakage, misdirection, or invagination of the device during vaginal intercourse probably results in the incidence of undesired pregnancy.
- Transmission of infection—failure of the device due to slippage, breakage, misdirection, or invagination, contact with infected semen or

vaginal secretions or vaginal/anal mucosa could result in the transmission of sexually transmitted infections (STIs).

- Adverse tissue reaction—when the patient-contacting materials of the device contact breached and compromised surfaces like vagina, cervix, anus, and external male and female genitalia and they are not biocompatible, the adverse reactions like cytotoxicity or systemic toxicity, local tissue irritation, skin sensitization occurs.
- Ulceration and other physical trauma—internal condom usage may cause abrasions, lacerations, bleeding, or other adverse effects in breached or compromised sites like vagina, anus, or penile tissue if the device is not designed appropriately.

The pregnancy and STI are the most common and clinically significant risks associated with the usage of single-use female condoms. To address these adversities, the following special controls were mentioned by the FDA, which has to be followed by the device for ensuring its safety and efficacy [26]:

- *Clinical testing*—is required to mitigate the risks occurred to female health. The following parameters can be assessed by clinical testing:
    - rate of total clinical failure of the device,
    - rate of individual failure modes (slippage, breakage, misdirection, invagination, and other failure modes as appropriate)

  when the device is used according to the intended usage (i.e., during vaginal and/or anal intercourse)
- *Nonclinical performance testing*—was conducted to determine the performance of the device as per the anticipated conditions of use
- *Contraceptive effectiveness study*—was conducted for evaluating the cumulative pregnancy rate, thus analyzing the contraception effect of the device indicated for vaginal intercourse
- *Cumulative pregnancy rate*—was determined based on contraceptive effectiveness study (when the intended use of the device is for vaginal intercourse)
- *Viral penetration study*—was conducted for demonstrating the effect of STIs, for analyzing the barrier property of the device
- *Mechanical testing*—was conducted to demonstrate the capacity of the device to withstand forces due to the anticipated usage. This can be helpful for the analysis of tensile, tear, and burst properties of the device
- *Compatibility testing*—the alterations in physical properties of the device that was adversely affected using additional lubricants were determined
- *Shelf-life testing*—conducted to analyze the performance characteristics and the packaging of the device that maintains its integrity for the proposed duration of shelf life.

Along with the above effects, the patient-contacting materials may cause adverse tissue reaction that was considered as an additional risk for the single-use condom. Hence, to mitigate the risk, the FDA has strictly proposed the *biocompatibility* testing for the device.

The FDA also suggested to list the following parameters to be mentioned on the label of the device [30]:

- associated risks and mitigation measures
- potential transmission of the infection
- adverse tissue reaction
- ulceration and/or other physical trauma
- personal and additional types of lubricants
- shelf-life of the device
- expiration date.

8.4 Toxicity of the devices—scientific evidences denoting their hazardous effect

However, OB/GYN devices have an ampoule amount of therapeutic effects, they are also showing a wide range of adverse effects. These adverse effects are life threatening occasionally. Some of the incidents reported were mentioned in this chapter. However, rather than mentioning all the adverse effects, only a few were documented in the lawsuit.

8.4.1 Urogynecologic surgical mesh implants

Surgical mesh is a kind of OB/GYN device, which is widely used in the females in the urbanized world. It provides support and repairs the weak and/or damaged tissue. The origin of the devices may be natural or synthetic.

Naturally, they are derived from animal tissues like intestine or skin, which was processed and disinfected for suitable use. The animals used is a pig (porcine) or cow (bovine). Most of the naturally prepared devices are absorbable.

Synthetically derived surgical meshes are made up of knitted mesh or nonknitted mesh sheet forms, and these materials may be absorbable or nonabsorbable or a combination of both.

The devices made of nonabsorbable materials remain in the body for a long time and considered as a permanent implant and they are responsible for providing permanent reinforcement and strength to the urogynecologic repair, whereas absorbable mesh degrades and loses its strength during the course of time, and is not intended to provide long-term reinforcement to the repair site. However, the degradation of material in absorbable mesh was intended to provide strength to the repair on the growth of the new tissue.

The major application of surgical mesh is to repair the pelvic organ prolapse (POP) and stress urinary incontinence (SUI). To repair the POP, support the urethra, and repair the SUI, surgical mesh was implanted permanently. The following are the three surgical procedures performed with surgical mesh for the treatment of pelvic floor disorders:

- transvaginal mesh to treat POP
- transabdominal mesh to treat POP
- mesh sling to treat SUI.

The above-mentioned individual procedures have their own risks and benefits. The following are the risks associated [31]:

- pain in the pelvic or vaginal area
- damage to the nerves
- a necessary revision surgery
- blockage of the urinary system
- ongoing incontinence
- mesh contraction or hardening
- organ perforation
- other possible consequences.

Due to the above consequences, the device was banned in New Zealand and Australia, but not in other countries, mainly the United States, as FDA has declined to outright the product. After several protests, on January 5, 2016, the FDA has reclassified the device into class III and required submission of PMA applications with more stringent review pathways. However, again, on April 16, 2019, the FDA has banned to sell these devices in the United States [32].

8.4.2 Contraceptive devices

The use of contraceptive devices reported many health complaints in females. On a wide-range analysis of clinical trial data, approximately 9% of women suffered from mild-to-moderate pain during the procedures, whereas 13% experienced delayed pain. The possible adverse effects reported on usage of contraceptive devices are as follows [33]:

- cramping
- vaginal bleeding
- nausea
- vomiting
- fainting
- pelvic or back pain for several days.

Long-term risks include the following:

- chronic pelvic pain
- allergic reactions
- ectopic pregnancies.

8.4.3 Intrauterine devices

IUD usage has resulted in the incidence of pelvic inflammatory diseases and subsequent tubal infertility. Many studies have proven their adversity. A study conducted by David, 2001, on pregnant and infertile controls, who has a previous history of contraceptive usage, has shown that IUDs cause tubular infertility along with *Chlamydia trachomatis* infection. The risk percentage was higher on the usage of copper IUDs [34].

There are many OB/GYN devices containing adverse effects; however, on considering the risk–benefit ratio and intended purpose, these devices were in the market and categorized under class II and class III depending on the rate of risk. Owing to this classification, the regulatory burden has increased on the devices for their acceptance, and the requirement of PMA is mandatory.

One such hormonal IUD that can be used for contraception, a long-term birth control, is *Mirena* [35], a T-shaped plastic frame that is inserted into the female uterus, where it releases a hormone called progestin. The following are the contraceptive mechanisms of Mirena:

- The mucus in the cervix is thickened by the progestin hormone to stop sperm reaching or fertilizing an egg.
- The device thins the uterine lining and suppress ovulation partially.

The device is effective for 5 years after its insertion and is approved by US-FDA. It can be used for the women of all ages, including teenagers, due to its following benefits:

- Usage of the device eliminates the need to interrupt sex for contraception.

- It does not require the participation of the partner.
- After insertion, the device stays for long term up to 5 years.
- Once the female's normal fertility was returned, it can be removed at any time.
- The device can be used during breastfeeding; however, waiting for 6–8 weeks after childbirth is recommended likely because earlier replacement may injure the uterus during the device placement.
- The device does not contain any side effects related to birth control methods containing estrogen.
- It can decrease menstrual bleeding after three or more months of its usage. After 1 year of its usage, the menstrual periods were stopped for 20% cases.
- It can decrease endometriosis pain and menstrual pain.
- It can decrease the risk of pelvic infection when compared to the other IUDs.
- It can decrease the risk of endometrial cancer when compared to the other IUDs.

The device can be prescribed for women with the following health complications:

- heavy menstrual bleeding
- cramping or pain with periods
- endometriosis
- endometrial hyperplasia or abnormal growth of the lining of the uterus
- adenomyosis or abnormal growth of uterine-lining tissue into the muscular wall of the uterus
- anemia
- fibroids.

The device can be prescribed for women with the following health complications:

- breast cancer
- uterine or cervical cancer
- abnormalities of the uterus, such as fibroids that interfere with the placement or retention of Mirena
- pelvic infection or current pelvic inflammatory disease
- unexplained vaginal bleeding.

Specific attention is needed in the following cases for device prescription:

- medications taking at present, including drugs without any prescription and herbal products

- having health complications like diabetes or high blood pressure
- a history of heart attack or feeble heart condition
- having migraine
- having hemorrhage or blood-clotting issues or stroke
- recent delivery or breastfeeding.

However, the device possesses its own risk. About 1% of females who are using Mirena may get conceived in a year, which may result in a higher risk of ectopic pregnancy where the fertilized egg gets implanted outside of the uterus, typically in a fallopian tube. However, the ectopic pregnancy risk was less in women using Mirena compared to the other women who are sexually active and not using contraception.

The other risks associated with Mirena are as follows:

- does not protect against STIs
- may cause perforation of the uterus during the device insertion and the risk was high during postpartum period.

The side effects associated with the device are as follows:

- headache
- acne
- breast tenderness
- irregular bleeding, which can improve after 6 months of use
- mood changes
- cramping or pelvic pain.

There is a risk of expelling the device from the uterus in the following conditions:

- have never been pregnant
- have heavy or prolonged periods
- have severe menstrual pain
- previously expelled an IUD
- age less than 20 years
- had Mirena inserted immediately after childbirth.

After insertion the healthcare provider may recommend for its removal if you develop the following complication:

- a pelvic infection
- inflammation of the endometrium (endometritis)
- endometrial or cervical cancer
- pelvic pain or pain during sex
- very severe migraine
- a significant increase in blood pressure, or have a stroke or heart attack
- possible exposure to an STI.

The device advised to be removed immediately if the above-mentioned complications were observed. During the removal, light bleeding and cramping are commonly observed, and the device removal can be more complicated.

The other IUD that is used for permanent birth control in women is *Essure* [36]. Once inserted, the birth control phenomena cannot be reversed. In this type of female sterilization, small metal and fiber coils were placed in fallopian tubes; this creates scar tissue preventing the sperm to reach the egg, thus inhibiting fertilization. During the procedure, along with Essure insertion, a flexible tube with a small camera (hysteroscope) was inserted through the vagina and cervix up to the uterus for doctor's observation to place the device at the right place in the fallopian tubule. For the prevention of pregnancy by showing its contraceptive activity it takes 3 months and, in some females, it may take even 6 months. Hence, during this time other forms of birth control procedures should be used. However, Essure cannot protect women from STIs.

The following are the benefits of using the Essure system:
- The risk of pregnancy is about 0.1% when the coils are placed at the proper place, indicating its efficiency of contraception.
- A little or no anesthesia is needed, and the procedure can be done in the doctor's office.
- Routine activities can be performed immediately.
- No incision or scarring of the skin will not be resulted.
- Usage of other contraceptive methods can be discontinued when the doctor assures the closure of fallopian tubes and working of the system.

No long-term side effects were observed in most of the women in spite of its contraceptive efficiency and long-term benefits, prescription of Essure is not suitable in certain cases, and opting other methods of contraception is recommended. The certain cases are as follows:
- if not sure to whether or not to become pregnant in future
- the materials used in manufacturing the device may contain traces of nickel or other metals; hence, metal allergy testing needs to be performed, and if it is positive, Essure should not be recommended
- if the female has a contrast (dye) allergy, the device should not be recommended as after insertion, a follow-up imaging test performed for functional monitoring of the device as the test use dye
- in conditions who are suffering from autoimmune diseases, which may trigger the excessive inflammation around the coil inserts

- in cases where abortion occurred within the past 6 weeks
- if recently had a pelvic infection
- if there is any health complication that blocks uterus or fallopian tubes openings, where the physician cannot insert the tube at proper place
- if the tubes are tied, that is, tubal ligation.

The research carried to identify the risks associated with the Essure found the following resulted in the following complications:

- pelvic pain
- allergic reaction, including hives, itching and face swelling
- heavy periods or spotting during ovulation
- infection from the procedure
- perforation of the uterus or fallopian tubes
- shifting of the coils to other places in the abdominal cavity.

In certain cases where the device is not placed properly or only one tube is blocked instead of two fallopian tubes, it may result in unintended pregnancy. However, it is very rare and only 1.5 out of 1000 people may get pregnant. Once the Essure system is implanted, pelvic procedures like electrosurgery and other types of endometrial ablation should not be done. Cramping, abdominal pain, and nausea or vomiting are common after the procedure, and the patient can return to their routine activities immediately.

However, these devices have long-term benefits, the safety is of primary concern, as they were in close contact with the biological system. Hence, the devices must clear PMA for their market approval.

8.5 Types of OB/GYN devices

The OB/GYN devices have a wide range of applications due to the growing gynecological complications in females. In the market, based on their applications, the gynecological devices were classified into the following types:

- *Surgical devices*
    - *Gynecological endoscopy devices*

        Hysteroscope

        Colposcope

        Resectoscope

Laparoscope
Endoscopic imaging systems
- *Female sterilization/contraceptive devices*
  Permanent birth control
  Intrauterine devices
  Intravaginal rings
  Subdermal contraceptive implants
- *Fluid management systems*
  - *Endometrial ablation devices*
    Hydrothermal ablation devices
    Radiofrequency ablation devices
    Balloon ablation devices
    Others (microwave, laser)
  - *Hand instruments*
    Vaginal speculum
    Tenaculum
    Curettes
    Trocars market
    Biopsy forceps
    Others
  - *Diagnostic imaging systems*
    MRI
    Ultrasound
    CT
    Radiology
    Mammography
    Others
  - *Gynecological chairs*
    Fixed—height
    Adjustable—height

8.6 Applications of OB/GYN devices [37]

OB/GYN devices have a wide range of applications associated. They are mainly designed for the management of the female's reproductive system, pregnancy, and childbirth.

The gynecological instruments used for implantation in the female reproductive system are as follows:

Vaginal dilator (variable rigidity)—it was inserted into the vaginal canal with pain-free vaginal dilation. The device was associated with an inflatable balloon that avoids insertion into the urethra. Air was introduced into the balloon initially; when the patient was confident about its usage, water was introduced and the balloon expands; thus, the vaginal canal expands, and the pressure was exerted. The vaginal contact with the device was continued for a period of 15 minutes and the pressure and/or contact time was increased gradually to a maximum of 12 atmospheres and 45 minutes of contact according to the regimen and instructions of a patient's health.

Stented anchoring of gastric space-occupying devices—these devices are provided with a stent configured with gastrointestinal tract, specifically the esophagus or the stomach for treating their deployment. To secure the stent, an expandable member with the stent that expands the patient's stomach was provided. On its expansion, the expandable member occupies a predefined volume in a patient's stomach, which is further tethered to deploy the stent, thus retaining or anchoring the expandable member within the stomach. Methods and systems for deploying the space-occupying devices are also provided.

Electrical detection of anatomic wall penetration and delineation of atomic structures during surgery—these are the devices and methods that are intended for the detection and/or prevention of intraoperative full-thickness penetration of anatomic walls and provide delineation of anatomic structures during surgery.

Minimally invasive rectal balloon apparatus—it was provided with a shaft along with a fluid passageway extension. At the end of the shaft, a balloon was provided; thus, the fluid passageway communicates with the interior of the balloon. When the balloon gets inflated, a laterally flat surface will be opened with the formation of a longitudinal groove. Upon its inflation, the balloon will possess a pair of bulges. Adjacent to the balloon, a ring was affixed to the shaft. The shaft has a plurality of holes formed thereon opening to an interior of the balloon.

Medical implant—they are the devices and methods intended to deliver and place a surgical sling without resorting to an abdominal incision.

Methods, systems, and devices for performing gynecological procedures—they are employed to perform gynecological procedures. For assessment of the peritoneal cavity of the patient, the device was inserted through the vaginal cavity, the cervix, and the uterus of the patient according to the embodiment.

Systems, an apparatus, and a method for treating a sexually dysfunctional female patient—a specific apparatus, as a system and a method is available for treating sexual dysfunction in a female patient. The apparatus provided with an expandable prosthesis that was adapted for implantation in the female erectile tissue and was adapted to be adjusted to temporarily achieve the enlarged status of the female erectile tissue.

Fallopian tube occlusion device—it is a device containing a retention member and a mesh material, which occludes a fallopian tube. The retention member has two properties: the first one is a lower profile configuration for delivery and the second one is expanded configuration for placement within the fallopian tube. The mesh material is specially designed with a configuration to block the passage of an egg through the tube. To secure the retention member to the fallopian tube, the member has a plurality of tube engagement members.

Method and apparatus for implanting an occlusive structure—it is a method to treat vein by implanting a bioabsorbable fibrous body into the vein through an access point spaced from a saphenofemoral junction. Toward the saphenofemoral junction, the body is moved in the vein.

Less traumatic method of delivery of mesh-based devices into the human body—a method including the extension of a dilator into the body of a patient in the first direction, such as a distal end portion of dilator extending from the body was included in some embodiments. The lament was defined through the lumen. When the distal end portion extends from the body, a portion of the dilator gets disposed of within the body. A small portion of the implant is passed through the lumen defined by the dilator. By moving the dilator in the first direction, the dilator is removed from the body.

Disposable gynecologic instrument for dilation of body cavities by fluid injection—a disposable kind of gynecological instrument used for dilation of body cavities of females by injecting fluid includes an instrument body—to which the bottom has fixed tightly with a fixed handle, a reservoir—which is in the frontal part of the instrument body, a projected trigger—which is positioned in a sliding manner and provided with a screw designed for pressing with two fingers, a main piston—where the screw is connected, the piston can be moved within a cylinder, where a bigger spring is placed around it and the outlet of the cylinder is connected to one branch of three-way pipeline and the remaining two are connected with an upper irreversible valve and lower irreversible valve, a front side of the instrument body that was attached to the screw thread and a sealingly attached main pipe and formed by longitudinal ribs, which were positioned crosswise and a series of ribs were placed in a slope of circular perimeter that increases the stiffness.

Balloon with a rigid tube for occluding the uterine artery—the apparatus is intended to be inserted in the subject's body regions vagina, vaginal fornix, uterus, and uterine artery. The apparatus was provided with a fornix-engaging structure that is inserted into the vagina, where it engages vaginal fornix. Through the fornix-engaging structure, a rod was inserted into the subject's body where it passes through the distal end of the rod through vaginal tissue at a first vaginal site until the distal end of the rod is at a first extrauterine site outside of the uterine artery, but in a vicinity of a portion of the uterine artery that supplies a uterine fibroid. To the fornix-engaging structure, a rod guide is a couple, and it guides the distal end of the rod to the first extrauterine site. At the distal end of the rod, a uterine artery compression device is disposed.

In situ materials formation—To deliver two or more fluent prepolymer solutions without premature crosslinking, a delivery system was configured and the methods and apparatus of hydrogel systems formation in situ were provided. The delivery system comprises the following—first and second *lumens* coupling first and second *inlet ports* and first and second *outlet ports*; they include a balloon, a flexible distal region, a mixing chamber, and a steerable distal end.

System and methods for preventing intravasation during intrauterine procedures—for improved gynecologic and urologic procedures, systems, methods, apparatus, and devices were designed. With the improved outcomes, reduction in pain, peri-procedural pain, and reduced recovery time patient benefit may be achieved. In a hospital setting, such as a doctor's office or clinic, various embodiments enabled procedures were performed. Rather than liquid distension media method, the mechanical distension method was employed and thus the risk of intravasation was eliminated.

Laparoscopic vaginal cuff occlude—for prevention of fluid flowing through the vagina, the embodiments comprised an apparatus and methodology. The apparatus comprised an introducer for insertion into the patient's vagina along with an expandable device coupled to the introducer. The expandable device was configured for expansion into substantially sealing engagement with an inner wall of the patient's vagina once the introducer is located within the patient's vagina. After expansion, the device can maintain fluid pressure in the abdominal cavity of the patient after a fluid connection that has been made with the vagina and the abdominal cavity.

Aneurysm sealing device—the device comprised first and second inflatable discs that are adjacent to each other with fluid communication. The discs were sized and constructed, which were inflated; thus, the aneurysm neck is engaged. The discs comprised a single wall that is inelastic and included with an internal member limiting the expansion in a direction parallel to the device axis. The aspect ratio is greater than 3 for the inflatable discs.

Canal dilation device—used for enlargement of the canal of a human or animal subject, including an elongate member and an inflatable body toward a distal end of the elongate member. In an uninflated or deflated state, the inflated body was delivered within the canal before inflation. With the inflatable body, the first lumen is in communication via one or more channels in between, thus enlarging the canal and it may include markings for sounding of, for example, uterine depth. One or more projections or other structure providing tactile cues were included during the positioning of the device within the canal and was configured to aid in the removal of cells from a tissue wall.

The other methods and apparatus/devices used for the treatment of female patients are as follows:

- Fallopian tube occlusion system
- Apparatus and method for preventing fluid transfer between on oviduct and a uterine cavity
- Delivery methods and devices for implantable bronchial isolation devices
- Treatment methods utilizing an inflatable dual balloon catheter
- Variable rigidity vaginal dilator and use thereof
- Cervical occluder
- Sexual stimulation devices and methods
- Methods of using in situ hydration of hydrogel articles for sealing or augmentation of tissue or vessels
- System and method for treating tissue wall prolapse
- Fibroid treatment apparatus and method
- High performance balloon catheter/component
- Composite flexible and conductive catheter electrode
- Devices and methods for occluding a fallopian tube
- Device and method for restricting blood flow to fibroids
- Erogenic stimulator with an expandable bulbous end
- Pessary device
- Single balloon ripening device with novel inserter and inflator

- Body canal dilation system
- Cervical dilator catheter
- Pelvic floor health articles and procedures
- Method of forming medical devices: intravascular occlusion devices
- Method and device for distending a gynecological cavity
- *Systems, methods, and devices for performing gynecological procedures*
- Vaginal dilator for use in vaginal rehabilitation and methods therefor
- Method and device for filtering body fluid
- Methods, systems, and devices for performing gynecological procedures
- Cryo balloon treatment for postpartum hemorrhage
- Methods and apparatus for intraluminal deposition of hydrogels
- Tissue electroperforation for enhanced drug delivery
- Cervical medical device, system, and method
- Inflatable dual balloon catheter
- System and method for treating urinary tract disorders
- Methods of using in situ hydration of hydrogel articles for sealing or augmentation of tissue or vessels
- In case of abnormal vaginal bleeding, vagina and cervix must be examined
- In case of cervical cancer screening, cervical smear must be taken
- High and well-experienced personnel is needed for insertion or removal of Intrauterine cervical devices
- For excluding infections, vaginal or cervical swab must be removed
- Allow the uterine sounds introduction.

8.7 Market range of the OB/GYN devices [38]

The global market size of the gynecological devices is valued at USD 8.9 billion in 2018. During the forecast period, it was anticipated to exhibit a CAGR of 8.4%. Advancement of the devices with an increased efficiency of minimally invasive procedures and imaging devices such as 3D endoscope has provided an intense boost to the growth of the market. Increased prevalence of obstetrics and gynecological diseases and conditions such as cervical cancer, uterine cancer, polycystic ovary syndrome, vaginal melanoma, extended bleeding, and irregular menstrual cycles

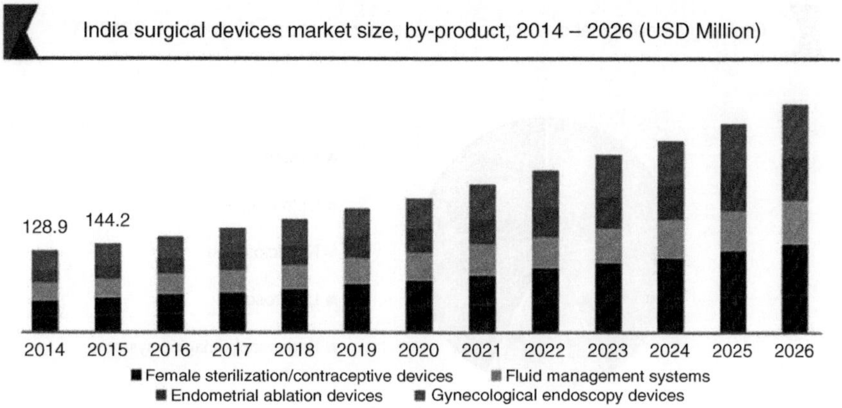

Figure 8.1 Market size of surgical devices in India, a by-product in the period of 2014–2026. *Based on www.grandviewresearch.com*

provided an increased demand for gynecological treatment. Despite this, growth in the number of new cases of feminine diseases and conditions is registered every year for raising awareness regarding the benefits of regular check-ups (Fig. 8.1).

As per the United Nations, published data of about 3.64 billion female population were accounted for various gynecological problems. The most common problems associated are menstrual problems and pregnancy. Increased awareness and frequent check-ups for the prevention of STDs have increased, which in turn stir up the demand for gynecological devices.

Demand for surgical devices has increased due to surgical procedures such as ablation, laparoscopy, endoscopy, and female sterilization. New innovations and technically advanced products add a spur to the growth of the market for a forecast period.

However, for product safety and restraining the growth of the market, stringent regulatory approval procedures were maintained. Alternative therapies such as personalized medicines and improved drug therapies are rapidly developing for inhibition of OB.GYN devices growth of the market (Fig. 8.2).

8.8 Conclusion

With the growing urbanized system and wide range of changes in daily life, there is an increased gynecological problem in females. Hence,

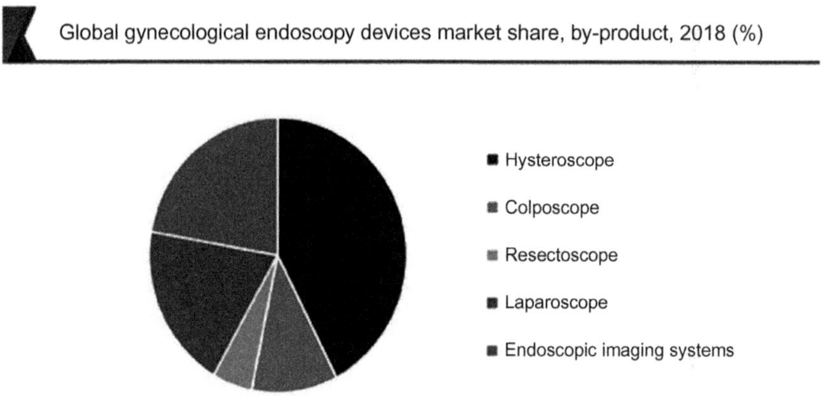

Figure 8.2 Market share of gynecological endoscopy devices globally, a by-product in 2018. *Based on www.grandviewresearch.com*

various types of treatment were in the market for the therapy of gynecological problems in females. OB/GYN devices were used for the treatment and diagnosis of gynecological problems. Most of the OB/GYN devices used are contraceptive devices and intrauterine devices. With the increasing demand, the complications and adverse effects associated with the devices are increasing. Hence, a stringent regulatory guideline is required for the approval of the devices. However, the present guidelines are more organized and require the device to pass through PMA before marketing the product.

References

[1] Obstrectics and gynaecology. Wikipedia. <https://en.wikipedia.org/wiki/Obstetrics_and gynaecology/>. Updated 20 August 2019.

[2] Medical device, recall and approval process: study recommends stricter FDA regulation. Recall center. <https://www.recallcenter.com/medical-device-recall-approval--process-study-recommend-stricter-fda-regulation/#2/>. Updated on June 2017.

[3] Obstrectics and gynecology devices panel. U.S. Food & Drug Administration. <https://www.fda.gov/advisory-committees/medical-devices-advisory-committee/obstetrics-and-gynecology-devices-panel/>. Updated on March 2018.

[4] Obstetrical and gynecological devices. Federal Register. <https://www.govinfo.gov/content/pkg/FR-2017-12-28/pdf/2017-28042.pdf/>. Published on December 2017.

[5] Teo ZWW, Schalock PC. Hypersensitivity reactions to implanted metal devices: facts and fictions. J Investig Allergol Clin Immunol 2016;26(5):279–94. Available from: https://doi.org/10.18176/jiaci.0095.

[6] D'Ambrosio F, Ricciardi L, Isola S, Gangemi S, Cilia M, Levanti C, et al. Systemic contact dermatitis to copper-containing IUD. Allergy 1996;51:658–9.

[7] Rongioletti F, Rivara G, Rebora A. Contact dermatitis to a copper-containing intrauterine device. Contact Dermat 1985;13:343.

[8] Pujol RM, Randazzo L, Miralles J, Alomar A. Perimenstrual dermatitis secondary to a copper-containing intrauterine contraceptive device. Contact Dermat 1998;38:288.

[9] Barkoff JR. Urticaria secondary to a copper intrauterine device. Int J Dermatol 1976;15:594–9.

[10] Barranco VP. Eczematous dermatitis caused by internal exposure to copper. Arch Dermatol 1972;106:386–7.

[11] Essure® is the only FDA-approved, minimally invasive procedure for permanent birth control. Essure. <https://www.hcp.essure-us.com/>. Updated December 2018.

[12] Meeting materials of the obstetrics and gynecology devices panel. U.S. Food and Drug Administration. <http://www.fda.gov/AdvisoryCommittees/CommitteesMeetingMaterials/MedicalDevices/MedicalDevicesAdvisoryCommittee/ObstetricsandGynecologyDevices/ucm463457.html/>.

[13] FDA activities: Essure. U.S. Food & Drug Administration. <https://www.fda.gov/medical-devices/essure-permanent-birth-control/fda-activities-essure/>. Published on June 2019.

[14] 21 CFR § 884.4350 – Fetal head elevator. Cornell Law School. <https://www.law.cornell.edu/cfr/text/21/884.4350/>.

[15] Medical devices; obstetrical and gynecological devices; classification of the fetal head elevator. Federal register. <https://www.federalregister.gov/documents/2017/12/19/2017-27277/medical-devices-obstetrical-and-gynecological-devices-classification-of-the-fetal-head-elevator/>. Updated December 2017.

[16] ISO 10993-1:2018. Biological evaluation of medical devices – Part 1: Evaluation and testing within a risk management process. <https://www.iso.org/standard/68936.html/>. Published on August 2018.

[17] ISO 10993-5:2009. Biological evaluation of medical devices – Part 1: Tests for in vitro cytotoxicity. Published on July 2009.

[18] ISO/AWI 10993-10:2009. Biological evaluation of medical devices—Part 10: Tests for skin sensitization. <www.iso.org/standard/75279.html/>.

[19] ISO 10993-11:2017. Biological evaluation of medical devices – Part 11: Tests for systemic toxicity. <www.iso.org/standard/68426.html/>. Published on September 2017.

[20] ISO 10993-6:2016. Biological evaluation of medical devices—Part 6: Tests for local effects after implantation. <www.iso.org/standard/61089.html/>. Published on December 2016.

[21] ISO 10993-3:2014. Biological evaluation of medical devices—Part 3: Tests for genotoxicity, carcinogenicity and reproductive toxicity. <www.iso.org/standard/55614./html/>. Published on October 2014.

[22] ISO 10993-4:2017. Biological evaluation of medical devices—Part 4: Selection of tests for interactions with blood. <www.iso.org/standard/63448.html/>. Published on April 2017.

[23] FDA tightening regulatory requirements for some medical devices. NPR. <https://www.npr.org/sections/health-shots/2019/03/04/689739642/fda-tightening-regulatory-requirements-for-some-medical-devices/>. Updated on March 2019.

[24] OB/GYN clinical service rules and regulations 2014. <www.sfdph.org/dph/hc/JCC/SFGH/Agendas/2015/Jan%2027/09c%20OBGYN%20Rules%20and%20Regulations%202014%20(3).pdf/>.

[25] Timothy MJ, Ghobadi Comeron W, Xu Shuai, Jessica RW. Overview of high-risk medical device recalls in obstetrics and gynecology from 2002 through 2016: implications for device safety. Am J Obstet Gynecol 2017;. Available from: https://doi.org/10.1016/j.ajog.2017.03.021.

[26] Federal register. <https://members.wto.org/crnattachments/2018/TBT/USA/18_0276_00_e.pdf/>. Updated on December 2017.

[27] What are 510(k) clearance and premarket approval?. Device watch. <https://www.devicewatch.org/reg/reg.shtml/>. Published on April 2008.

[28] Walter Jessica R, Hayman Emily, Tsai Shelun, Ghobadi Comeron W, Shuai X. Medical device approvals through the premarket approval pathway in obstetrics and gynecology from 2000 to 2015 process and problems. Obstet Gynecol 2016;127 (6):1–8.

[29] General hospital and personal use devices; reclassification of sharps needle destruction device. Federal register. <https://www.federalregister.gov/documents/2017/11/07/2017-24191/general-hospital-and-personal-use-devices-reclassification-of-sharps-needle-destruction-device/>. Published on July 2017.

[30] Gynecological mesh: the medical device that has 100,000 women suing. Pharma Watch Dog.<https://www.pharmawatchdog.com/gynecological-mesh-medical-device-100000-women-suing/>.

[31] Urogynecologic surgical mesh implants. U.S. Food & Drug Administration. <https://www.fda.gov/medical-devices/implants-and-prosthetics/urogynecologic-surgical-mesh-implants/>. Updated October 2019.

[32] FDA to take another look at Essure contraceptive device after health complaints. NPR. <https://www.npr.org/sections/health-shots/2015/07/14/421745255/safety-worries-lead-fda-to-take-another-look-at-essure-contraceptive/>. Updated July 2015.

[33] David H, Roger LR, Douglas JT, Fernando GI, Raymundo GR. Use of copper intrauterine devices and the risk of tubal infertility among nulligravid women. N Engl J Med 2001;345:561–7.

[34] Inserted in female reproductive system patents (Class 606/193). Justia patents. <https://patents.justia.com/patents-by-us-classification/606/193?page = 2/>.

[35] Mirena (hormonal IUD). Mayo clinic. <https://www.mayoclinic.org/tests-procedures/mirena/about/pac-20391354/>.

[36] Essure. Mayo clinic. <https://www.mayoclinic.org/tests-procedures/essure/about/pac-20394017/>.

[37] Gynecological devices market analysis report by product (handheld instruments, diagnostic imaging devices, surgical devices, software), by region, competitive landscape, and segment forecasts, 2019–2026. <https://www.grandviewresearch.com/industry-analysis/gynecological-device-market/>. Published on February 2019.

[38] Global OB-GYN ultrasound systems detailed analysis report 2017–2022. <https://marketdesk.org/report/global-ob-gyn-ultrasound-systems-market-2017-dar/>. Published on December 2019.

CHAPTER NINE

Urology and nephrology

Pralhad Wangikar*, Praveen Kumar Gupta, Bhagyashree Choudhari and Rajeev Sharma
PRADO, Preclinical Research and Development Organization, Pvt. Ltd., Pune, Maharashtra, India
*Corresponding author

Abstract

The use of implants in urology has experienced exponential growth in the recent past. Urological implants are used for the correction of functional deficits and to improve the quality of lives of affected patients. The urological implants varied from little more than a silicone tube using single biomaterial to a combination of biomaterials such as polymer on metal, metal stents, and biodegradable stents and to active energy emitting implants that have energy sources or are designed to selectively absorb or respond to energy like brachytherapy seeds used in prostate cancer. The development of implantable genitourinary prostheses has similarly grown from simple testicular substitutes to the large group of implantable penile prostheses, artificial urinary sphincters and possible future developments of the artificial bladder, urethral materials, and artificial implantable kidneys. Growing awareness about the benefits of implantable devices, in terms of abridged treatment and recovery time and advanced technology, is propelling the market in developing various devices for urological diseases.

Although these devices and implants provide great benefits to patients, they also present risks associated with the anatomic site as well as the host's immunologic response. Therefore toxicological testing plays a very important role in accelerating the discovery of new implants by supporting product development and validation, enhancing the quality of the product, and getting the regulatory approvals within stipulated timelines. This chapter presents a brief overview of urological implants used in some of the commonly observed urological diseases and their toxicological evaluation. The basic pathophysiology of each disease has been discussed considering that the development of respective implants might have some correlations with stages of the disease. The tests employed in toxicological assessment of the urological implants have some links with complications associated with their use; hence, complications are briefly touched upon. One section has been devoted to describing various models, assays, or tests employed for assessment of efficacy, implant performance, and safety. The chapter concludes with summarizing the aspects of the toxicological evaluation of urological implants, the role of pathology in the safety evaluation of urology implants, and future trends in the development of urological implants.

Keywords: Urological implants; toxicological assessment; urinary incontinence; prostate cancer; ureteral obstruction; penile prosthesis

Toxicological Aspects of Medical Device Implants.
DOI: https://doi.org/10.1016/B978-0-12-820728-4.00009-5
© 2020 Elsevier Inc.
All rights reserved.

9.1 Introduction

9.1.1 Urology diseases and incidence

Historically, the urinary tract is divided into an upper tract, consisting of the collecting duct, renal pelvis, and ureters and lower tract consisting of urinary bladder and urethra. From the urodynamic point, this system is considered as one unit that is completely interdependent [1]. According to the American Urological Association Foundation (AUAF), kidney and ureteral stones, urinary incontinence (UI), benign prostatic hyperplasia, cancer of the prostate, and urinary tract infections (UTIs) are among the most common urological diseases. Annually, more than 661,000 Americans suffer from kidney failure and 468,000 patients are given dialysis. UTIs are one of the most common microbial diseases affecting people of all age groups. Globally, UTIs affect around 150 million people every year. Diabetic patients have a higher risk of developing UTIs and complications associated with it. With a global increase in the diabetic population, complications, like dysuria and organ damage that are associated with UTIs, are also on the rise.

There are many urologic disorders and diseases. The urologic diseases describe a wide variety of conditions, all related to the filtering and carrying of urine out of the body. These diseases can affect men, women, and children of all ages. Some of the diseases identified as common by the AUAF are kidney and ureteral stones, urinary incontinence, prostate cancer, and erectile dysfunction [2]. With high incidence rates and health complications associated with urological diseases, there is an increasing demand for healthcare interventions to manage them, which, in turn, is propelling the market of urology healthcare products including surgical and diagnostic devices.

9.1.2 Importance of medical devices and implants

Medical devices play a crucial role in the treatment and diagnosis of illness and disease. New medical devices are being developed to save lives, treat disease and injury, and improve the quality of life for patients around the world. They range from common medical supplies (bandages, hospital gowns) to complex instruments that help to save and sustain life (heart valves, artificial pancreas). They include tools that aid in the detection of disease (MRIs, in vitro diagnostics) and digital technology that is driving a revolution in healthcare (medical apps, surgical planning tools, closed-loop drug-delivery devices).

Medical implants are devices or tissues when they are partly or totally introduced, surgically or medically, into the human body or on the surface of the body and are intended to remain there after the procedure. Many implants are prosthetics, which are intended to replace missing body parts. Some implants are made from skin, bone, or other body tissues. Others are made from metal, plastic, ceramic, or other materials. Many implants deliver medications, monitor body functions, or provide support to organs and tissues [3,4].

In the past six decades, implantable medical devices or systems have been advanced through developments in science and engineering, especially in microelectronics, biotechnology, and materials. Medical experts have exerted honorable efforts to improve the quality of patients' lives with various medical devices, such as the implantable cardiac defibrillator, cochlear implants, implanted bladder stimulator, and implantable wireless pressure sensors [5].

9.1.3 Development of implants

Spurring innovation to develop safer, more effective devices and implants that address unmet needs is also about improving patient safety. Thus speeding up the development of medical devices/implants has a great number of potential benefits such as abridged recovery and treatment time, gaining more easy access to patients and physicians. At the same time, the pathway from ideation to widespread patient use is highly regulated, complicated, time consuming, and expensive. As device technology continues to evolve and the types of medical devices expand exponentially, it is important to assure that reasonable device safety must also keep pace. We must be vigilant in protecting and promoting public health by minimizing unnecessary risks at all stages of a device's development, evaluation, and marketing, as innovation and safety of medical devices are two sides of the same coin.

9.1.4 Toxicological testing and its importance

Toxicological testing plays a very important role in accelerating the discovery and development of medical devices, enhancing the quality of the product and getting the regulatory approvals within stipulated timelines by supporting product development and validation. A toxicological risk assessment or biological risk assessment will provide an acceptable level of reassurance to the patients in a clinical investigation. Urology has seen dramatic changes over the past 20 years. It has moved from an open surgical specialty with few drug treatments to a specialty that has enthusiastically embraced endoscopic (minimally invasive) techniques for common conditions such as erectile dysfunction and urinary incontinence. The advances that have occurred in the past few years have been mainly in the treatment of diseases that are becoming more common as the population ages. These include urological malignancies, prostate and bladder cancer, as well as lower urinary tract symptoms in older men and urinary incontinence and urinary tract infections, particularly in older women.

The pathway of development of urology implants from ideation to widespread patient use is highly regulated, complicated, time consuming, and expensive. It involves many steps, each requiring specialized knowledge and expertise. The main aim of the toxicological assessment of urological implants is that the device will not compromise the clinical condition or safety of the patient or user or other persons.

Analysis of risks associated with the use of urological implants should be weighed against the benefits to the patient. An appropriate toxicological risk assessment and state of the art risk-benefit analysis must be carried out by qualified personnel so that it can ensure that public health is not endangered. In this chapter, we have identified commonly occurring urology diseases, explained the pathophysiology of each disease as the development of implants might be related to the stages of the disease, and reported complications associated with the use of implants and tests, and assays employed in the assessment of the toxicological or biological risk of these urological implants. The consideration has been given to the toxic endpoints based on the specifics of the individual implants. Already available data from other sources that allowed evaluation of the hazard have been studied.

Although there are various disease conditions affecting the urinary system, we have presented the following commonly found urological diseases and implants used in their treatment:

- ureteral obstruction
- urinary incontinence
- prostate cancer
- erectile dysfunction.

9.2 Ureteral obstruction

9.2.1 Etiology

A ureteral obstruction, impairment in urine flow within the upper urinary tract, is a blockage in one or both of the tubes (ureters) that carry urine from the kidneys to the urinary bladder. This impairment may result from either mechanical or functional obstruction in the kidney or ureters. Mechanical obstruction might be due to foreign bodies, tumors, inflammation, congenital, or acquired abnormalities, while functional obstruction might be related to ureterovesical reflux and neurological bladder [6].

The etiology of ureteral obstruction might be due to the anatomic relationship of the obstruction to the ureteral wall—either intrinsic or extrinsic. Intrinsic obstruction describes obstruction within the kidney or in the lumen of the urinary tract due to ureteropelvic junction stenosis, stone, ureteral stricture, or secondary to genitourinary malignancies. Extrinsic obstruction is due to a benign or malignant process originating outside the urinary tract. A ureteral stricture is characterized by a narrowing of the ureteral lumen, causing a functional obstruction. Ureteric strictures (narrowing) can develop at different locations. They are more frequent in the lower third of the ureter. However, they can be located at multiple sites, may extend over a long segment, and can be bilateral [7–9].

9.2.2 Pathophysiology of ureteral obstructions

The ureters are approximately 25 cm in length and allow transport of urine from the kidney to the bladder via peristalsis. The wall of the ureter is composed of three layers: the mucosa, muscularis, and adventitia. Different from other transport tubules such as the GI tract, the ureter lacks the connective tissue layer known as the submucosa. The innermost mucosa layer is further divided into the transitional epithelium, which prevents urine absorption, and the lamina propria, a relatively thick layer of connective tissue. The mucosa typically exhibits a folded morphology. However, as peristaltic waves travel the ureter, the folds can stretch and increase the diameter of the ureter dramatically. The muscularis responsible for peristaltic motion is composed of two bands of smooth muscle orthogonally oriented in longitudinal and circular directions. This muscle contracts in a wave-like motion to form boluses of urine that move along the ureter in the inferior direction. It has been reported that the pressure generated by the peristalsis can be as high as 1.9 kgf/cm^2. The outermost adventitia layer is composed of areolar connective tissue, and its primary purpose is to anchor the ureter to the posterior abdominal wall. It has been observed that the ureter has three physiologic narrowings: first, where the ureter connects to the kidney, the ureteropelvic junction; second, where it crosses over the iliac vessel; finally, where it connects to the bladder, the ureterovesical junction. The ureteropelvic junction and ureterovesical junction are the locations where stones are most likely to be trapped. These three narrowings also limit retrograde instrumentation such as placement of a ureteral stent [10–12].

Ureteral obstruction may become life threatening, either due to increased intrarenal pressure (which may stop urine production and over time cause kidney failure) or by causing an infection. To remove the obstruction, the pressure must be relieved. This may be done by direct drainage of the kidney (a nephrostomy) or via the insertion of a stent [13].

9.2.3 Implants used to treat ureteral obstruction

Ureteral stents are minimally invasive tools to preserve the drainage of renal pelvis whenever ureteral patency is at risk to be obstructed due to extrinsic or intrinsic etiologies. FDA regulation, 21 CFR 876.4620 (a), describes ureteral stent or ureteric stent as a tube-like implanted device that is inserted into the ureter to provide ureteral rigidity and allow the passage of urine.

Indications that determine when to use a ureteral stent can be broadly organized under six main classifications: (1) relief of a ureteral obstruction; (2) adjunct to stone therapy; (3) perioperative placement to provide a mold around which healing can occur, where they act as scaffold over which epithelium grows; (4) management of urolithiasis where they are used for obstruction and hydronephrosis relief; (5) relief of ureteral strictures, may be ureteropelvic junction obstruction and to relieve pain; and (6) for relief of extrinsic malignant ureteral obstruction [14].

Ideal characteristics of perfect stent shall include the following: ability and strength to hold in position, radio-opaque material, surface coating and design of stent, easy manipulation of its shape, and excellent tensile strength. The stent should be able to present in ureter without degradation of its structure and function (biodurability) and without influencing urothelium (biocompatibility). Furthermore, from a clinician's point, an ideal stent should be easy to implant, maintain ureter patency with no additional interventions, allow longer intervals between stent exchange, be easy to remove, be patient comfort, and be resistant to bacterial colonization.

As its first description in the literature in 1952, the ureteral stent has undergone a plethora of evolutionary changes to become the ubiquitous tool urologists use today. The first stent described was little more than a silicone tube, while it provided adequate drainage; it frequently migrated into the bladder. However, in 1967, ureter specific stent was designed by Gibbons. This stent was barbed on the exterior and had a "C" shaped bend at the proximal end to prevent the stent from moving up or down the ureter. In 1978 there was the introduction of the double-pigtail and double-J stents; since this modern-day stent, the development of stents has evolved to include softer biomaterials that are more resistant to encrustation and infection [15].

There are three main classes of materials that are employed to fabricate ureteric stents: polymers, metals, and biodegradable/bioabsorbable materials.

1. Polymeric stents

Polymeric stents are manufactured with synthetic polymeric compounds. Many materials have been proposed for use in ureteral stents such as the following: *polyethylene*, a synthetic polymer, was one of the first materials to be used. It has good rigidity for stent placement but was discarded due to the tendency to fragment as well as its stiffness and brittleness properties. *Silicone* is considered as "gold standard" material for ureteral stents, its uniform surface makes it less prone to encrustation and its inertness makes it ideal for long implantation. However, its high coefficient of friction makes implantation difficult; therefore, silicone is almost never used without some sort of surface coating. In addition, it is difficult to handle because of its softness and elasticity, particularly in the presence of tortuous ureters and extrinsic compression. *Polyurethane (PU)* is a polymer composed of an organic group attached via carbamate groups ($-NHCO_2-$). It combines the elastic properties of silicone with the rigidity of polyethylene. However, still, PU is not the ideal biomaterial to be used in ureteral stents because of its stiffness, prone to encrustation, reported ureteral erosion and ulceration, and discomfort in patients. *Silitek*, produced by ACMI, property of Surgitek (Racine, WI), is a proprietary polyester copolymer made to replace silicone. It is firm and has a high radial stiffness to resist compression. Studies have shown that it has an encrustation profile similar to silicone. It has relatively weak coil retention strength that may make it more likely to migrate. *C-flex*, the property of Consolidated Polymer Technologies (Clearwater, FL), is a polymer made up of styrene/ethylene-butylene/styrene block copolymers. It has thermoplastic properties; however, it is a comparatively weak stent and is more prone to encrustation. *Percuflex* is a proprietary olefinic block copolymer and is another thermosetting PU. Percuflex softens in the body and has better physical properties than PU. However, encrustation is similar to standard PU and can easily get compressed [16–18].

2. Metal stents

Metal stents are first applied in urology in 1988 and have a longer dwell time and less stent change-associated morbidities. Four general types of metal stents are currently available: self-expandable, balloon-expandable, covered, and thermoexpandable shape-memory stents. Metal stents have been designed with the objective to overcome the disadvantages of polymeric stents, to preserve long-term urinary drainage avoiding the need for frequent exchange. Metallic stents are much cheaper than polymeric stents; however, a common problem of the metal stent is that it induces local tissue hyperplasia, with ingrowth of urothelial tissue through the structure of the stent that in a long term may result in recurrent obstruction [9].

3. Biodegradable stents

These stents get absorbed over time, obviating the need for cystoscopic removal, and thus mitigating procedure-related complications, cost, and patient discomfort. Their reliability of complete dissolution and controllability of degradation rate remains to be perfected. The benefit of the biodegradable ureteral stent is due to its physical properties of change in the surface as the stent degrades due to erosion, decreasing the bacterial adhesion and encrustation development. Additionally, biodegradable materials being softer give more patient comfort [19]. Biodegradable stents are made with high molecular weight polymers such as polyglycolide, polylactide, and uriprene. Materials used in the design of biodegradable ureteral stents can be divided into synthetic materials such as polylactic acid and poly(lactic-coglycolic acid) blends and natural origin materials (alginate, gellan gum, and gelatin blends). Absorbable metals, also known as biodegradable metals, are metals that corrode gradually in vivo with an appropriate host response, and then they dissolve completely while assisting tissue healing. More recent research has reported the use of biodegradable metal materials such as magnesium [20,21,22,23]. Iron (Fe), magnesium (Mg), zinc (Zn), and their alloys are among the studied absorbable metals and have shown their safety and efficacy when tested in animals [24,25].

To prevent the encrustation and bacterial adhesions and for easier implantation, various coatings have been tried. Hyaluronic acid is a glycosaminoglycan that inhibits the nucleation, growth, and aggregation of salts. Heparin is a highly sulfated glycosaminoglycan that is known as an anticoagulant, and it prevents biofilm formation due to its electronegativity repelling proteins and microorganisms. Polyvinylpyrrolidone is a water-absorbing polymer. Owing to its excellent wetting properties, it is used for coating ureteral stents, and the water layer prevents bacterial adhesion [26,27].

9.2.4 Complications of ureteral stents used

Ureteral stenting is the most common procedure in urology; despite their extensive use, these ureteral stents are fraught with a wide array of complications. Understanding these complications will help to identify how stent design and its clinical use can be improved. The following are some of the complications of ureteral stents.

9.2.4.1 Stent discomfort (irritative bladder symptom)

The most common adverse effect of both acute and chronic stenting is stent-related discomfort. Patients who are stented for benign disease experience irritative voiding symptoms, as well as pain and discomfort that is not restricted to the urinary tract but involves the whole body [28,29]. Giannarini et al. [30] and Al-Kandari et al. [31], in different experiments, identified that positioning of the distal stent loop within the bladder as a cause for stent-associated discomfort and also excessive stent length in the bladder that contributed to severe dysuria, urgency, and more impaired quality of life than correct stent length. Pain often worsens during micturition and can radiate to the ipsilateral flank secondary to ureteral pressure reflux and stent movement, both of which act via different mechanisms. Chew et al. [32] examined stent and ureteral movement with changes in patient body position and found that indwelling stents moving within the urinary tract during normal daily activities cause physical irritation and inflammation of the urothelium at the location of the stent curls in the bladder and kidney, likely resulting in additional pain and discomfort.

9.2.4.2 Ureteral peristalsis

Kinn and Lykkeskov-Andersen [33] and Venkatesh et al. [34] studied the effect of stents on ureteral peristalsis and reported that indwelling stents affect ureteral peristalsis by triggering a period of hyperperistalsis, in which the ureter attempts to expel the stent (a partial obstruction), shortly after stent insertion and eventual cessation of peristaltic activity (aperistalsis). This might cause pain and discomfort, as the absence of ureter peristalsis may cause hydronephrosis.

9.2.4.3 Stent migration

Stent migration or stent movement is common even with an appropriately positioned stent. The factors that affect stent movement within the urinary tract include length and diameter of the stent, the material used, stent dwell time, and renal movement with respiration. Jeon et al. [35]

studied the procedures for determination of ideal stent length for endourologic surgery and found that determination of stent length according to patient height does not correlate well with the length needed for endoscopic procedures; however, radiographic assessment of the distance between the ureteropelvic and ureterovesicular junction is more accurate and associated with a lower frequency of distal migration.

9.2.4.4 Stent-induced urinary tract infections

After the introduction of the stent into the ureter, the risk of infection in the urinary tract increases; proteins start adsorbing to the stent surface rapidly enabling deposition of minerals and other urine components as well as the attachment of bacteria. The most common bacteria seen in UTIs are *Escherichia coli* (*E. coli*), Staphylococcus, and Pseudomonas. The deposition of a urinary conditioning film on the surface of stents increases bacterial adhesion and biofilm formation [36]. Patients with the systemic disease have a high risk of UTIs, and the most effective antibiotic prophylaxis protocol has to be patient-specific and must be designed with careful consideration of the patient's medical history and previous antibiotic use [19]. To overcome the stent-induced UTI, it has been recommended to shorten the stent dwell times and antimicrobial prophylaxis for high-risk patients. Currently, urine culture is the most frequently used method to determine stent colonization and infection status while the stent is indwelling [37].

9.2.4.5 Stent encrustation

Similar to bacterial colonization, stent encrustation increases with dwell time. All stents elicit different forms and degrees of encrustation after insertion. The presence of the stent provides a substrate for the deposition of minerals including calcium oxalate, struvite, apatite, and uric acid along with organic macromolecules. Risk factors for encrustation include stone disease, urinary sepsis, chemotherapy, pregnancy, chronic renal failure, and metabolic or hormonal abnormalities, and the most important being the indwelling time. The most common location of encrustation is the proximal end at the anchor that sits in the kidney [38] and the distal pigtails because the curls are constantly in contact with urine in the kidney and bladder, the section within the ureteral lumen is usually the last to encrust, and it might be because of the "wiping" effect of ureteral peristalsis [39]. None of the materials used for manufacturing of stent are resistant to crystal deposition and eventual encrustation; however, of all materials available, silicone is least prone to struvite and hydroxyapatite encrustation [17,40,41].

9.2.5 Toxicological evaluation of ureteral stents

Liatsikos et al. [9] studied ureteral patency in malignant ureteral obstruction cases for 10 years. They used tests such as urinalysis, blood biochemistry tests, and transabdominal ultrasound or intravenous urography to detect hydronephrosis, hyperplastic reaction and/or encrustation or tumor ingrowth, stent migration. Tunney et al., in two different studies [17,42], assessed ureteral stent biomaterial encrustation. They employed a model representing upper urinary tract conditions to compare the long-term struvite and hydroxyapatite encrustation of five materials used in the fabrication of ureteral stents. They reported that silicone was least prone to struvite encrustation, followed by polyurethane, silitek, percuflex, and hydrogel-coated polyurethane, in rank order. In another study, they assessed urinary tract biomaterial encrustation using a modified Robbins device continuous flow model. They used artificial urine in conjunction with 5% CO_2 to simulate the physiological environment within the upper urinary tract. The widely used urinary device biomaterials, including silicone and polyurethane, were investigated in the model for hydroxyapatite and struvite encrustation. Scanning electron microscopy, energy dispersive X-ray analysis, and atomic absorption spectroscopy all showed that silicone was less prone to encrustation than polyurethane and that hydroxyapatite deposition was predominant on both surfaces.

Antiencrustation characteristics of the stent material have been assessed by using in vitro and in vivo models. Lock et al. [43] studied the degradation and antibacterial properties in artificial urine of Mg, Mg−Y, and Mg−3Al−1Zn (AZ31) that was the first to show the potential of absorbable metals for urological applications. Zhang et al. [44,45] assessed pure Mg and Mg-6wt.% Zn alloy implants for their biodegradable potential by using in vitro and in vivo models. The in vitro corrosion behavior was studied by potentiodynamic polarization and immersion tests in simulated body fluid (SBF) at 37°C. The degradation tests demonstrated that the pure Mg consistently corroded faster than the alloys in simulated body fluids, artificial urine, and in the bladder. Wang et al. [46] designed two in vitro bladder models to evaluate the ability of whole coated catheters to (1) impede bacterial migration along external surfaces of the catheter and (2) inhibit encrustation. An in vitro bladder model consisted of a glass vessel maintained at 37°C by a water heating jacket ("bladder"), an acrylic tube ("urethra"), and two peristaltic pumps. The source of infection was pumped into the urethra allowing bacteria to attach and colonize on the catheters; when bacteriuria developed, the catheter was removed and the biofilm formation on these segments was determined using crystal violet staining.

9.3 Urinary incontinence

9.3.1 Etiology

UI is one of the priority health issues recognized by WHO, which is also known as involuntary urination or any uncontrolled leakage of urine. Control over the urinary sphincter is either lost or weakened. Urinary incontinence is not just a medical problem. It can affect emotional, psychological, and social life. Many people who have urinary incontinence are afraid to do normal daily activities. It is a common and distressing medical condition that severely affects the quality of life [47,48].

Factors linked to urinary incontinence include increasing age, increasing parity, vaginal deliveries, obesity, pelvic surgery, diabetes mellitus, depression, constipation, chronic respiratory problems, and menopause. Urinary incontinence is more common in females than in males [49]. Urinary incontinence can result from both urologic and nonurologic causes. Urologic causes can be classified as either bladder or urethral dysfunction and may include detrusor overactivity, poor bladder compliance, urethral hypermobility, or intrinsic sphincter deficiency. Nonurologic causes may include infection, medication or drugs, psychological factors, polyuria, stool impaction, and restricted mobility [50]. As the treatment of incontinence may vary with the type of incontinence, it is important to identify the specific type of incontinence.

9.3.2 Pathophysiology of urinary incontinence

The system providing urinary continence is a complex network of subsystems, each contributing to the overall goal of maintaining continence. Understanding the pathophysiology of incontinence on the anatomic level will help to identify specific defects and the mechanistic information about the pathophysiology of urinary incontinence and will help guide research into prevention and treatment selection for the individualized treatment to the incontinent patients [51].

1. Urethrovesical pressure dynamics

To retain the urine in the bladder, urethral closure pressure must be greater than bladder pressure, both at rest and during increases in abdominal pressure. The resting tone of the urethral muscles maintains a favorable pressure relative to the bladder when urethral pressure exceeds bladder pressure. When bladder pressure increases several times higher than urethral pressure, such as during coughing, a dynamic process increases urethral closure pressure to enhance urethral closure and maintain continence. Thus increased intraabdominal pressure is transmitted to both urethra and bladder equally leaving the pressure differential unchanged [52]. Normal voiding is the result of changes in both of these pressure factors: urethral pressure falls and bladder pressure rises. Both the magnitude of the resting pressure in the urethra and the increase in pressure generated during a cough determine the pressure at which leakage of urine occurs [53].

Relationship between the functioning of each element of the continence mechanism, resting urethral pressure, pressure transmission, and the pressure needed to cause leakage of urine are central to understanding urinary continence. It requires an examination of the effects on urethral closure of pressure dynamics in relation to the anatomy of the continence structures. The constrictive effect of the urethral sphincter establishes urethral pressure above bladder pressure, and this pressure differential keeps urine in the bladder at rest. Thus normally, continence involves a balance between urethral closure and detrusor muscle activity.

2. Urethral support system

The urethral support system consists of all the structures extrinsic to the urethra that provide a supportive layer on which the proximal urethra and midurethra rest. The major components of this supportive structure are the anterior vagina, the endopelvic fascia, the arcus tendineus fasciae pelvis, and the levator ani muscles. Functionally, the levator ani muscle and the endopelvic fascia play an interactive role in maintaining continence and pelvic support. Impairments usually become evident when the system is stressed [51]. If there are breaks in the continuity of the endopelvic fascia or if the levator ani muscle is damaged, the supportive layer under the urethra will be more compliant and will provide reduced resistance during transient increase in abdominal pressure so that closure of the urethral lumen cannot be ensured and stress incontinence becomes possible [54].

If the nerves to the levator ani muscle are damaged (such as during childbirth), the denervated muscles would undergo atrophy, leading to paravaginal defect damaging the urethral support system [55]. When this occurs, an increase in abdominal pressure can no longer effectively compress the urethra against the supporting endopelvic fascia to close it during an increase in abdominal pressure leading to incontinence. The paravaginal defect can be repaired surgically, and normal anatomy can thus be restored.

3. The sphincteric closure system

Sphincteric closure of the urethra is normally provided by the urethral striated muscles, the urethral smooth muscle, and the vascular elements within the submucosa. Each believed to contribute equally to resting urethral closure pressure [56–58]. The total number of striated muscle fibers within the ventral wall of the urethra has been found to decrease with age. The concomitant age-related loss of nerve fibers in these striated urogenital sphincters is directly correlated with the loss in striated muscle fibers. Thus age-related deterioration of the urethral musculature might result in loss of urethral closure pressure [59], and this correlation also supports the hypothesis of a neurogenic source for stress urinary incontinence and helps to explain why faulty innervation could affect continence [60,61].

4. Continence control system (Fig. 9.1)

The levator ani muscles, endopelvic fascia, and muscular structures of the urethra comprise a system that helps to prevent loss of urine during stress. The coordinated action of these elements depends on the central nervous system. The nerve dysfunction or denervation of the pelvic musculature indicating neurologic injury after vaginal birth might be related to stress incontinence [55]. It is well established that the urethra and bladder neck in women have an abundance of both estrogen and α-adrenergic receptors [62].

Thus alterations in the anatomy and/or function of either the bladder or urethra during the filling/storage or emptying phases of urination may result in urinary incontinence. Simply stated, urinary incontinence occurs as a result of abnormalities of the urethra (i.e., the bladder outlet and urinary sphincter) or the bladder or a combination of abnormalities of both of these structures. Abnormalities may result in either overfunction or underfunction of the bladder and/or urethra, resulting in the development of urinary incontinence.

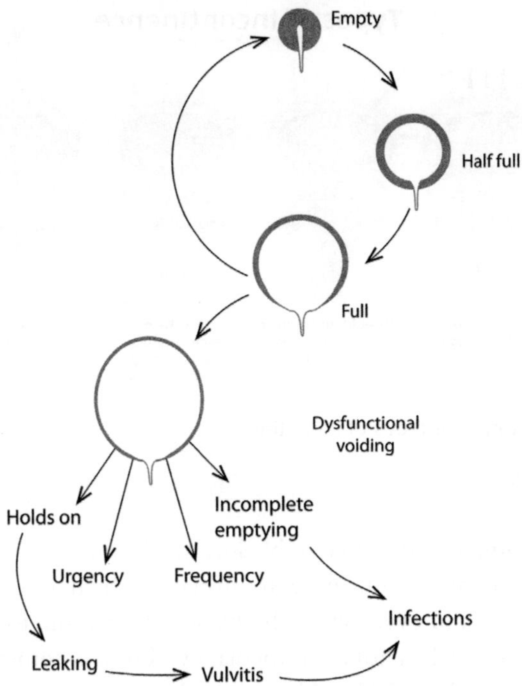

Figure 9.1 Continence control system.

9.3.3 Types of urinary incontinence (Fig. 9.2)

There are four main types of urinary incontinence.

1. Stress urinary incontinence

   Urinary incontinence that occurs because of a poorly functioning urethra is designated as stress urinary incontinence (SUI). This condition occurs when a compromised urethral sphincter is no longer able to resist the flow of urine from the bladder during periods of increased intraabdominal pressure. Stress incontinence is caused by impaired sphincter function due to pelvic floor weakness and nerve malfunction. It can happen when pressure on the bladder increases such as during exercise, laughing, sneezing, or coughing.

   Risk factor for SUI in women includes physical changes resulting from aging, pregnancy, childbirth, gynecological surgery, lowered estrogen levels, menopause, and neurological disorders [63]. Although SUI is usually considered a female disorder, it can also occur in men after prostate surgery called postprostatectomy SUI [64,65].

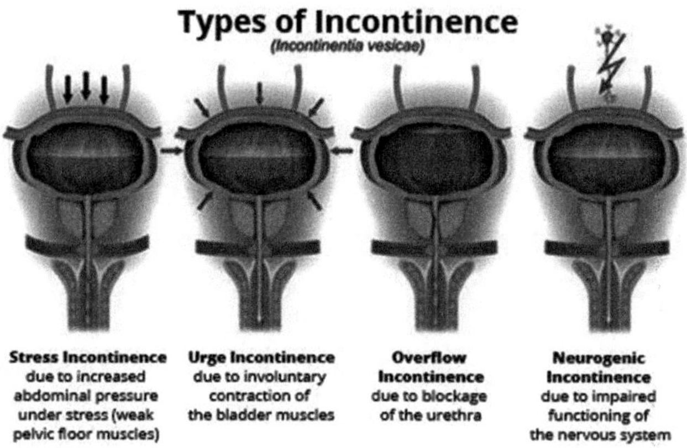

Figure 9.2 Illustration of types of incontinence.

2. Urge incontinence (overactive bladder syndrome)

   A sudden, irresistible urge to urinate, which can often occur at short intervals and even when the bladder is not full, forces the person concerned to seek a toilet immediately. UUI is sometimes called as overactive bladder (OAB). However, the terms are not interchangeable because about two-thirds of patients with OAB do not have UI [66,67]. The urgency urinary incontinence involves physiological perturbations to bladder functions such as detrusor overactivity, poor detrusor compliance, and bladder hypersensitivity. The detrusor muscle overactivity results in uninhibited or involuntary muscle contractions [68].

3. Overflow incontinence

   If the pressure in the urinary bladder exceeds the pressure of the bladder sphincter, a continuous trickle of urine is discharged, this is known as overflow incontinence. It is a condition of paradoxical incontinence caused by chronic urinary retention. In this situation, the intravesical pressure eventually equals the urethral resistance, resulting in periodic leakage or dribbling. Overflow incontinence may be caused by obstructive processes anywhere in the lower urinary tract or by impaired disorders of bladder emptying. The most common cause of this type of UI is bladder outlet obstruction due to benign prostatic hyperplasia, urethral stricture disease, postprostatectomy bladder neck contracture, pelvic organ prolapse, and impaired contractility. Men are more affected by this type of incontinence than women [69].

4. Reflex incontinence

   Reflex incontinence is caused by a dysfunction in the detrusor muscle. Even if the bladder is not full, this muscle contracts and squeezes, signaling the body to urinate. The risk factor for reflex incontinence includes serious neurological impairment either from spinal cord injuries or multiple sclerosis or radiation treatment or surgical damage. There are two types of reflex incontinence: supraspinal reflex incontinence—brain performance is impaired by diseases such as Alzheimer's, Parkinson's, Dementia, or by a stroke; spinal reflex incontinence—the connection from the brain to the spinal cord is interrupted. The cause is a disease or injury to the spinal cord (e.g., paraplegia, multiple sclerosis). There is no control over the function of the bladder or sphincters.
5. Mixed urinary incontinence

   The International Continence Society defines mixed urinary incontinence as involuntary leakage associated with exertion and urgency [70]. Stress and urge incontinence can also occur in combination; thus, it includes both components of urge incontinence and stress incontinence. In mixed incontinence condition, overactive bladder combined with a disorder of the closure system is involved [71].

9.3.4 Implants used for urinary incontinence

Treatment options for urinary incontinence in women are designed to prevent the involuntary loss of urine from the urethra. Current therapies include nonsurgical such as behavioral therapy, for example, bladder training, fluid and dietary modification, and drug therapy; with surgical therapy, more than 200 different surgical procedures are currently available.

There are many factors that should be considered when determining the optimal therapy for a patient with urinary incontinence. These include the etiology and type of urinary incontinence; bladder capacity; renal function; sexual function; severity of the leakage and degree of bother to the patient; the presence of associated conditions, such as vaginal prolapse, or concurrent abdominal or pelvic pathology requiring surgical correction; prior abdominal and/or pelvic surgery; and finally, the patient's suitability for and willingness to accept, the costs, risks, morbidity, and success (and failure) rates associated with each intervention.

No single procedure or intervention is optimal for all patients. Interventions for one type of urinary incontinence may not be applicable to other types of urinary incontinence. The key to an optimal therapeutic outcome is an accurate diagnosis combined with the selection of an appropriate intervention that is acceptable to the patient after balancing multiple factors [72,73].

The following implants are used for various conditions of urinary incontinence.

1. Vaginal cones—weighted cone devices attached to vaginal muscles and are intended to strengthen the pelvic floor musculature. The vaginal cone is a tampon-like device made up of ABS Plastic and Medical grade silicone that is inserted into the vagina and kept in place by active muscle contraction of the pelvic floor [74]. It is believed that the sensation that the cone is slipping out of the vagina triggers a strong sensory feedback mechanism that results in the contraction of the pelvic floor muscles to keep the cone in place [75].
2. Occlusive devices—they are extraurethral and intraurethral occlusive devices. Extraurethral devices include Miniguard, which is a disposable, single-use, triangular foam device that is held in the perimeatal area with an adhesive hydrogel. FemAssist is a hat-shaped silicone device that is placed over the urethral meatus. the product is designed to be placed directly over urethra where it will be held in place by its vacuum action. It can be worn for a maximum of 4 hours or until voiding and then washed with hot soapy water and reinserted. It can be reused for a week [76]. CapSure is a reusable device to which a lubricant is applied before it is kept in place by suction. It can be reused for up to 2 weeks. Intraurethral devices are single-use, disposable, and thin and flexible. Some of the devices such as Reliance (UroMed Corporation, Needham, MA), VIVA (B. Braun Melsungen AG, Melsungen, Germany), and FemSoft (Rochester Medical Corporation, Stewartville, MN) have several features that enhance its retention within the urethra.
3. Colpexin sphere is placed in the vaginal canal to provide support for pelvic floor muscles. This device improves prolapse defects and the utility of pelvic floor exercises [77].
4. Pessaries provide support for the bladder neck at the urogenital angle [78]. The type of pessary should be chosen based on the severity of SUI, the presence of prolapse, and sexual activity. Incontinence pessaries are silicone or rubber devices that are placed transvaginally. They are designed to support the urethra and bladder wall, increase urethral length, and provide gentle compression of the urethra against

the pubic bone. This structural arrangement reduces and often prevents leakage when intraabdominal pressure increases, essentially resolving the problem of incontinence [79]. Different types of pessaries are available and some have been designed specifically to treat SUI. The latter group includes incontinence ring pessary, ring pessary with support (common size 2–7, characterized by ease of insertion), incontinence dish (common size 3–5, medium ease of insertion and removal), and the Uresta device. All of them exert their action by stabilizing the urethra and increasing urethral resistance. The pessary is made of a medical-grade rubber that has been extensively tested for biocompatibility and safety in medical applications and meets the criteria for use in class II medical devices.

5. Electrical stimulation units—a rectal or vaginal probe is used to apply electrical stimulation to the pelvic floor, with the aim of inhibiting the micturition reflex and improving contraction of the pelvic floor musculature [73]. Zeng et al. [80] evaluated the biological effects of electrical stimulation on pelvic floor muscle strength and neuropeptide Y expression of SUI. They have shown that electrical stimulation increases the release of neuropeptide Y as a neurotransmitter, which reflects the recovery of the damaged nerve to increase the muscle strength and concluded that electrical stimulation may be ideal physiotherapy for SUI patients in clinical conditions. The only commercially available neuromodulation systems include implantable sacral nerve modulation and percutaneous tibial nerve stimulation (PTNS). RENOVA iStim System is an implantable tibial neurostimulation device for the patients with refractory OAB. A clinician programmer (CP) unit is used to set individual stimulation parameters for each patient to optimize therapeutic outcomes [81].
6. Artificial urinary sphincter—AUS-800 is an implantable, fluid-filled solid silicone elastomer device used to treat stress urinary incontinence. It restores the natural process of urinary control by stimulating normal sphincter function by opening and closing urethra at the patient's control. The expected lifespan of an AUS-800 is around 10 years, with a likely need for revision due to either mechanical failure or urethral atrophy [82].
7. FlowSecure TM (RBM-Med)is a new prosthesis for the management of urinary incontinence due to ISD. It is an adjustable prosthesis filled with normal saline without contrast. It is a one-piece device consisting of two reservoirs placed in the paravesical space, a cuff that surrounds

the urethra and a control pump with a self-sealant port that is placed in the patient's scrotum.

8. Male perineal slings

Male perineal slings have been developed to provide treatment for men who have mild-to-moderate leakage, not severe enough for an AUS, but enough to restrict day-to-day activities. Invance is the first generation of male perineal slings. It is anchored to the inferior pubic rami with bone screws and achieves continence by providing fixed compression of a urethral segment. Argus and the AdVance sling systems are the second generation of male perineal slings. The Argus consists of a padded foam cushion fixed to the bulbar urethra and provides "adjustable" compression of a urethral segment. The AdVance is a "transobturator" sling that aims to correct the "urethral hypermobility" that results from a radical prostatectomy where the membranous urethral supports through the prostate and puboprostatic ligaments are lost. The sling lifts the bulbomembranous urethra vertically. The ProAct incontinence device is a novel implantable device consisting of two separate balloons that are placed just distal to the bladder neck. Reinjectable ports are located in the scrotum, which allows adjustments to balloon pressure. ProAct may be considered as an alternative to an AUS [83].

9.3.5 Complications of implants for the urinary incontinence

Complications resulting from either a male sling or AUS implantation may be categorized as occurring intraoperative, early postop (<90 days) or late postop (> 90 days). Intraoperative complications may include urethral injury occurring at the time of urethral dissection or passage of a trocar for male sling placement. Bladder injuries including bladder perforation occur during trocar passage with retropubic sling placements. Early postoperative complications include urinary retention, infection and/or erosion, perineal pain, and de novo detrusor overactivity. Infections of the AUS device or sling material may be secondary to unrecognized urethral erosion, repeated device placements, prior erosions, or radiation therapy. The most commonly isolated organisms with infection include *S. aureus*, *S. epidermidis*, Enterococcus, Methicillin-resistant *S. aureus*, and gram-negative bacilli [84]. Postoperative perineal pain is more common with male sling placement than AUS, and mechanical failure is unique to AUS devices [85].

The reported complications or adverse effects of occlusive devices such as FemAssist usually been transient; however, they included vulvar and lower urinary tract irritation, vaginal irritation, and urinary tract infections [75]. Some of the devices like Reliance, VIVA, and FemSoft reported hematuria, UTIs, and discomfort. Vaginal pessaries have been reported to cause vaginal soreness or irritation and development of UTIs during the clinical trials.

Adverse effects of artificial urinary sphincter such as FlowSecure TM (RBM-Med) may include acute urinary tract infection leading to erosion, tissue damage, and misplacement of device. Poor bladder compliance, damage to urethra due to faulty insertion methods, and fibrotic bladder have also been reported. Complications of male perineal slings such as Invance, Argus, and the AdVance sling systems included osteomyelitis and pain related to the bone screws, urethral erosion, infection, and transient dysuria.

Dmochowski et al. [81] reported long-term (3-year follow-up) results of safety, efficacy, quality of life, and satisfaction of patients treated for refractory OAB using an implantable tibial neurostimulation (Renova Istim) system. A wireless peripheral neurostimulator device (BlueWind Medical Ltd.) was implanted in patients with refractory OAB, on the posterior tibial nerve, approximately 5 cm above the medial malleolus. The implant electrically stimulates the tibial nerve and is wirelessly powered by a wearable external control unit that controls the therapeutic parameters and is worn by the patient on the lower leg during specified treatment periods in home settings. A CP unit is used to set individual stimulation parameters for each patient to optimize therapeutic outcomes. The authors concluded that the BlueWind Medical RENOVA iStim System for the treatment of OAB demonstrated long-term safety and efficacy as well as a sustainable significant improvement in the quality of life of patients.

Porpiglia et al. [86] reported feasibility, safety, and functional results at 1-year follow-up of temporary implantable nitinol device (TIND) used for relief of lower urinary tract symptoms. A temporary implantable nitinol device (TIND; Medi-Tate) was implanted within the bladder neck and the prostatic urethra. The device was removed 5 days later in an outpatient setting. Demographics, perioperative results, complications (according to the Clavien system), functional results, and quality of life (QoL) were evaluated. Four complications were recorded, including urinary retention, transient incontinence due to device displacement, prostatic abscess, and urinary tract infection. The author concluded that the functional results are encouraging and the treatment significantly improved patient QoL.

9.4 Prostate cancer

9.4.1 Etiology

Worldwide, prostate cancer is the most commonly diagnosed malignancy and the sixth leading cause of cancer death in men with more than one million cases currently diagnosed annually. Prostate cancer risk factors include male gender, older age, positive family history, increased height, obesity, hypertension, lack of exercise, persistently elevated testosterone levels, Agent Orange exposure, and ethnicity. Fortunately, prostate cancer primarily impacts older men as many prostate cancers are slow-growing, low grade with relatively low risk, and limited aggressiveness [87]. Monitoring and observation can often suffice until mortality arrives via senescence. Over the past few years, the improvement of treatments, together with the early diagnosis, allowed an increasing survival rate from 69% to almost 99%. The therapies available for the treatment of prostate cancer are also associated with considerable morbidity, particularly in genitourinary dysfunction. Therefore clinicians and patients need to assess together the balance of risks and benefits of therapies with the aim to treat prostate cancer with the lowest risk of recurrence and at the same time, with minimal morbidity from side effects or complications [88,89].

9.4.2 Pathophysiology of prostate cancer

The prostate is roughly 3 cm long, about the size of a walnut and weighs approximately 20 g. The prostate gland is located below the urinary bladder at the base of the penis and immediately anterior to the rectum in the male pelvis. It surrounds the posterior part of the urethra; however, there is no difference in the internal lining of the proximal, prostatic, and posterior urethra. The prostate is primarily made up of glandular tissue that produces fluid that constitutes about 30%–35% of the semen. This prostatic portion of the semen nourishes the sperm and provides alkalinity that helps to maintain a high pH. The prostate gland requires androgen (testosterone) to function optimally. Cancer begins with a mutation in normal prostate glandular cells, usually beginning with the peripheral basal cells [90,91].

Prostate cancer is most common in the peripheral zone and the types of prostate cancer are based on the type of the cell that the cancer has started in. With this information, the doctor can decide the treatment that is needed [92].

1. Acinar adenocarcinoma—it develops in the gland cells that line the prostate gland and shows typical glandular patterns on microscopic examination. They are the most common type of prostate cancer. Nearly everyone with prostate cancer has this type.
2. Ductal adenocarcinoma—ductal adenocarcinoma starts in the cells that line the ducts (tubes) of the prostate gland. It tends to grow and spread more quickly than acinar adenocarcinoma.
3. Transitional cell (or urothelial) cancer—it starts in the cells that line the urethral tube. This type of cancer usually starts in the bladder and spreads into the prostate. However, rarely it can start in the prostate and may spread into the bladder entrance and nearby tissues.
4. Squamous cell cancer—these cancers develop from flat cells that cover the prostate. They tend to grow and spread more quickly than adenocarcinoma of the prostate.
5. Small cell prostate cancer—it is made up of small round cells. It is a type of neuroendocrine cancer.

The Gleason prostate cancer score has been shown over time, to be the most reliable and predictive histological grading system available. It has stood the test of time and has been universally adopted for all prostate cancer pathological descriptions [90,93].

9.4.3 Implants used in the prostate cancer

Treatment for prostate cancer is complex, driving demand for better and more innovative medical technology. The first decision in managing prostate cancer is determining whether any treatment at all is needed. The best option depends on the cancer stage, Gleason score and the PSA level as well as individual patient preferences, health, comorbidities, quality of life, and age. Prostate cancer, especially low-grade tumor, often grows so slowly that frequently no treatment is required. Many low-risk cases can now be followed with active surveillance. A number of treatment options are available to men diagnosed with prostate cancer, including watchful waiting, hormonal therapy, surgery, and radiation therapy.

Focal therapy is an emerging treatment option that involves the focal ablation of prostate cancer with the preservation of surrounding healthy tissue. Focal therapy has been proposed as the next major change in the way prostate cancer is treated, with only subregions of the prostate receiving high doses of radiation. There is the potential for significant reductions in treatment-related toxicity compared with conventional, whole gland treatments. Focal therapy modalities include cryotherapy, high-intensity focused ultrasound, laser ablation, photodynamic therapy, irreversible electroporation, radiofrequency ablation, and focal brachytherapy [94–97].

The most significant inroads for prostate cancer have been made by medical device firms specializing in three areas: External radiation therapy, internal radiation therapy, and laparoscopic robotic surgery.

9.4.3.1 External beam radiation therapy

In this, the beams of radiation are focused on the prostate gland from an equipment outside the body. Older external beam radiation therapy (EBRT) techniques were not able to focus radiation on the tumor within the prostate gland; healthy tissues were often exposed to radiation. A newer EBRT uses an intensity-modulated radiation therapy technique, uses a computer-driven machine that moves around the patient as it delivers radiation. It shapes the beams and aims them at the prostate from several angles, allowing the radiation dose to conform more precisely to the three-dimensional shape of the tumor. The intensity of the beams can be adjusted to deliver a higher dose to cancer while avoiding normal tissue. It was approved for use in Australia and Japan in 2017 and in Taiwan in January 2018. Proton beam therapy is also a type of external beam radiation. It uses protons rather than X-rays. The use of protons may allow a very high dose of radiation to reach the prostate while reducing the amount of normal tissue that is affected [98–100].

Following approved systems are available:

1. Halcyon, launched by Palo Alto, Varian Medical Systems California.
2. Calypso, used in conjunction with the Halycon system, is a system of soft transponders.
3. CyberKnife, by Accuray, Inc., Sunnyvale, California. CyberKnife destroys tumors by aiming beams of radiation from multiple directions.

9.4.3.2 Internal radiation therapy (brachytherapy)

Internal radiation therapy, also called brachytherapy, allows a higher dose of radiation in a smaller area than might be possible with external radiation treatment. Brachytherapy is a treatment at a short distance, radioactive material (radiation source), sealed in a smallholder, is implanted directly into the prostate gland very close to or inside the tumor.

Different types of implants may be called pellets, seeds, ribbons, wires, needles, capsules, balloons, or tubes are used.

The length of time an implant is left in place depends on the type of brachytherapy. Some implants are permanent, while others are taken out after a few minutes or days. It depends upon the type of cancer, location, general health of the patient, and other treatments. In high-dose-rate brachytherapy, a powerful radioactive source is used and treatment is given only for a few minutes and maybe repeated over the course of a few days to weeks. The radioactive material is not left in the body. In low-dose-rate brachytherapy, the implant gives off lower doses of radiation over a longer period. Some implants are left in for few days and then removed and while some smaller implants are left in place permanently [101,102].

There are various companies manufacturing the radioactive seeds as implants, some examples are as follows:

- UroMed Corporation, Bebig GmbH (Germany) Symmetra-125.S06: Titanium capsule-sealed laser, containing a radio-opaque gold wire inside and a ceramic layer with iodine-125.
- Best Medical International (USA), Model 2301: Double encapsulated titanium, interior accommodates a marker of tungsten and iodine-125 adsorbed on an unspecified substrate.
- BARD, SourceTech Medical (USA), BrachySource STMIodine-125: The capsule is titanium welded by laser equipment. Inside of the seed has a gold wire as a marker, a layer of aluminum, and a coating of copper. Iodine-125 is deposited in a cylinder of aluminum with a gold core and a layer of nickel.

Clinical studies have provided the evidence that focal therapy treatments can decrease the dose and toxicity over current whole gland therapy [103] and have advantages over other options such as avoiding overtreatment of low-risk prostate cancers, sparing the bladder, sphincter, neurovascular bundles, and bowel. It prevents continence, erectile dysfunction, and is cost saving, and overall it improves the quality of life. However, focal therapy has some disadvantages. The major obstacle lies in the proper identification of the ideal patient for focal therapy. The consequences of improperly designating a patient for focal therapy may be profound [104]. Improper designation of patient for focal therapy depends upon the use of proper diagnostic tools. Each diagnostic tool has its own disadvantages including the difficulty of diagnosing central cancer, recent biopsies often present with hemorrhage, limits diagnostic accuracy, further, tumor characterization and risk estimation remain imperfect. Thus focal therapy will be problematic as some tissue may be left untreated [105].

Hypofractionation schemes and associated higher rectal doses have evoked the need for improved protection of the rectum during prostate cancer irradiation. Ben-Yosef et al. [106] and Levy et al. [107] developed an inflatable balloon that is implanted via a minimally invasive procedure. The balloon is made of a biodegradable polymer called poly(lactide-co-ε-caprolactone). The implant is inserted rolled throughout the perineum; inflated in situ with physiological saline; sealed and placed between the rectum wall and the prostate gland.

9.4.4 Complications of implants used

Complications from external beam radiation therapy include prostate size and potential radiation side effects to the bowel and bladder (radiation proctitis and cystitis). There is an increased risk of hematuria, and erectile dysfunction is another relatively common complication. Other complications may be fatigue, increased fracture risk, and higher incidence of secondary malignancies [108,109].

Mallick et al. [108] explained the pathogenesis of radiation-induced cystitis and proctitis. Radiation causes single and double-stranded DNA breaks that lead to activation of DNA damage, gene repair, and apoptosis. Additionally DNA penetrates the deeper muscle of urinary bladder causing endarteritis and compromised blood supply and inadequate supply of nutrients to bladder tissue. These damaged blood vessels can survive from months to years after damage, which makes it difficult to predict when radiation cystitis will develop.

Brachytherapy is an option for the treatment of T1 and early T2 prostate cancers only. Contraindications may include an earlier transurethral resection of the prostate, poor general health, obesity, bowel disease, previous abdominal surgery, pubic arch interference, and urinary retention. The potential side effects of brachytherapy include acute side effects from the radiation, such as urine retention due to swelling from the procedure or radiation, radiation urethritis, and prostatitis. There may be slight bleeding under the scrotum where the needles were placed. These potential side effects will decrease as the seeds lose their potency. Erectile dysfunction and seed migration have also been reported. There is a small chance of long-term or permanent side effects as dysuria at 1 year decreased sexual potency [110].

9.4.5 Testing of implants used for prostate cancer

Complications are related to the type of implants used; therefore, the testing paradigm shall be based on the careful study of the implants in use and complications associated with it. The studies for implants used for prostate cancers mainly concentrate on radiation safety along with routine biocompatibility testing. On one hand, biological individualization of treatment is important; on the other hand, identification of molecules that can serve as targets for radiosensitization is also fundamental in prostate cancer treatment. Biological individualization of treatment in personalized radiation oncology includes pretreatment identification of patient subgroups with radioresistant tumors that would have a high risk of recurrence after standard radiotherapy alone; pretreatment identification of subgroups that have a high chance of tumor cure after radiotherapy alone and identification of subgroups with a high risk of distant metastasis after local treatment. Cancer radiotherapy needs to consider the selection of appropriate radioactive molecule as some of the tumor-selective targets influence the radiosensitivity of some tumor cells, but not others: the relationship between a molecule and the radiosensitivity of given tumor cell line and determination of selectivity of radiosensitization of tumor cells over normal cells [111,112]. Tang et al. [113] have also described the role of metabolism in cancer cell radioresistance and radiosensitization methods. The toxicology models that can be used for testing safety and efficacy of radiation implants include in vitro cell culture assays as well as in vivo ectopic and orthotopic xenograft models. In vitro testing attempts to understand potential tumor selectivity and to predict possible tissue toxicity; however, many of the cell types that are relevant for studies of normal tissue toxicity will fail to reflect the true radiosensitivity. Studies that show that the radioactive agent is capable of hitting the target molecule in relevant cell line systems should be selected. Ideally, In vitro studies should support the mechanistic basis of the targeted approach, including evidence that target knockdown is associated with modulation of the radiation response [114].

Cox et al. [115], described the toxicity criteria of the Radiation Therapy Oncology Group and the European Organization for Research and Treatment of Cancer. They have categorized the toxicity of radiation therapy as Grade 0—no symptoms, Grade 1—minor symptoms requiring no treatment, Grade 2—symptoms responding to simple outpatient management, Grade 3—distressing symptoms altering radiotherapy, hospitalization for diagnosis or minor surgical intervention may be required, Grade 4—major surgical intervention or prolonged hospitalization required, Grade 5—fatal complication.

Assessment of commonly described complications of implants used for prostate cancer includes ruling out the other causes of complications before the start of the treatment, which includes tests on blood, urine and serum, cystoscopy and imaging for hematuria, urinary calculi, tumors, infections, and bleeding anomalies [108]. Ben-Yosef et al. [106] reported that an implantable, biodegradable, inflatable, preshaped triangular balloon of commercially used poly(L-lactide-co-ε-caprolactone) copolymer material developed to provide separation between prostate and rectum was safe and effective for its intended use of separating tissues for the desired duration.

9.5 Erectile dysfunction

9.5.1 Etiology

Erectile dysfunction (ED), also known as impotence, is a type of sexual dysfunction characterized by the inability to develop or maintain an erection of the penis during sexual activity. The condition is also on occasion called phallic impotence. The reality is that ED is a natural part of aging and that the prevalence increases with age; however, the Massachusetts Male Aging Study (MMAS) found that 52% of men between 40 and 70 years old reported having some form of ED. In the MMAS, they found that roughly 50% of men at 50 years old, 60% of men at 60 years old, and 70% of men at 70 years old had ED [116].

Male sexual arousal is a complex process that involves the brain, hormones, emotions, nerves, muscles, and blood vessels. Erectile dysfunction can result from a problem with any of these. Similarly, stress and mental health concerns can cause or worsen erectile dysfunction; sometimes a combination of physical and psychological issues also causes erectile dysfunction. Many factors contribute to erectile dysfunction: physical causes include heart disease, high cholesterol, diabetes, obesity, drugs, neurogenic disorders, cavernosal disorders, surgery, aging, lifestyle habits such as smoking, alcoholism, and other substance abuse, and sleep disorders; psychological causes include depression, anxiety or other mental health conditions, stress, relationship problems, and poor communication [117–120].

9.5.2 Pathophysiology of erectile dysfunction

Knowledge of the physiological processes underlying erection is essential to understand erectile dysfunction. The process of achieving penile erection involves the integration of psychological, neurological, and vascular processes, which combine to initiate a physiologic response within the penile vasculature. Pathophysiology of erectile dysfunction has been studied and reviewed in detail by many scientists [121–123]. They have classified erectile dysfunction as developing from psychological, neurological, hormonal, and vascular pathologies, drug induced, or combinations of these factors.

The pathophysiology of erectile dysfunction varies because psychological erectile dysfunction might be due to loss of libido, overinhibition, or impaired nitric oxide release; neurogenic erectile dysfunction might be related to failure of initiation of nerve impulse or interrupted neural transmission; hormonal might be due to loss of libido and inadequate nitric oxide release; vasculogenic (arterial or cavernosal) might be because of inadequate arterial flow or impaired venoocclusion; drug-induced erectile dysfunction might be due to central suppression and systemic diseases [124–127]. In both cases, an intact neural system is required for a successful and complete erection. Stimulation of the penile shaft by the nervous system leads to the secretion of nitric oxide, which causes the relaxation of smooth muscles of corpora cavernosa (the main erectile tissue of penis) and subsequently penile erection. Additionally, adequate levels of testosterone (produced by the testes) and an intact pituitary gland are required for the development of a healthy erectile system [128].

9.5.3 Implants used to treat erectile dysfunction

A penile prosthesis is a device, either external or implanted surgically within the corpora cavernosa of the penis, that substitutes for or supplements the function of the erectile bodies to achieve penile rigidity, thus simulating an erection. The earliest documentation of an artificial penis for medical use dates to the 16th century. Yet penile implants to treat erectile dysfunction did not occur until 1973. Dr. Scott and colleagues described a novel penile prosthetic device that used inflatable silicone cylinders. Although more invasive than some of the other currently available therapies, penile prosthesis surgery has the advantages of high patient satisfaction rates and avoidance of systemic adverse events in the vast majority of cases. The device is indicated for use in men with organic or treatment-resistant impotence or erectile dysfunction that is the result of various physical conditions such as cardiovascular disease, diabetes, and pelvic trauma. Penile implants can also be used in men who experience other types of erectile problems, such as those caused by Peyronie's disease, or because of prostate cancer treatments [129]. As such, the ideal penile prosthetic device for

ED treatment would mimic a native physiologic erection as closely as possible, both in function and appearance, would mimic the flaccid state of the penis and be discreet when not in use and would not interfere with urination or other activities of daily living [130].

There are two types of penile implants: inflatable implants and noninflatable implants. The inflatable implants are either two-piece implants or three-piece implants, which are filled with fluid from a fluid reservoir that is implanted in the scrotum. Three-piece implants are more complex; however, they perform better than that of two-piece implants. Noninflatable implants are semirigid tubes that can be bent to shape. There are several different types of noninflatable implants with varying trade-offs. The biggest advantages of noninflatable implants are cost and ease of insertion. The surgery to implant these devices is much simpler than for inflatables [131–133]. Le et al. [134] described a novel physiologic penile prosthesis that uses shape memory alloy properties to mimic the transition between a flaccid and erect penis using magnetic induction instead of hydraulic pressure. They prototyped an implantable penile prosthesis cylinder using temperature-tuned nickel-titanium alloy tubes laser cut to specifications and activating it using an external inducer wand (handheld magnetic inductor).

9.5.4 Complications of penile prosthesis

Surgical techniques and antibiotic coverage of the newer prosthesis implants have improved safety and both patient and partner satisfaction; however, operative complications can be severe and include increased morbidity and hospitalization cost. Jain et al. [135] reported that the complications seen after penile prosthesis insertion are mechanical failure, infection, and problems related to migration or incorrect sizing of the prosthesis. They attributed the mechanical failure of inflatable prostheses to a large number of different types of devices used. It usually occurs with inflatable prostheses and is a rare complication for a modern semirigid device. Lewis [136] studied long-term results of penile prosthetic implants and reported that there is a 5% mechanical failure rate at 5 years. Infection is the most feared complication of penile prosthetic surgery. Patients at particular risk of infection are diabetics and those who have had previous penile prosthetic surgery. Pineda and Burnett [137] reviewed the penile prosthesis infections and explained that there are two types of inflatable penile prosthesis (IPP) infections: coagulase-negative Staphylococcus species and those caused by organisms that are more virulent and systemically toxic.

Factors responsible for infection include spinal cord injury, IPP revision, and longer operative times; other factors are diabetes, immunosuppression, and concomitant surgeries. The correct size of implanted prostheses is essential for long-term success; too short implants cause supersonic transport deformity. Overlong prostheses can produce an S-shaped deformity and with semirigid rods, erosion can occur. Vakalopoulos et al. [138] explained the postoperative complications reporting system for inflatable penile prostheses implantation that is classified according to the Modified Clavien System in terms of postoperative morbidity, costs, and patient satisfaction. This modified system includes seven grades (Grades I–V) with two subgroups for Grades III and IV. Grade I includes any deviation from the normal postoperative course, Grade II includes complications requiring special pharmacological treatment, Grade III (a and b) includes complications that need special surgical, endoscopic, or radiological intervention, Grade IV (a and b) includes life-threatening complications, and Grade V is patient death.

9.5.5 Toxicological evaluation of penile prosthesis

Infections associated with penile implants result in serious medical consequences. Mansouri et al. [139] assessed the antimicrobial activities of penile prostheses, InhibiZone implants preimpregnated with minocycline and rifampin, and Titan implants dipped in vancomycin. Darouiche et al. [140] assessed the efficacy of minocycline/rifampin-impregnated silicone pump bulb sections from penile implants. They inoculated these implants with *S. aureus* for 8 hours at room temperature, and the test devices were allowed to dry for 30 minutes. They reported that all impregnated implants produced zones of inhibition against *S. aureus* and protected against staphylococcal colonization of devices.

Le et al. [134] tested the penile prosthesis (temperature-tuned nickel-titanium alloy) by implantation in cadaveric tissue and tested temperature change in middle and surface probes that never exceeded 28°C from a baseline at room temperature ~25°C. Wang et al. [141] evaluated the hardness of penile prosthesis with a Shore Durimeter and the buckling force of the prosthesis determined by a push-pull gauge and a specially designed sampling table. Henry et al. [142] used the Fastsize EQM device to measure penile axial rigidity by monitoring the strength of erections through noninvasive pressure measurements.

Table 9.1 shows the details of implants used for various urology and nephrology diseases.

Table 9.1 Devices used for treatment of urology and nephrology diseases.

Sr. No	Disease condition	Devices used	Material used	Key comments
1	Stress urinary incontinence in females	Vaginal pessary (ring pessary, ring pessary with support, incontinence dish, and Uresta device, Introl, a bladder neck support prosthesis)	Silicone and rubber	Structural arrangement reduces and often prevents leak-age when intraabdominal pressure increases
		Vaginal cones	Acrylonitrile butadiene styrene (ABS) plastic frame and silicone rubber	Strengthening of the pelvic floor muscles
		Occlusive devices Extraurethral—Miniguard	Miniguard is a foam device held in the perimeatal area with an adhesive hydrogel	Provide occlusion of urinary opening by creating a seal
		Electrical stimulation units	Tampon-shaped exerciser (electrode) with the channel switch	Electrical stimulation of the pelvic floor nerve and muscle tissues
	Postprostatectomy stress urinary incontinence (PPSUI)	The artificial urinary sphincter (AUS800)—three components: cuff, pump, and pressure-regulating balloon	Silicone elastomer and fluorosilicone lubricant	Implantable fluid-filled device. simulates normal sphincter function by opening and closing urethra
	Male mild urinary incontinence	Male perineal slings; Invance, AdVance, Argus, ProACT	Padded foam cushion fixed to the bulbar urethra	Achieves continence by providing fixed compression of a urethral segment
2	Prostate cancer	Halcyon, Calypso, CyberKnife	External beam radiation therapy device	Beams of radiation are focused on the prostate gland from an equipment outside the body
		Symmetra-125.S06, Model 2301, STMIodine-125	Brachytherapy—ceramic layer with iodine-125; titanium capsule	Higher dose of radiation in a smaller area

3	Urethral stricture	Permanent Urolume Wallstent	Stainless steel alloy woven into a 42 French lumen tubular mesh	To support the repair of the urethral wall and to achieve urinary drainage. The mode of action of the urethral stents used so far is based on their mechanical properties
		Urolume prostatic stents	Elgiloy conatins cobalt, chromium, nickel, molybdenum, iron, traces of manganese, carbon, silicon phosphorus, sulfur, and beryllium	
		Thermoexpandable Memotherm	Metal mesh stent of nitinol (nickel and titanium)	These stents help to prevent the edges of the cut stricture from adhering together and forming a shrinking mass of scar tissue
		Urospiral	Coiled stainless steel wire	
		Prostakath	Gold-plated wire	
		UroCoil system	Nickel–titanium alloy (nitinol) and expanded to 24–30°F	
		Memokath	Thermoexpandable and made of nitinol	
		Covered metallic temporary stent, for example, Song urethral stent	Single thread of 0.1 mm-diameter nitinol filament in a tubular configuration and it is covered with polyurethane or polytetrafluoroethylene	
		Allium urethral stents	Nitinol wire skeleton covered with a biocompatible polymer	
		SR biodegradable stents	Poly-L-lacticacid, Polylactide, polyglycolide, Vicryl	

(Continued)

Table 9.1 (Continued)

Sr. No	Disease condition	Devices used	Material used	Key comments
		Self-expandable spiral prostatic stents	SR-PGA, SR-PLLA, SR-PLA 96/4 with barium and SR-PLGA	
		Barnes stent	Polyurethane	
		Spanner	Polyurethane	
4	Ureteral obstruction	Fluoro-4 (Bard, USA)	Silicone	Highly biocompatible when compared to other materials, uniform surface, less prone to encrustation High-coefficient of friction makes implantation difficult, difficult to handle due to its softness and elasticity, particularly in the presence of tortuous ureters and extrinsic compression
		Bardex (Bard, USA)	Polyurethane	Combines the elastic properties of silicone with the rigidity of polyethylene Stiffness, prone to encrustation Ureteral erosion and ulceration in animal studies and discomfort in patients
		Silitek (Medical Engineering©, Argentina)	Polyester copolymer	High radial stiffness to resist compression, High tensile

		strength, relatively weak coil retention Encrustation profile similar to silicone, relatively weak coil retention strength more likely to migrate, the high incident rate of edema
C-Flex (Cook© Medical, USA)	Styrene/ethylene-butylene/styrene block copolymers	Lower surface friction allowing less particle adhesion, lower Mechanical strength compared to polyurethane and PureFlex thermoplastic properties Comparatively weak hydrogel coated stents are more prone to encrustation
Percuflex (Boston Scientific, USA)	Olefinic block copolymer	Another thermosetting Polyurethane softens in the body, better physical properties than polyurethane, low coil, and tensile strength Encrustation is similar to standard PU and can easily get compressed

(Continued)

Table 9.1 (Continued)

Sr. No	Disease condition	Devices used	Material used	Key comments
		Resonance (Cook Medical, Bloomington, IN)	Nonmagnetic nickel–cobalt–chromium—molybdenum alloy	In reality is a solid JJ stent, applied in malignant ureteral cases to provide long-term urinary function Metallic double pigtail stent, high tensile strength, corrosion resistant
		Memokath 051 (PNN© medical, Denmark)	Nickel titanium (Nitinol)	Soft and strong, not indicated for patients with functional stenosis or stone formation
		Wall Stent (Boston Scientific, USA)	Stainless steel wire mesh	Segmental metallic stents, Simplicity of fabrication Stent occlusion due to tumor ingrowth as well as overgrowth. Removal of these stents is difficult
		Uriprene (Poly-Med Inc., USA)	Biodegradable polymer composed of L-lactide, glycolide, and copolyester components	Reduction of secondary procedures 80% of the stents degraded within 2–3 weeks and 100% of stents were eliminated by week 4

9.6 Aspects of toxicological evaluation of urological implants

Medical expenditures for devices are increasing along with the aging of human populations and are reflected by a shift in venture capital funding into medical device technology [143]. Contrasted to pharmaceuticals or biologics, medical devices lack chemical action and do not depend on being metabolized [144]. In general, medical devices are progressively regulated based on complexity and associated risk factors of invasiveness, duration of contact, affected body system, or local versus systemic effects. The risk to the user or patient determines the amount of testing required for approval. Class I and II devices have minimal potential for harm and are generally simpler, claim substantial equivalence to similar marketed devices hence may require limited testing but no or limited clinical testing. A 510-K application of premarket notification is generally required for approval of Class II devices. Class III or surgically implantable devices have the highest risk and are subject to the most extensive testing and highly regulated premarketing approval or equivalent. Once marketed, devices can be reclassified into lower or higher categories based on positive or negative clinical experiences [145].

Safety evaluation of medical devices usually involves all aspects including composition, manufacturing, packaging, and safety testing. These aspects of the planning process are intertwined and interdependent. The level of focus each aspect requires can be affected by the history of use of the materials, the target population, and the intended use of the device [144]. The material selected is tested for "fit to purpose" of the device, such as mechanical, physical, chemical, and toxicological characteristics. New or novel materials and additives are continually involved in the applications and hence, if the product is made up of a new material that has not been used in healthcare applications before, a full suite of testing may be required.

9.6.1 Efficacy or performance testing of urological implants

We have seen, urological implants varied from little more than a silicone tube using single biomaterial to the combination of biomaterials, biodegradable stents, to active energy emitting implants like brachytherapy seeds used in prostate cancer. Furthermore, urology implants are nonresorbable (permanent) or resorbable (biodegradable stents), and the rate of resorption by the body can usually be tuned to the desired period. Thus urology implants, as per classification of medical devices are from class I to class III, that is. minimal risk to high risk to active implants. Therefore for evaluation of performance, nonclinical and clinical safety of the urological implants, basic understanding of complex reactions involving specific implant characteristics (chemical, physical, and thermal), as well as cellular and secretory factors is required. The successful toxicological assessment also recommends knowledge of molecular, cellular, tissue, and organ pathobiology. In addition, understanding of principles of healing, selection of host testing model, surgical techniques, healing time, clinical endpoints, techniques of specimen collection, and preparation are all pivotal in the evaluation of the implant and host response [146].

For testing the functionality or efficacy of urological implants, various models were used. This model development requires a proper understanding of the pathophysiology of the disease for which the urology implants are being manufactured. Performance testing of urology implants varies with the diversity of devices and components and a variety of the clinical conditions of the devices. Specific techniques routinely employed in assessment to understand the implant's performance and host response to implants include the use of imaging techniques, computer-assisted analysis, and morphologic analysis (macroscopic, microscopic, and ultrastructural). There was the use of various models for the assessment of the efficacy of the urology implants. With regard to the testing of the efficacy of prostate cancer, Tang et al. [113] have described the role of metabolism in cancer cell radioresistance and radiosensitization methods. The models that can be used for testing safety and efficacy of radiation implants include in vitro cell culture assays as well as in vivo ectopic and orthotopic xenograft models. In the case of ureteral stents, Tunney et al. [17,27] employed a model representing upper urinary tract conditions, using artificial urine and modified Robbins device continuous flow model to assess ureteral stent biomaterial encrustation. Efficacy of penile prosthesis have been studied in cadavers and using in vitro and in vivo models, as described in previous sections.

9.6.2 Toxicity testing of urological implants

In general, urology implants shall be tested for evidence of biocompatibility (absence of localized irritation or toxicity) and if urology implants elute the drug, then additional tissues and organs in the body shall be evaluated for systemic effects. The material used for urological implants may cause systemic effects such as those occurring in the tissues distant from the site of contact, which can be associated with leachable chemicals or degradation products released from implants, following exposure to biological fluids, inflammatory cells, or both. Mechanisms associated with systemic effects may include chemical toxicity, nonspecific cytokine activation with systemic inflammation, vasoactive effects associated with complement activation, or specific immune-mediated response. The examiner must be aware of organ structures where implants are placed, background findings that are uniquely associated with the particular host, and general responses of urological devices to physical and chemical injury to determine if microscopic findings are of toxicological importance.

9.6.3 Role of pathology in safety evaluation of urology implants

Pathologic evaluation of the safety of medical devices has a central position in regulatory testing programs. The device pathology is typically a necessity in the prelude for regulatory submission of medical devices. A pathologic analysis is tailored to the type of device and involves gross and microscopic evaluation of the medical device and associated tissues [147,148]. Although the migration of test materials has been cited as a cause of abnormal placement of materials [149], inappropriate initial placement into target sites or completely missing the target site is more probable. Therefore gross examination of implants in situ is important; various imaging techniques, including gross photography, microcomputed tomography (Micro-CT) scanning, radiography, and microradiography, are used in the macroscopic examination of implants are well described by Rousselle and Wicks [150].

Primary biological responses to biomaterials and medical devices involves typical of a response to any foreign body such as activation of the immune and vascular systems, degeneration and necrosis. These responses may be directly induced by the biomaterial or implant or tissue proliferation or vascular activity. Use of pathological techniques help to define tissue response to biomaterial both locally and systemically, by evaluating tissues grossly and their sections under a light microscope. The gross pathology examination is very critical for extraction, dissection of implants, and obtaining optimal samples for subsequent histopathological examination. The sections obtained then can be stained with hematoxylin and eosin stain routinely or special stains, histochemistry, immunohistochemistry, and cryomicrotometry may be required as per the type of implant and tissue involved. For studying the detailed effects of implant and tissue reaction at molecular levels, electron microscopy (transmission and scanning) can be used. Special procedures may also be required for energy-based medical devices such as prostate implants or nanoparticles intended to receive specific light frequencies and transmit heat [151]. Thus device pathology plays a very important role in the integration of new technologies to viewing interactions with patient bodies and contributing to the toxicological assessment of medical devices including urological implants [152]. There are various types of urological implants; therefore, implant-specific techniques can be used to understand the efficacy, implant performance, and safety of particular urology implants.

9.7 Future trends in the development of urology and nephrology implants and conclusions

Currently, we are in an era where new technology in medicine is fast growing and quickly becoming applicable. Urology, as a specialty, has always been at the forefront of rapidly embracing innovation and research and, improved upon to achieve better patient outcomes. Because of these technological advances, more options will be available for the treatment of urology diseases in the years to come. Great efforts are being made in the fields of tissue engineering and regenerative medicine to provide alternative cell-based approaches for the treatment of renal failure, including bioartificial renal systems and the implantation of bioengineered kidney constructs [153]. Recent advances have been made in the generation of kidney organoids in vitro that engraft in vivo [154]. In the future, much will have changed in imaging, diagnostics, and the utilization of new techniques currently under development. Emerging technologies derived from artificial intelligence and machine learning are increasingly transforming medical procedures and devices and will offer great opportunities. There is currently a focus on portable, wearable devices and self-care systems to improve the quality of life of renal patients [155,156]. The most recent trends in the development of computer-based intelligent decision support systems and expert systems applied to dialysis are based on artificial neural networks and genetic algorithms.

3D bioprinting is a promising additive manufacturing technology based on the deposition of biomaterials and cells in the micrometer scale (with a printing resolution of 10–10,000 μm) to form precise structures comparable to the tissue [157]. Another interesting approach is the wearable artificial kidney, a 5-kg wearable, miniaturized device with a sorbent-based hemodialysis system that is worn on the waist like a toolkit belt and is currently under development at the University of Washington, USA. Similarly, a new mechanical device called "Erektor" has been introduced recently. The device is applied externally and no surgical intervention is required. Erectile technologies may revolutionize ED treatment, and in the very near future, ED may become a curable condition [158]. A variety of minimally invasive therapies (MITs) have been developed to address the limitations and shortcomings of surgery and medical therapy for the management of lower urinary tract symptoms (LUTS) due to benign prostatic obstruction (BPO). Narrowband imaging (NBI) is one of the new techniques, using specific blue and green wavelengths in endoscopy to enhance mucosal detail [159]. Hsueh and Chiu [160] reported that the use of NBI in transurethral resection of bladder tumors reduced tumor recurrence.

Developments in fields of imaging, diagnostics, robotics, minimally invasive techniques, nanotechnology, tissue engineering, and artificial intelligence, likely hold the key to a new era for urology and nephrology. However, the time and high-quality toxicological evaluation studies will decide which of these therapies will be accepted by patients and urologists.

References

[1] Hickling DR, Sun TT, Wu XR. Anatomy and physiology of the urinary tract: relation to host defense and microbial infection. Microbiol Spectr 2015;3(4):1–28.

[2] Kim S. Urologic diseases. Written by Krista O'Connell (Internet), <https://www.healthline.com/health/renal-and-urological-disorders/>; 2016 [cited 20.01.16].

[3] Maitz MF. Applications of synthetic polymers in clinical medicine. Biosurf Biotribol 2015;1(3):161–76.

[4] USFDA. Medical devices, products and medical procedures, implants and prosthetics (Internet), <https://www.fda.gov/medical-devices/products-and-medical-procedures/implants-and-prosthetics/>; 2018 [cited 28.08.18].

[5] Joung YH. Development of implantable medical devices: from an engineering perspective. Int Neurourol J 2013;17:98–106.

[6] Rose JG, Gillenwater JY. Effects of obstruction on ureteral function. Urology 1973;12:139.

[7] Lawrentschuk N, Russell JM. Ureteric stenting 25 years on: routine or risky? ANZ J Surg 2004;74(4):243–7.

[8] Yachia D. Recent advances in ureteral stents. Curr Opin Urol 2008;18(2):241–6.

[9] Liatsikos EN, Karnabatidis D, Katsanos K, Kallidonis P, Katsakiori P, Kagadis GC, et al. Ureteral metal stents: 10-year experience with malignant ureteral obstruction treatment. J Urol 2009;182:2613–17.

[10] Nakagawa Y. Mechanical property of the human ureter. Japanese J Urol 1989;80 (10):1481–8.
[11] Simeone C, Zanotelli T, Tralce L, Cancarini G, Tosana M, Da Pozzo GP. Structure, physiology and physiopathology of the ureter. Arch Ital Urol Nefrol Androl 1993;65 (1):21–5.
[12] Rassoli A, Shafigh M, Seddighi A, Seddighi A, Daneshparvar H, Fatouraee N. Biaxial mechanical properties of human ureter under tension. Urol J 2014;11 (3):1678–86.
[13] Asakawa J, Iguchi T, Tamada S, Ninomiya N, Kato M, Yamasaki T, et al. Treatment outcomes of ureteral stenting for malignant extrinsic ureteral obstruction: a comparison between polymeric and metallic stents. Cancer Manag Res 2018;10:2977–82.
[14] Lam JS, Gupta M. Update on ureteral stents. Urology 2004;64:9–15.
[15] Richter S, Ringel A, Shalev M, Nissenkorn I. The indwelling ureteric stent: a 'friendly' procedure with unfriendly high morbidity. BJU Int 2000;85:408–41.
[16] Mardis HK, Kroeger RM, Morton JJ, Donovan JM. Comparative evaluation of materials used for internal ureteral stents. J Endourol 1993;7(2):105–15.
[17] Tunney MM, Keane PF, Jones DS, Gorman SP. Comparative assessment of ureteral stent biomaterial encrustation. Biomaterials 1996;17(15):1541–6.
[18] Al-Aown A, Kyriazis I, Kallidonis P, Kraniotis P, Rigopoulos C, Karnabatidis D, et al. Ureteral stents: new ideas, new designs. Ther Adv Urol 2010;2:85–92.
[19] Lange D, Bidnur S, Hoag N, Chew BH. Ureteral stent-associated complications—where we are and where we are going. Nat Rev Urol 2015;12:17–25.
[20] Olweny EO, Landman J, Andreoni C, Collyer W, Kerbl K, Onciu M, et al. Evaluation of the use of a biodegradable ureteral stent after retrograde endopyelotomy in a porcine model. J Urol 2002;167(5):2198–202.
[21] Barros AA, Rita A, Duarte C, Pires RA, Sampaio-Marques B, Ludovico P, et al. Bioresorbable ureteral stents from natural origin polymers. J Biomed Mater Res B 2015;103:608–17.
[22] Wang H, Liu J, Zeng J, Zeng C, Zhou Y. Expression of TβR-2, Smad3 and Smad7 in the vaginal anterior wall of postpartum rats with stress urinary incontinence. Arch Gynecol Obstet 2015;291:869–76.
[23] Hermawan H. Updates on the research and development of absorbable metals for biomedical applications. Prog Biomater 2018;7:93–110.
[24] Francis A, Yang Y, Virtanen S, Boccaccini AR. Iron and iron-based alloys for temporary cardiovascular applications. J Mater Sci Mater Med 2015;26:138.
[25] Haude M, Ince H, Kische S, Abizai A, Tölg R, Alves LP, et al. Sustained safety and clinical performance of a drug-eluting absorbable metal scaffold up to 24 months: pooled outcomes of BIOSOLVE-II and BIOSOLVE-III. EuroIntervention 2017;20:432–9.
[26] Riedl CR, Witkowski M, Plas E, Pflueger H. Heparin coating reduces encrustation of ureteral stents: a preliminary report. Int J Antimicrob Agents 2002;19(6):507–10.
[27] Tunney MM, Gorman SP. Evaluation of a poly(vinyl pyrollidone)-coated biomaterial for urological use. Biomaterials 2002;23(23):4601–8.
[28] Joshi HB, Newns N, Stainthorpe A, MacDonagh RP, Keeley Jr FX, Timoney AG. Ureteral stent symptom questionnaire: development and validation of a multidimensional quality of life measure. J Urol 2003;169:1060–4.
[29] Miyaoka R, Monga M. Ureteral stent discomfort: etiology and management. Indian J Urol 2009;25(4):455–60.
[30] Giannarini G, Keeley Jr FX, Valent F, Manassero F, Mogorovich A, Autorino R, et al. Predictors of morbidity in patients with indwelling ureteric stents: results of a prospective study using the validated ureteric stent symptoms questionnaire. BJU Int 2011;107(4):648–54.

[31] Al-Kandari AM, Al-Shaiji TF, Shaaban H, Ibrahim HM, Elshebiny YH, Shokeir AA. Effects of proximal and distal ends of double-J ureteral stent position on postprocedural symptoms and quality of life: a randomized clinical trial. J Endourol 2007;2:698–702.

[32] Chew BH, Knudsen BE, Nott L, Pautler SE, Razvi H, Amann J, et al. Pilot study of ureteral movement in stented patients: first step in understanding dynamic ureteral anatomy to improve stent comfort. J Endourol 2007;21:1069–75.

[33] Kinn AC, Lykkeskov-Andersen H. Impact on ureteral peristalsis in a stented ureter. An Exp Study Pig Urol Res 2002;30:213–18.

[34] Venkatesh R, Landman J, Minor SD, Lee DI, Rehman J, Vanlangendonck R, et al. Impact of a double-pigtail stent on ureteral peristalsis in the porcine model: initial studies using a novel implantable magnetic sensor. J Endourol 2005;19:170–6.

[35] Jeon SS, Choi YS, Hong JH. Determination of ideal stent length for endourologic surgery. J Endourol 2007;21(8):906–10.

[36] Elwood CN, Lo J, Chou E, Crowe A, Arsovska O, Adomat H, et al. Understanding urinary conditioning film components on ureteral stents: profiling protein components and evaluating their role in bacterial colonization. Biofouling 2013;29:1115–22.

[37] Farsi HM, Mosli HA, Al-Zemaity MF, Bahnassy AA, Alvarez M. Bacteriuria and colonization of double-pigtail ureteral stents: long-term experience with 237 patients. J Endourol 1995;9:469–72.

[38] Kawahara T, Ito H, Terao H, Yoshida M, Matsuzaki J. Ureteral stent encrustation, incrustation, and coloring: morbidity related to indwelling times. J Endourol 2012;26(2):178–82.

[39] Singh I, Gupta NP, Hemal AK, Aron M, Seth A, Dogra PN. Severely encrusted polyurethane ureteral stents: management and analysis of potential risk factors. Urology 2001;58:526–31.

[40] Gorman SP, Tunney MM. Assessment of encrustation behavior on urinary tract biomaterials. J Biomater Appl 1997;12(2):136–66.

[41] Shaw GL, Choong SK, Fry C. Encrustation of biomaterials in the urinary tract. Urol Res 2005;33:17–22.

[42] Tunney MM, Keane PF, Gorman SP. Assessment of urinary tract biomaterial encrustation using a modified Robbins device continuous flow model. J Biomed Mater Res (Appl Biomater) 1997;38:87–93.

[43] Lock JY, Wyatt E, Upadhyayula S, Whall A, Nuñez V, Vullev VI, et al. Degradation and antibacterial properties of magnesium alloys in artificial urine for potential resorbable ureteral stent applications. J Biomed Mater Res A 2014;102:781–92.

[44] Zhang S, Zheng Y, Zhang L, Bi Y, Li J, Liu J, et al. In vitro and in vivo corrosion and histocompatibility of pure Mg and a Mg-6Zn alloy as urinary implants in rat model. Mater Sci Eng C 2016;68:414–22.

[45] Zhang S, Bi Y, Li J, Wang Z, Yan J, Song J, et al. Biodegradation behavior of magnesium and ZK60 alloy in artificial urine and rat models. Bioact Mater 2017;2:53–62.

[46] Wang L, Zhang S, Keatch R, Corner G, Nabi G, Murdoch S, et al. In-vitro antibacterial and anti-encrustation performance of silver-polytetrafluoroethylene nanocomposite coated urinary catheters. J Hosp Infect 2019;103(1):55–63.

[47] Abrams P, Blaivas JG, Stanton SL, Anderson JT. The standardisation of terminology of lower urinary tract function. Scand J Url Nephrol 1988;114(suppl):5–19.

[48] Sandvik H, Kveine E, Hunskaar S. Female urinaryincontinence. phychosocial impact, self-care and consultations. Scand J Caring Sci 1993;7:53–6.

[49] Agarwal BK, Agarwal N. Urinary incontinence: prevalence, risk factors, impact on quality of life and treatment seeking behaviour among middle aged women. Int Surg J 2017;4(6):1953–8.

[50] Currie CJ, McEwan P, Poole CD, Odeyemi IA, Datta SN, Morgan CI. The impact of the overactive bladder on health-related utility and quality of life. BJU Int 2006;97:1267–72.

[51] Delancey JO, Ashton-Miller JA. Pathophysiology of adult urinary incontinence. Gastroenterology 2004;126(1 Suppl 1):S23–32.

[52] Enhörning G. Simultaneous recording of intravesical and intraurethral pressure. Acta Chir Scand 1961;276(suppl):1–68.

[53] Kim K-J, Ashton-Miller JA, Strohbehn K, DeLancey JOL, Schultz AB. The vesico-urethral pressuregram analysis of urethral func-tion under stress. J Biomech 1997;30:19–25.

[54] Richardson AC, Edmonds PB, Williams NL. Treatment of stressurinary incontinence due to paravaginal fascial defect. Obstet Gynecol 1981;57:357–62.

[55] Allen RE, Hosker GL, Smith ARB, Warrell DW. Pelvic floor damage and childbirth: a neurophysiological study. Br J Obstet Gynaecol 1990;97:770–9.

[56] Strobehn K, Quint LE, Wojno EJ, DeLancey JOL. Magnetic resonance imaging anatomy of the female urethra: a direct histologic comparison. Obstet Gynecol 1996;88:750–6.

[57] Strohbehn K, DeLancey JOL. The anatomy of stress incontinence. Oper Tech Gynecol Surg 1999;2:15–16.

[58] Rud T, Anderson KE, Asmussen M, Hunting A, Ulmsten U. Factors maintaining the intraurethral pressure in women. Invest Urol 1980;17:343–7.

[59] Perucchini D, DeLancey JOL, Ashton-Miller JA, Pechers U, Kataria T. Age effects on urethral striated muscle: I. Changes in number and diameter of striated muscle fibers in the ventral urethra. Am J Obstet Gynecol 2002;186:351–5.

[60] Smith ARB, Hosker GL, Warrell DW. The role of partial denervation of the pelvic floor in the aetiology of genitourinary prolapse and stress incontinence of urine: a neurophysiological study. Br J Obstet Gynaecol 1989;96:24–8.

[61] Pandit M, DeLancey JO, Ashton-Miller JA, Iyengar J, Blaivas M, Perucchini D. Quantification of intramuscular nerves within the female striated urogenital sphincter muscle. Obstet Gynecol 2000;95(6.1):797–800.

[62] Cardozo L. Discussion: the effect of estrogens. Urology 1997;50(6A suppl):85.

[63] Townsend MK, Danforth KN, Rosner B. Body mass index, weight gain, and incident urinary incontinence in middle-aged women. Obstet Gynecol 2007;110(2 Part 1):346–53.

[64] Dorey G. A clinical overview of the treatment of post-prostatectomy incontinence. Br J Nurs 2007;16:1194–9.

[65] Smith IA. Postprostatectomy stress urinary incontinence. Aust Fam Phys 2009;38 (6):399–404.

[66] Abrams P, Cardozo L, Fall M, Griffiths D, Rosier P, Ulmsten U, et al. Standardization sub-committee of the international continence society: the standardization of terminology in lower urinary tract function: report from the standardization sub-committee of the international continence society. Urology 2003;61(1):37–49.

[67] Abrams P, Andersson K-E, Birder L, Brubaker L, Cardozo L, Chapple C, et al. Evaluation and treatment of urinary incontinence, pelvic organ prolapse, and fecal incontinence. Neurourol Urodyn 2010;29(1):213–40.

[68] Abrams P. Describing bladder storage function: overactive bladder syndrome and detrusor overactivity. Urology 2003;62:28–37.

[69] Smith DR, Tanagho EA, McAninch JW. Smith's general urology. 17th ed. New York: Lange Medical Books/McGraw-Hill; 2008.

[70] Brubaker L, Stoddard A, Richter H, Zimmern P, Moalli P, Kraus SR, et al. Mixed incontinence comparing definitions in women having stress incontinence surgery. Neurourol Urodyn 2009;28(4):268–73.

[71] DeMaagd GA, Davenport TC. Management of urinary incontinence. Pharmacol Ther 2012;37(6):345–61 361B-361H.

[72] Wein AJ, Rovner ES. Pharmacologic management of urinary incontinence in women. Urol Clin North Am 2002;29:537–50.
[73] Rovner ES, Wein AJ. Treatment options for stress urinary incontinence. Rev Urol 2004;6(Suppl 3):S29–47.
[74] Peeker I, Peeker R. Early diagnosis and treatment of genuine stress urinary incontinence in women after pregnancy: midwives as detectives. J Midwifery Womens Health 2003;48(1):60–6.
[75] Wilson PD, Bo K, Hay-Smith J, Nygaard I, Staskin D, Wyman J. Conservative treatment in women. In: Abrams P, Cardozo L, Khoury S, Wein A, editors. Incontinence. 2nd ed. Plymouth, UK: Health Publication Ltd; 2002. p. 571–624.
[76] Bachmann G, Wiita B. External occlusive devices for management of female urinary incontinence. J Womens Health (Larchmt) 2002;11(9):793–800.
[77] Sasso KM. The Colpexin sphere: a new conservative management option for pelvic organ prolapse. Urol Nurs 2006;26(6):433–40.
[78] Richter HE, Burgio KL, Brubaker L. Continence pessary compared with behavioral therapy or combined therapy for stress incontinence: a randomized controlled trial. Obstet Gynecol 2010;115(3):609–17.
[79] Wood LN, Anger JT. Urinary incontinence in women. BMJ 2014;349:g4531.
[80] Zeng J, Liu J, Zeng C, Chen D. Biological effects of electrical stimulation on pelvic floor muscle strength and neuropeptide Y expression. Int J Clin Exp Med 2019;12 (3):2427–34.
[81] Dmochowski RR, Kerrebroeck PV, Digesu GA, Heesakkers JPFA. Long-term results of safety, efficacy, quality of life and satisfaction of patients treated for refractory OAB using an implantable tibial neurostimulation system: Renova Istim™ System. J Urol 2019;201(Suppl. 4) PD31-02, e565–e566.
[82] Smith IA, Shaw E, Rashid P. Postprostatectomy stress urinary incontinence - current and evolving therapies. Aust Fam Physician 2009;38(6):399–404.
[83] Gilling PJ, Bell DF, Wilson LC, Westenberg AM, Reuther R, Fraundorfer MR. An adjustable continence therapy device for treating incontinence after prostatectomy: a minimum 2-year follow-up. BJU Int 2008;102(10):1426–30.
[84] Magera JS, Elliott DS. Artificial urinary sphincter infection: causative organisms in a contemporary series. J Urol 2008;180(6):2475–8.
[85] Trost L, Elliott DS. Male stress urinary incontinence: a review of surgical treatment options and outcomes. Adv Urol 2012;1–13.
[86] Porpiglia F, Fiori C, Bertolo R, Garrou D, Cattaneo G, Amparore D. Temporary implantable nitinol device (TIND): a novel, minimally invasive treatment for relief of lower urinary tract symptoms (LUTS) related to benign prostatic hyperplasia (BPH): feasibility, safety and functional results at 1 year of follow-up. BJU Int 2015;116(2):278–87.
[87] Leslie SW, Siref LE. Cancer, prostate. Stat Pearls. Treasure Island (FL): Stat Pearls Publishing; 2018. Available from: <http://www.ncbi.nlm.nih.gov/books/NBK470550/>.
[88] Bass EJ, Ahmed HU. Focal therapy in prostate cancer: a review of seven common controversies. Cancer Treat Rev 2016;51:27–34.
[89] Cooperberg MR, Chan JM. Epidemiology of prostate cancer. World J Urol 2017;35 (6):849.
[90] Lee SH, Shen MM. Cell types of origin for prostate cancer. Curr Opin Cell Biol 2015;37:35–41.
[91] Toivanen R, Shen MM. Prostate organogenesis: tissue induction, hormonal regulation and cell type specification. Development 2017;144(8):1382–98.
[92] Tobias J, Hochhauser WD. Cancer and its management. 7th ed. John Wiley & Sons, Ltd.; 2014Copyright © 2015. Available from: https://doi.org/10.1002/9781118468753.
[93] Chen N, Zhou Q. The evolving Gleason grading system. Chin J Cancer Res 2016;28(1):58–64.

[94] Ahmed HU, Pendse D, Illing R, Allen C, van der Meulen JH, Emberton M. Will focal therapy become a standard of care for men with localized prostate cancer? Nat Clin Pract Oncol 2007;4(11):632–42.
[95] Lindner U, Trachtenberg J, Lawrentschuk N. Focal therapy in prostate cancer: modalities, findings and future considerations. Nat Rev Urol 2010;7(10):562–71.
[96] Ouzzane A, Betrouni N, Valerio M, Rastinehad A, Colin P, Ploussard G. Focal therapy as primary treatment for localized prostate cancer: definition, needs and future. Future Oncol 2017;13(8):727–41.
[97] Pesapane F, Patella F, Fumarola EM, Zanchetta E, Floridi C, Carrafiello G, et al. The prostate cancerfocaltherapy. Gland Surg 2018;7(2):89–102.
[98] Niehoff P, Loch T, Nürnberg N, Galalae R, Egberts J, Kohr P, et al. Feasibility and preliminary outcome of salvage combined HDR brachytherapy and external beam radiotherapy (EBRT) for local recurrences after radical prostatectomy. Brachytherapy 2005;4(2):141–5.
[99] èyczek J, Kawczyńska MM, Garmol D, Kasprowicz A, Kulik A, Dąbkowski M, et al. HDR brachytherapy as a solution in recurrences of locally advanced prostate cancer. J Contemp Brachyther 2009;1(2):105–8.
[100] Abreha SK. Model-based cost-effectiveness analysis of external beam radiation therapy for the treatment of localized prostate cancer: a systematic review. Cost Eff Resour Alloc 2019;17:10.
[101] Brumm J. Brachytherapy as a treatment option for prostate cancer: overview and nursing considerations. Proc (Bayl Univ Med Cent) 2000;13(3):227–9.
[102] Stish BJ, Davis BJ, Mynderse LA, Deufel CL, Choo R. Brachytherapy in the management of prostate cancer. Surg Oncol Clin N Am 2017;26(3):491–513.
[103] Peach MS, Trifiletti DM, Libby B. Systematic review of focal prostate brachytherapy and the future implementation of image-guided prostate HDR brachytherapy using MR-ultrasound fusion. Prostate Cancer 2016;1–13.
[104] Gburek BM, Kollmorgen TA, Qian J, D'Souza-Gburek SM, Lieber MM, Jenkins RB. Chromosomal anomalies in stage D1 prostate adenocarcinoma primary in situ hybridization. J Urol 1997;157(1):223–7.
[105] Mearini L, Porena M. Pros and cons of focal therapy for localised prostate cancer. Prostate Cancer 2011;1–8. Available from: https://doi.org/10.1155/2011/584784.
[106] Ben-Yosef R, Paz A, Levy Y, Alani S, Muncher Y, Shohat S, et al. A novel device for protecting rectum during prostate cancer irradiation: in vivo data on a large mammal model. J Urol 2009;181(3):1401–6.
[107] Levy Y, Paz A, Yosef RB, Corn BW, Vaisman B, Shuhat S, et al. Biodegradable inflatable balloon for reducing radiation adverse effects in prostate cancer. J Biomed Mater Res B Appl Biomater 2009;91(2):855–67.
[108] Mallick S, Madan R, Julka PK, Rath GK. Radiation induced cystitis and proctitis - prediction, assessment and management. Asian Pac J Cancer Prev 2015;16 (14):5589–94.
[109] Wortel RC, Incrocci L, Mulhall JP. Reporting erectile function outcomes after radiation therapy for prostate cancer: challenges in data interpretation. J Sex Med 2017;.
[110] Dutta SW, Alonso CE, Libby B, Showalter TN. Prostate cancer high dose-rate brachytherapy: review of evidence and current perspectives. Expert Rev Med Dev 2018;15(1):71–9.
[111] Tofilon PJ, Camphausen K. Molecular targets for tumor radiosensitization. Chem Rev 2009;109(7):2974–88.
[112] Krause M, Dubrovska A, Linge A, Baumann M. Cancer stem cells: radioresistance, prediction of radiotherapy outcome and specific targets for combined treatments. Adv Drug Deliv Rev 2017;109:63–73.

[113] Tang L, Wei F, Wu Y, He Y, Shi L, Xiong F, et al. Role of metabolism in cancer cell radioresistance and radiosensitization methods. J Exp Clin Cancer Res 2018;37(1):87.

[114] Torrance CJ, Agrawal V, Vogelstein B, Kinzler KW. Use of isogenic human cancer cells for high-throughput screening and drug discovery. Nat Biotechnol 2001;19:940–5.

[115] Cox JD, Stetz J, Pajak TF. Toxicity criteria of the radiation therapy oncology group (RTOG) and the European organization for research and treatment of cancer (EORTC). Int J Radiat Oncol Biol Phys 1995;31(5):1341–6.

[116] Feldman HA, Goldstein I, Hatzichristou DG. Impotence and its medical and psychosocial correlates: results of the Massachusetts male aging study. J Urol 1994;151:54–61.

[117] Klein R, Klein BE, Lee KE, Moss SE, Cruickshanks KJ. Prevalence of self-reported erectile dysfunction in people with long-term IDDM. Diabetes Care 1996;19:135–41.

[118] Araujo AB, Esche GR, Kupelian V. Prevalence of symptomatic androgen deficiency in men. J Clin Endocrinol Metab 2007;92:4241–7.

[119] Aksam A, Yassin A, Saad F. Testosterone and erectile dysfunction. J Androl 2008;29.

[120] Langer R, Sharma E, Langer B, Gupta RK, Kumari R, Majeed M. Erectile dysfunction: prevalence and determinants among T2DM men attending a tertiary care hospital in northern India. Int Surg J 2019;6(4):1115–19.

[121] Lue TF. Erectile dysfunction. N Engl J Med 2000;342(24):1802–13.

[122] Dean RC, Lue TF. Physiology of penile erection and pathophysiology of erectile dysfunction. Urol Clin North Am 2005;32(4):379–95.

[123] Lasker GF, Maley JH, Kadowitz PJ. A review of the pathophysiology and novel treatments for erectile dysfunction. Adv Pharmacol Sci 2010;2010:1–10.

[124] Bancroft J, Wu FC. Changes in erectile responsiveness during androgen replacement therapy. Arch Sex Behav 1983;12:59–66.

[125] Levine FJ, Greenfield AJ, Goldstein I. Arteriographically determined occlusive disease within the hypogastric-cavernous bed in impotent patients following blunt perineal and pelvic trauma. J Urol 1990;144:1147–53.

[126] Rosen MP, Greenfield AJ, Walker TG, Grant P, Dubrow J, Bettmann MA, et al. Cigarette smoking: an independent risk factor for atherosclerosis in the hypogastric-cavernous arterial bed of men with arteriogenic impotence. J Urol 1991;145:759–63.

[127] Hsieh JT, Lue TF, Muller SC, Aboseif SR, Orvis BR, Tanagho EA. The influence of blood flow and blood pressure on penile erection. Int J Impot Res 1989;1:35–42.

[128] Shamloul R, Bella AJ. Erectile dysfunction. Biota Publishing; 2014, ISBN: 978-1-61504-653-9. p. 6.

[129] Sadeghi-Nejad H. Penile prosthesis surgery: a review of prosthetic devices and associated complications. J Sex Med 2007;4:296–309.

[130] Le B, Burnett AL. Evolution of penile prosthetic devices. Korean J Urol 2015;56(3):179–86.

[131] Iwatsubo E, Tanaka M, Takahashi K, Akatsu T. Non-inflatablepenile prosthesis for the management of urinary incontinence and sexual disability of patients with spinal cord injury. Paraplegia 1986;24(5):307–10.

[132] Hartman RP, Kawashima A, Takahashi N, LeRoy AJ, King BF. Inflatable penile prosthesis (IPP): diagnosis of complications. Abdom Radiol 2016;41(6):1187–96.

[133] Chung E. Penile prosthesis implant: scientific advances and technological innovations over the last four decades. Transl Androl Urol 2017;6(1):37–45.

[134] Le BV, McVary KT, McKenna K, Colombo A. Use of magnetic induction to activate a "touchless" shape memory alloy implantable penile prosthesis. J Sex Med 2019;16(4):596–601.

[135] Jain S, Bhojwani A, Terry TR. The role of penile prosthetic surgery in the modern management of erectile dysfunction. Postgrad Med J 2000;76:22–5.

[136] Lewis RW. Long-term results of penile prosthetic implants. Urol Clin North Am 1995;22(4):847–56.

[137] Pineda M, Burnett AL. Penile prosthesis infections-a review of risk factors, prevention, and treatment. Sex Med Rev 2016;4(4):389–98.
[138] Vakalopoulos I, Kampantais S, Gkagkalidis K, et al. Complications of inflatable penile prostheses implantation classified according to the modified Clavien system. Adv Urol 2014;14:5.
[139] Mansouri MD, Boone TB, Darouiche RO. Comparative assessment of antimicrobial activities of antibiotic-treated penile prostheses. Eur Urol 2009;56(6):1039–45.
[140] Darouiche RO, Mansouri MD, Raad II. Efficacy of antimicrobial-impregnated silicone sections from penile implants in preventing device colonization in an animal model. Urology 2002;59(2):303–7.
[141] Wang SJ, Chen KK, Lin AT, Young ST, Chang LS. Hardness evaluation of penile prostheses. Int J Urol 2006;13(5):569–72.
[142] Henry GD, Jennermann C, Eid J. Evaluation of satisfaction and axial rigidity with titan XL cylinders. Adv Urol 2012;.
[143] Richtel M. What's the flavor of the month? Medical devices. New York Times; 2007. p. 11.
[144] Schuh JCL. Medical device regulations and testing for toxicologic pathologists. Toxicol Pathol 2008;36:63–9.
[145] Food and Drug Administration (FDA). Medical devices; reclassification of six cardiovascular preamendments class III devices into class II. final rule. Fed Registry 2001;66:18540–2.
[146] Alves A, Metz A, Render J. Microscopic and ultrastructural pathology in medical devices. In: Boutrand J-P, editor. Biocompatibility and performance of medical devices. Oxford Woodhead Publishing Limited.; 2012. p. 457–99.
[147] Gad SC, Gad-McDonald S. Biomaterials, medical devices, and combination products: biocompatibility testing and safety assessment. Boca Raton, FL: CRC Press; 2016.
[148] Kirchhof N. What is "preclinical device pathology": an introduction of the unfamiliar. Toxicol Pathol 2019;47(3):205–12.
[149] Friedemann MC, Mehta NA, Jessen SL, Charara FH, Ginn-Hedman AM, Kaulfus CN, et al. Introduction to currently applied device pathology. Toxicol Pathol 2019;47(3):221–34.
[150] Gad S. Implantation biology and studies. In: Gad S, editor. Safety evaluation of medical devices. New York: Marcel Dekker, Inc; 2002. p. 269–93.
[151] Rousselle S, Wicks J. Preparation of medical devices for evaluation. Toxicol Pathol 2008;36(1):81–4.
[152] Gad SC, Schuh CL. Toxicologic pathology forum opinion paper: considerations for toxicologic pathologists evaluating the safety of biomaterials and finished medical devices. Toxicol Pathol 2018;46(4):366–71.
[153] Chung HC, Ko IK, Atala A, Yoo JJ. Cell-based therapy for kidney disease. Korean J Urol 2015;56(6):412–21.
[154] Bantounas I, Ranjzad P, Tengku F, Silajdžić E, Forster D, Asselin MC, et al. Generation of functioning nephrons by implanting human pluripotent stem cell-derived kidney progenitors. Stem Cell Rep 2018;10(3):766–79.
[155] Hueso M, Navarro E, Sandoval D, Cruzado JM. Progress in the development and challenges for the use of artificial kidneys and wearable dialysis devices. Kid Dis 2019;5:3–10.
[156] Khan W, Muntimadugu E, Jaffe M, Domb AJ. Implantable medical devices, in book- advances in delivery science and technology- focal controlled. Drug Deliv 2014;33–60.

[157] Derakhshanfar S, Mbeleck R, Xu K, Zhang X, Zhong W, Xing M. 3D bioprinting for biomedical devices and tissue engineering: a review of recent trends and advances. Bioact Mater 2018;3(2):144–56.
[158] Stein MJ, Lin H, Wang R. New advances in erectile technology. Ther Adv Urol 2014;6(1):15–24.
[159] Bernstein DE, Bernstein BS. Urological technology: where will we be in 20 years' time? Ther Adv Urol 2018;10(8):235–42.
[160] Hsueh TY, Chiu AW. Narrow band imaging for bladder cancer. Asian J Urol 2016;3:126–9.

CHAPTER TEN

Orthopedics

Nobel Bhasin[1,*] and Manish Ranjan[2]
[1]Department of Medicine, University of Chicago, Chicago, IL, United States
[2]Department of Surgery, Northwestern University, Chicago, IL, United States
*Corresponding author

Abstract

Several approaches have been used to address the age-old problem of joint fractures and spine ailments. The first excision joint arthroplasty was recorded in 1886 performed by Anthony White in London. Challenges to successful implant in the early days were presented in the form of infection, corrosion, and lack of tensile strength of implants. With the evolution of surgical techniques and the invention of stainless steel in 1924, metals began to be routinely used in joint implants. It was not until the late 1950s that the spinal implants began to be performed to treat scoliosis. Modern metallic implants now comprise cobalt—chromium alloys, stainless steel, and titanium alloys. The human body forms an aqueous environment that constantly attacks the metal implant leading to corrosion. This electrochemical degradation and the wear of implants present major clinical concern. The eroded metal ions can be deposited in the vicinity of distal organs with severe cytotoxic, genotoxic, and immunologic effects. Due to the small size of metal ions released by corrosion, they can be ingested by macrophages or distributed systemically via lymphatics to lymph nodes, liver, and spleen. From spleen metal, ions can further find a way into the bloodstream and be circulated across different tissues in the body.
The high morbidity associated with metal implants in joints and spine has prompted research in biomaterials. Other metals, ceramics, and polymers have also been used as implants due to their ability to resist mechanical stress. Capacity building in the area of biomaterials could help mitigate the wear and corrosion-induced toxicities in joint and spinal implants.

Keywords: Metal implant; metal toxicology; biomaterials

10.1 Introduction

Orthopedic implants have been in use for over a hundred years to aid the condition of bone loss and trauma. Orthopedic implants can be temporary in the form of plates, screws pins, wires, and nails to aid recovery from fractures or they could be permanent in cases of inflammatory and degenerative diseases

Toxicological Aspects of Medical Device Implants.
DOI: https://doi.org/10.1016/B978-0-12-820728-4.00010-1
© 2020 Elsevier Inc.
All rights reserved.

requiring joint replacements. An ideal orthopedic implant needs to have excellent stability, tensile strength, and flexibility, resistance to corrosion, aseptic loosening, and bioactivity [1,2]. Metals, ceramics, and polymers are the most common biomaterial implants to address the varying needs of the patients [1,2]. With more than 7 years of exposure, an abnormally high local and systemic concentration of the biomaterial could be observed with associated deleterious effects [2,3]. With an increase in life expectancy and a rise in the number of people with bone disease, human exposure to orthopedic implants has risen necessitating attention to implant-induced toxicity [3].

Total hip replacement is one of the most common of total joint arthroplasties [4]. The currently used bearing surfaces of hip implants can be classified into two major categories: hard on soft and hard on hard. The hard-on-soft bearing comprises ultra-high molecular weight polyethylene (UHMWPE) [5]. UHMWPE remains the current gold standard as a bearing surface for total hip arthroplasty due to its biocompatibility and high resistance to fracture [1,5]. UHMWPE can undergo oxidative degeneration and cause the collection of wear debris leading to osteolysis [1,5]. A multitude of approaches have been adopted to address the problem of wear including radiation crosslinking, different processing, and sterilization microstructural tailoring of UHMPE [1,5]. The problem of wear has persisted despite the capacity development in the prosthesis and the technique. The polyethylene wear particles induce a chronic-inflammatory response ultimately leading to failure of the metal on polyethylene (MOP) implants [1,6]. Improvements in the design of the next generation of metal on metal (MOM) implants have improved stability and durability, but a higher local and circulating concentration of metal products has been observed [1,7]. The use of ceramic head on cross-linked polyethylene has shown promising results with lower wear rates in the ceramic on polyethylene bearing relative to the MOP bearing [1,8]. Osteolysis associated with the large particle size generated from hard-on-soft bearing prosthesis is its major flaw. MOM and ceramic-on-ceramic implants generate smaller particles, but the osteolysis is induced by larger particles [9]. This chapter will focus on MOM implant-induced adverse effects, associated mechanisms, clinical manifestation, and management.

10.2 Factors affecting metal-induced toxicity

MOM hip prosthesis is primarily composed of cobalt–chromium alloys combined with molybdenum and titanium alloys in combination with vanadium and aluminum where manganese, iron, tungsten, and zirconium may also be included [1,10]. Although wear associated with MOM implants produces smaller particles, there is still significant concern over the corrosion of the metals that lead to high exposure to metal ions in the patient. Metal particles generated from wear are released into the vicinity of the implant and systemically induce toxicity. Cr-containing debris is constantly found, but Co is not discovered after a few weeks. MOM prostheses generate metallic wear particles, corrosion products, metal ions, and nanoparticles lower than MOP implants [1,9]. Wear particles undergo corrosion and increase the metal ion levels [11]. Cr–Co release is the quickest and has proven the most detrimental in the context of the orthopedic implant [1,9].

10.2.1 Wear

The nature of wear particles can vary depending on the source of the wear particles [12]. Three main wear mechanisms have been recognized fatigue induced by cyclic stress that leads to microfracture, surface delamination, and abrasion from wear particles derived from softer materials [12]. Other mechanisms of wear particle generation like mechanically assisted fretting have also been reported and are mostly attributable to the mechanical microenvironment at the interface between surfaces [12]. *Size of wear particles:* The MOP implants generate faster wear debris, corrosion products, metal ions, and nanoparticles compared to the MOM implants. For this reason, MOM made a comeback in the 1990s [1]. The size of debris is one of the major determinants of osteolytic loosening and the most common reason for implant failure [1]. In a successfully functioning implant, the wear volume is often low ($<5\ mm^3$ per million cycles or per year) with an average of particle below 100 nm primarily composed of Cr [1,13]. However, if the implant happens to be malpositioned, wear volume and particle size can dramatically increase 100 mm^3 per million cycles or per year and up to 1000 nm, respectively [1,13]. Results from in vitro experiments using hip simulators often underestimate the wear; it is advisable to combine the in vivo data to get realistic potential detriment before introduction to humans [14,15]. Regular histological examinations of periprosthetic tissue often cannot detect the wear particles below 100 nm, which may be present more than one billion particles per gram of tissue [1,16]. The impact of the size on biomolecules adsorbed is still being examined; it appears that structural variation, surface charge, and surface chemistry would be important to gain a deeper understanding [1].

10.2.2 Composition of wear particles

Once released, metal particles interact with biomolecules and often protein gets absorbed to the surface of the particle [1]. Different structures of oligomers emerging from protein ion complex emerge based on affinity [1,17]. A human serum can more easily interact with Cr derived from Co-based alloys relative to its ability to interact with titanium-based alloys [17–19]. The inflammatory response generated in the microenvironment depends on the adsorbed proteins [1]. Serum albumin adsorption increases tumor necrosis α (TNFα) signaling, and IgG adsorption leads to interleukin (IL) 1β. Additionally, bacterial remnants on the surface of the implant can have severe consequences leading to aseptic loosing and implant failure [20]. Toll-like receptor (TLRs) on the macrophages would recognize the pathogen-associated molecular patterns leading to the production of several inflammatory cytokines [20]. In an aseptic pathology, the effect of wear particles on proinflammatory signaling is also increased leading to osteoclast differentiation and osteolysis [1,21]. Excessive production corrosion products also induce macrophage production, and it has been demonstrated that macrophages ingest/disseminate corrosion products collected in a synovial-like interface membrane irrespective of nature of the particle [1,22]. The highest concentration of the metal particles is observed in the periimplant tissue; a high concentration of necrotic and apoptotic macrophages is observed near the implant tissue [1,22]. Surface ulceration and synovial necrosis can occur if CoCr particles are present in the vicinity even if the implant is not loose [1]. Examining the chemical nature of the particles is a developing field, and we do not fully understand the composition of the particles in wear debris. It has been observed that Cr(III)PO4 but no Cr(VI) was present in the periprosthetic tissue of patients who underwent MOM implant surgery along with Co(II) and Mo(VI) when Cr was abundant [1,22].

10.2.3 Metal ions shape and chemistry

Studies examining the shape of metal ions have shown round and oval shapes of Cr ions that are mostly observed in MOM implants [1]. In vitro data suggest that a high concentration of ions is necessary to be cytotoxic irrespective of the size of the ions. It has also been demonstrated that larger and irregular CoCr particles induce IL1β production mediated by lysosomal damage [1,23]. Smaller particles generated are readily ingested by osteoclast, macrophages, and dendritic cells; the larger ones induce an inflammatory response by damaging the lysosomal membrane. Prosthetic wear debris activates NALP3 protein. Once activated, NALP3 and its protein PYCARD recruit capase 1 that cleaves and activates pro-IL-1β and pro-IL-18 [24]. Smaller particles ($<10\ \mu m$) though capable of inducing inflammatory response have been known to be either phagocytosed or diffused to be distributed systemically; the concentration of particles needed to induce the inflammatory repose is however not clear [25]. Data from clinical studies have shown conflicting results on the correlation between wear volume and induction of inflammatory response leading to implant failure in the form of pseudotumor [26–28]. The correlation between wear rate and ion concentration in blood has been debated in clinical studies, but it is evident from in vitro data that exposure to Co ions is likely to induce inflammatory signaling mediated by IL-6 and TNFα [29]. The concentration of metal ions in circulation varies with duration of implant, the wear volume including the micro and nanoparticles in the periprosthetic tissue and the surface area of the device. MOM implants have smaller wear volume but smaller than 100 nm; wear particles that are produced are susceptible to corrosion reaction [1]. MOM with fretting/crevice is associated with larger wear volume attributed to its large head. Metal implants including total hip arthroplasty (THA) and hip resurfacing arthroplasty (HRA) have been shown to have led to a higher concentration of metal ions in blood compared to the patient who underwent ceramic-on-ceramic or MOP implant [1].

10.3 Adverse effect of metal ions

10.3.1 Local adverse effect of metal debris

The periprosthetic tissue in both THA-MOM implants and other metal implants experiences microscopic abnormalities that can be detected upon histological testing for THA. These microscopic abnormalities are referred to as adverse local tissue reaction (ALTR) and adverse reactions to metal debris (ARMD) as umbrella terms for cell damage, and inflammatory response to wear particles [1,30].

10.3.2 Cell damage due to metal debris

Cell debris from Co, Cr, Ti, Ni, and Mo products have causally implicated in cell damage in the tissue surrounding the implant. The cell damage is categorized into programmed cell death, autophagy, necrosis, and necroptosis [31]. Apoptosis is also known as programmed cell death induced by external and internal stress. Apoptosis signaling in cells is highly regulated and is often triggered in response to disease, inflammation, and malignancy [32]. Autophagy is a cellular mechanism for recycling cytosolic constituents, and it allows for degradation and recycling of cellular organelles and proteins [33]. Necrosis has been described as an injury to cells due to extrinsic factors like toxic metal debris. This pathology is marked by induction of strong inflammatory response to surrounding tissue which prevents phagocytosis of damaged cells. Necroptosis is a newer term used to describe the programmed cellular response to extrinsic stress in the form of cell death. This form of cellular damage shows histological features resembling necrosis, and the cell death signaling is induced via stimulation of cell death receptors [33–35].

Cell damage due to the wear debris is greatly affected by the type of metal, its concentration, and duration of exposure in the tissue surrounding the implant. Cell death by apoptosis is observed more often in MOM implants than non-MOM implants [36]. With shorter exposure to implants capable of producing corrosion-prone debris like MOM implants, minimum damage to tissue is observed. However, a longer duration of exposure and the massive phagocytosis of nanoparticles can lead to secondary ion release and an increase in reactive oxygen species (ROS) [37]. Such pathology is consistent with exposure to Cr, Ni, and Co. Co has been shown to stabilize transcriptional activator hypoxia-inducible factor and mimic hypoxic conditions to induce necrosis in periprosthetic tissue [38]. Additionally, $CoCl_2$ has been shown to induce muscle atrophy and apoptosis in myotubes by deregulation of the phosphoinositide 3-kinase/protein kinase B (PI3K/AKT) and NF-kB pathways [39,40]. Low-dose exposure to Ti oxide nanoparticles over time has been shown to induce autophagic effect [41]. Ni nanoparticles have been shown to cause blockage of autophagy by oxidation of methionine and accumulation of modified proteins. The blockage of autophagy can upset the cellular homeostasis and osteointegration of the metal implant. Autophagy has been shown to play a complex role both in osteointegration and osteolysis [42]. In Ti-based metal implants, it enabled osteointegration, but autophagy signaling induced by CoCr can induce osteoblast apoptosis [42]. Further research is needed to fully understand the response to different metals in the implant microenvironment.

10.3.3 Periprosthetic immune response

There are pathologic differences in the immune response to wear debris derived from MOP and MOM implants. Polymeric wear particles derived from MOP implants have been associated with the occurrence of granuloma in the synovial pseudomembrane surrounding the implant. Wear particles are often discovered trapped in the extracellular matrix and also intracellularly in immune cells that infiltrate the implant microenvironment [43]. The progression of this condition characterized by macrophagic phagocytosis of the wear particles is central to the development of osteolysis [43]. Immune response to MOM implants can show both THA and HRA, and even non-MOM THA implants with CoCr have displayed "mixed" etiology. MOM periprostatic histologies could range from displaying only macrophage infiltration to some showing a mix of lymphocytes, macrophages, and sacriod-like granulomas [1,44]. It has been suggested that the necrotic and inflammatory profile observed after MOM implants correlated with component loosening and formation of pseudotumor [1,45]. Cytotoxicity and hypersensitivity to metals are believed to be the two primary contributing factors for the creation of this etiology. Factors contributing to the variation in patient response are yet not well understood, and it can be suggested that patient's factors such as weight and lifestyle choices may play an important role in the manifestation of varied etiology [45]. The primary immune cells in contact with implant wear debris are the osteoblasts and the macrophages present in the surrounding tissue. These cells secrete cytokines and chemokines to induce proinflammatory response and attract monocytes and dendritic cells to the microenvironment [46]. Upon receiving the chemotactic signal circulating cells adhere to vascular endothelium and extravasate to implant microenvironment [47]. Receptor activator of nuclear factor-κB (RANK), expressed by macrophages/monocytes, allows them to be precursors to osteoclasts [46,47]. RANK ligand and macrophage colony-stimulating factor (M-CSF) expression allows de novo osteoclastogenesis that ends up increasing bone resorption [47–50]. Additionally, any therapeutic initiatives directed toward the immune reactivity of macrophages are rendered useless once they differentiate into osteoclasts [1]. Macrophages that ingested the metal wear particles and the free metals escape the synovial-like membrane in the periprosthetic tissue and infiltrate the bone marrow. Co(II) and Cr(III) ions resulting from the corrosion of metal particles or from the phagocytosis upon reaching the bone marrow niche may disable the differentiation function of osteogenic precursors, thus inhibiting further osteogenesis [1,36]. Another mechanism contributing to the inflammatory microenvironment of the implant is macrophage polarization [51]. It is believed that the initial contact with metal wear particles activates M0 macrophages that are polarized toward M1 macrophages [52,53]. M1 macrophages induce inflammatory signaling and cause cytokine release (interferon-c(IFN-c), granulocyte-M-CSF, IL-4, or IL-13, as well as IL-17α) eventually manifesting as chronic inflammation. Chronic inflammation at the implant site often leads to fibrosis, and it is believed that M2 and/or Mreg macrophages appear at the site to repair the damaged tissue [53]. However, molecular data from MOP THA show that polarizing cytokines were discovered at the time of revision surgery for aseptic loosening and the implant site could potentially express both M1 and M2 macrophages [54]. Examining the immune response to metal particles is difficult without accounting for the proteins adsorbed on the metal surface. It has been suggested that proteins such as heat shock proteins, heparin sulfate oxidized low-density lipoprotein, serum amyloid A, versican, biglycan, tenascin C, and lactoferrin must be adsorbed on the metal surface to form what has been referred to as "protein corona layer" [55]. It is believed that the protein layer is a soft outer layer and a hard inner layer and the composition may vary depending on size, surface topography, and the charge of the metal particle [56]. This protein corona is believed to alter the signaling pathways and cell's innate immune response [56]. Toll-like receptor 4 (TL4R4) is an important component of the innate immune response of the cell; it has been reposted that Co and Ni ions derived from the metal debris could activate inflammatory signaling mediated by this molecule [57]. Ti particles phagocytosed by bone marrow-derived monocytes are capable of altering the TLR4 signaling pathway and the signaling of other TLRs molecules [58]. Several factors influence the innate immune response of the cells leading to a chronic inflammatory state in the periprostatic tissue, eventually bone resorption manifesting in osteolysis and implant failure [1].

ALVAL reaction aseptic lymphocytic vasculitis associated lesion (ALVAL) falls under ARMDs specific to lymphocyte-mediated immunological response present at the time of revision surgery of THA in the tissue surrounding the prosthetic [59]. ALVAL has now been adapted as a semiquantitative measure of estimating tissue damage as correlated with the presence of wear debris [60]. Clinically, ALVAL score has found more use in patients with MOM implants [61,62]. Several different methods of scoring are available; it has been observed that a high ALVAL score correlated with lesser metal debris and low ALVAL score is detected in patients with a high metal quantity of debris. It has been suggested that high metal wear may induce a macrophagic reaction, and lower metal present may induce lymphoidogenesis [60,63]. Reports examining the histological profile of the MOM hip arthroplasties have shown a mixture of features including surface necrosis, macrophagic response, and granuloma formation and evolving ALVAL [64]. A significant number of cases undergoing revision surgery for MOM hip arthroplasties show diffuse chronic lymphocytic synovitis and several display lymphoid aggregates with germinal centers. ALVAL is discovered in other arthroplasties as well; however, MOM arthroplasties carry surface necrosis, loss of architecture, and metal debris in macrophages [1,63]. ALVAL has also been discovered in patients who underwent revision surgery for unexplained pain, along with indicators of an adaptive immune response. B and T lymphocyte aggregates were distributed along the vasculature and intramurally in these patients [1]. Non-MOM also displays similar characteristics in cases of hip arthroplasty revision surgery including perivascular lymphocytes and the presence of metal debris [1]. Similar to MOM-THA fretting corrosion is the primary source of metal ion debris. Two primary sources of the metal particles have been identified: the head–neck and the neck–stem taper junctions [1,65,66]. The presence of T lymphocytes is discovered regardless of the implant constitution. T-cell lymphocyte subpopulations coexist with perivascular aggregates, modular implants often show B lymphocytes and germinal centers [1,67]. A key factor in the generation of proinflammatory environment regardless of the design of the implant is the recruitment of osteoclast precursors and ensuing periprosthetic osteolysis [1].

10.3.4 Pseudotumor

Pseudotumors represent a neosinovial proliferation that could be present in soft tissue or bone with necrosis and a variable amount of fluid present. Different histological profiles have been recorded in patients with pseudotumors comprising macrophages and lymphocytes [1,36]. Continuous exposure to metal wear, and chronic inflammation and cytotoxicity that follow has been cited as the main mechanism leading to pseudotumors [1,68]. Clinical studies have not discovered a direct correlation between pseudotumor incidence and volume of exposure to the metals [1,69]. Hypersensitivity to metal has also been suggested as a reason for pseudotumor formation in patients with MOM-THA [68,69]. A lower proportion of memory T lymphocytes was discovered in patients with pseudotumors and has been suggested as a biomarker of diagnosis for pseudotumors [68]. Other reports have also suggested that other signs of metal hypersensitivity be included as indicators of pseudotumors. Tertiary lymphoid organ-like features consisting of lymphoid aggregates of T and B cells have also been reported suggesting the involvement of the autoimmune mechanism [70]. Multiple risk factors have been identified for pseudotumors comprising gender, implant design, and head size of the implant and abnormal position of acetabular component [71,72]. Larger heads in MOM have been associated with a higher incidence of pseudotumors [71,72]. An eightfold higher occurrence of pseudotumors has been observed in women compared to men. The reason for this difference is not fully understood. It has however been suggested that different ranges of motion and differences in hydrodynamic lubrication put women at a higher risk for pseudotumors than men [26,71]. It is particularly hard to diagnose patients with pseudotumors because several patients may display common symptoms of pain; others may be asymptomatic [1,73]. Formation of pseudotumor mass causes compression of surrounding muscles and nerves causing pain. Psuedotumors may mimic infections and patients often need to go through a revision surgery [74]. Detection of pseudotumors remains difficult because a lot of patients are asymptomatic. Ultrasound can be used to detect pseudotumors in both MOM-THA and MOM-HRA patients, and magnetic resonance imaging can be used on MOM-HRA patients [73]. Revision arthroplasty is highly recommended in patients with pseudotumor with elevated metal ion levels, and patients with lower metal ion levels are recommended for regular monitoring [74]. Pseudotumors with dangerous levels of circulating metals present danger of systemic toxicity, and THA revision is highly recommended in such patients [74].

10.4 Metal ion-associated systemic toxicity

Metal ion released after the surgery other than being deposited periprosthetically is also found in circulation and several organs such as kidney, liver, and bladder [75,76]. Several patients of MOM surgeries display no adverse effects with high serum concentrations of metal, and the management of potential hazards due to systemic exposure to metal ions is currently being debated [77,78]. In systemic exposure to metals from the implant, researchers are unable to find a parallel from the existing exposure data because large bodies of toxicological data are derived from exogenous intermittent exposure [76]. Currently, there is no acceptable "standard" concentration of circulating metal particles derived from the prosthesis. Cellular and molecular studies have demonstrated time and again the relationship between inflammation, cytotoxicity, DNA damage, and even lymphocyte concentrations [79–82]. Epidemiologic data suggest no potential damage to the kidney, heart, and nervous system in patients with MOM-THA [1]. Case studies with cardiomyopathy and impact on the nervous system and thyroid gland have been reported where the symptoms may not have been reduced by the removal of the prosthesis [83–85]. Association between cancer incidence and MOM prosthesis has also not been shown in any epidemiologic study although they may have been underpowered [86–89]. Co and Cr ions have been shown to induce signaling across barriers to induce genetic instability on the other side of the barrier. This becomes particularly relevant for younger patients and with the possibility of transplacental transfer of metals. The concentration of metal ion discovered in fetal blood is lower than the mothers due to the modulatory effect of the placenta. However, Co and Cr ions transferred could have a teratogenic impact on the fetus [90,91]. Co and Cr ions produce ROS that has been shown to induce DNA damage and lipid peroxidation [91]. The development of oxidative stress has been causally implicated in several diseases [92–94]. Additionally, several reports have indicated the risk of development of renal dysfunction due to the inability of the kidney to clear out excess metal ions. Our current clinical knowledge on endogenous systemic exposure to metals is lacking, and it prevents us from establishing a risk marker of excessive exposure [1]. Longer epidemiologic studies with younger patients need to be undertaken to enhance our understanding of risk from endogenous exposure to metal ions [1].

10.5 Immunotoxicity

Metals have long been known to adversely impact the immune system and have been described as immune toxicants by the Food and Drug Administration guideline (FDA1999) [1]. Principles and methods for immunological testing of medical device testing (ISO/TS 10993–20:2006) include adaptive immune response including immunosuppression, immunostimulation, autoimmunity, and hypersensitivity as a potential impact of metal implants including THA [1,95]. Metal implants give endogenous exposure to metals and can lead to acute or chronic inflammation and adversely impact adaptive immunity. Due to the nature of exposure being endogenous and systemic has presented the researcher with a challenge in examining the immunotoxicity [1]. Additionally, since no clear association has been drawn between the dose of exposure or volume of metal debris and adverse outcomes, a standardization of the recommendation has been difficult. Further, due to overlap in symptoms, it can be difficult to determine the nature of toxicity [1,96].

Studies have shown that Cr released from the prosthesis is associated with reduction lymphocyte subpopulations, and in vitro data have shown that clinically relevant concentrations of Co and Cr can initiate apoptosis by inhibiting the Il2 receptor release in a dose-dependent manner [97–99]. The data suggest that higher levels of Cr could impair cell-mediated immune response [100,101]. An immune-suppressive effect of Cr exposure has also been reported in the mortem study of THA patients [75]. Other in vitro studies reported the proliferation of lymphocyte upon exposure to Cr. It has been suggested by researchers that impaired cell-mediated immune response exposes the patient to a greater threat of bacterial infections [102].

10.5.1 Immune hyporeactivity or immune suppression

According to Grandchi et al., "The hypersensitivity reactions are abnormal or pathologic immune responses to repeated exposure to an antigen in predisposed individuals" [1]. Case studies of patients with metal implants have displayed excessive and uncontrolled immune response in patients with metal implants. The body treats a "self" substance as a foreign and continues to attack it in the form of self-directed T cells and autoantibodies [1,103]. Due to technical difficulties in the identification of self-directed antibodies and T cells, clinical data on the subject remain scarce [103]. Type IV hypersensitivity to the reaction to metals has been widely studied [1]. Ni, Co, Cr, and V have been implicated most often in inducing hypersensitivity, and reaction to Al and Ti has been rare. The metal ions and the debris clearing from phagocytosis, upon contact with body fluids form haptens with proteins [1]. The formation of this complex alters the secondary and tertiary structure of proteins. These proteins can signal as "nonself" to the body's immune system and induce excessive immune response [1]. These metal protein complexes can be discovered in the synovial fluid or far from the site of the implant after being distributed by the lymphatic system [104,105]. Metal and protein complexes are transported via satellite lymph nodes by antigen-presenting cells (APC) [1]. The exposure of APC with captured antigen stimulates T lymphocytes to proliferate and cause tissue damage [1]. Lymphocyte stimulation particularly CD4 + Th lymphocyte stimulation causes the cytokine production and activation of CD8 + Tcy lymphocytes [1]. This pathology is often accompanied by a local adverse immune response like ALVAL and pseudotumors [30]. The hypersensitivity reaction often requires the removal of the implant due to severe tissue damage [106,107].

Patients suffering from a metal allergy often display symptoms after many years. Common symptoms have been observed to mimic infection and implant loosening. It is also possible that a patient may display local euthymia, eczema, and vasculitis and hair loss [108]. For patients of metal allergy having undergone THA, adverse effect on mental health has also been reported [109]. It is important to undertake several large-scale epidemiologic studies and conduct clinical trials and meta-analysis of existing data to arrive at reliable data on the prevalence of metal sensitization. Currently, no laboratory test exists to predict the possible clinical outcome of the implant [1]. The prevalence of metal sensitivity is 31% in patients compared to the general population at 9%, but a person who tests positive for metal sensitivity can have good clinical outcomes just as a person who tested negative for metal sensitivity may develop hypersensitivity to the metal exposure [1,110]. Metal sensitization occurring due to implants can be mediated by soluble factors released by T lymphocytes that allow osteolysis [19]. The macrophages in the periprosthetic tissue have been shown to differentiate into osteoclast upon induction by RANKL or by other cytokines and growth factors. The activity of RANKL and differentiation into osteoclast is regulated by the balance between the expression of RANK and osteoprotegerin (OPG) [111]. RANKL binds to RANK expressed on preosteoclasts to induce signaling cascade that allows differentiation to osteoclast [111]. OPG is a decoy receptor upon binding RANK; it prevents the differentiation of osteoclast [111–113]. No difference in the expression of RANK and OPG has been reported in THA patients with osteolytic loosing suggesting the role of noncanonical signaling via RANK induced by other cytokines and growth factors [113]. The people with metal allergy needing an implant may be at a higher risk for hypersensitivity and osteolytic loosening. The dose needed to induce the response cannot be ascertained [1]. Oxidized zirconium has been used to prevent hypersensitivity. The femoral component of TKA has the main candidate of zirconium oxide use due to its hardness and resistance to friction. Zirconium oxide use in revision surgery has also been shown to be useful in relieving the patient of metal-induced sensitivity symptoms [114]. Epidemiologic study with a cohort of 17,000 people showed no difference in revision rate in the TKA femoral component made out of hypoallergenic zirconium versus CoCr alloy [115].

Our current knowledge base is insufficient to distinguish between different forms of toxicity symptomatically and neither do we have the information to determine who may endure excessive inflammatory response due to metal allergy. A concerted effort on part of laboratory scientists in conjunction with clinicians is needed to fully understand the complex biological mechanism at play. Such insight along with large-scale epidemiologic data would be needed to make reliable recommendations for patients before surgery and for the management of postsurgery complications. It is also important to make the patient aware of the potential signs of osteolysis for timely treatment potential adverse reactions [1].

10.6 Patient management

MOM implants have a 5-year revision rate of 3%–6% compared to 1.5% revision rate of MOP implants [1]. This discrepancy raises serious concerns for the safety of MOM implants. This concern becomes more important for younger patients because longer exposure to implant is expected. Regular patient screening for surgery-associated complications has been suggested to clinicians [1]. People who have undergone the surgery with large MOM implants fare worse but regular screening is highly recommended for all patients with MOM implants [1]. National and international organizations have come up with guidelines for clinicians for the management of patients with MOM bearings [1,116]. After the data from Australian national joint replacement surgery showed high revision rates for Depuy ASR hip implant, Australia's Therapeutic Goods Administration facilitated its withdrawal from use [1]. Regular screening for higher circulating metal ion concentrations and imaging for potential local adverse reactions along with imaging have been very helpful in early detection of failing implant [1]. It has been suggested if imaging results show abnormalities and blood metal ion concentration is greater than and part per billion and rising, a revision surgery should be recommended. The scientific community on emerging and newly identified health risks (SCENIHR) has extended this recommendation for MOM implants combined with recommendations on follow-up and technical issues. American Academy of orthopedic surgeons and orthopedic surgeons of the European Federation of National still have several discrepancies in recommendations for the management of MOM-THA. Arriving at a consensus on recommendations will allow scientific community to come up with implementable strategies managing MOM implants [1].

10.7 Conclusion

MOM hip implants are cost-effective options for most patients in need of hip replacement surgery. Due to the potential adverse impact of metal exposure, it is advisable to review the recommendation of MOM implants based on individual patient needs. Additionally, the use of CoCr-based hip implants for patients of child-bearing age may be contraindicated. Patient awareness of potential signs of implant failure combined with regular screening can be used as a potential tool for measure for early detection of adverse reaction to the implant. The consensus in regulatory agencies based on systematic data from revision surgeries and clinical trials on outcome should enable the development of patient management strategies for clinicians. Lastly, cellular and molecular studies need to be undertaken to further our understanding of the adverse reaction. Data from these studies will enable identification of markers for early diagnosis with specificity for the nature of the condition.

References

[1] Granchi D, Savarino LM, Ciapetti G, Baldini N. Biological effects of metal degradation in hip arthroplasties. Crit Rev Toxicol 2018;48(2):170–93.

[2] Drummond J, Tran P, Fary C. Metal-on-metal hip arthroplasty: a review of adverse reactions and patient management. J Funct Biomater 2015;6(3):486–99.

[3] Lavernia CJ, Iacobelli DA, Brooks L, Villa JM. The cost-utility of total hip arthroplasty: earlier intervention, improved economics. J Arthroplasty 2015;30(6):945–9.

[4] Maradit Kremers H, Larson DR, Crowson CS, Kremers WK, Washington RE, Steiner CA, et al. Prevalence of total hip and knee replacement in the united states. J Bone Joint Surg Am 2015;97(17):1386–97.

[5] Brach Del Prever EM, Bistolfi A, Bracco P, Costa L. UHMWPE for arthroplasty: past or future? J Orthop Traumatol 2009;10(1):1–8.
[6] Kandahari AM, Yang X, Laroche KA, Dighe AS, Pan D, Cui Q. A review of UHMWPE wear-induced osteolysis: the role for early detection of the immune response. Bone Res 2016;4:16014.
[7] Ansari F, Ries MD, Pruitt L. Effect of processing, sterilization and crosslinking on UHMWPE fatigue fracture and fatigue wear mechanisms in joint arthroplasty. J Mech Behav Biomed Mater 2016;53:329–40.
[8] Kumar N, Arora GN, Datta B. Bearing surfaces in hip replacement - evolution and likely future. Med J Armed Forces India 2014;70(4):371–6.
[9] Amstutz HC, Campbell P, Kossovsky N, Clarke IC. Mechanism and clinical significance of wear debris-induced osteolysis. Clin Orthop Relat Res 1992;276:7–18.
[10] Tolan NV, Sierra RJ, Moyer TP:. Evidence against implant-derived cobalt toxicity: case report and retrospective study of serum cobalt concentrations in an orthopedic implant population. Clin Biochem 2015;48(3):130–4.
[11] Billi F, Campbell P. Nanotoxicology of metal wear particles in total joint arthroplasty: a review of current concepts. J Appl Biomater Biomech 2010;8(1):1–6.
[12] Prokopovich P. Interactions between mammalian cells and nano- or micro-sized wear particles: physico-chemical views against biological approaches. Adv Colloid Interface Sci 2014;213:36–47.
[13] Madl AK, Liong M, Kovochich M, Finley BL, Paustenbach DJ, Oberdorster G. Toxicology of wear particles of cobalt-chromium alloy metal-on-metal hip implants Part I: physicochemical properties in patient and simulator studies. Nanomedicine 2015;11(5):1201–15.
[14] Bowsher JG, Hussain A, Williams PA, Shelton JC. Metal-on-metal hip simulator study of increased wear particle surface area due to 'severe' patient activity. Proc Inst Mech Eng H 2006;220(2):279–87.
[15] Jacobs JJ, Urban RM, Hallab NJ, Skipor AK, Fischer A, Wimmer MA. Metal-on-metal bearing surfaces. J Am Acad Orthop Surg 2009;17(2):69–76.
[16] Maloney WJ, Sun DH, Nakashima Y, James R, Smith RL. Effects of serum protein opsonization on cytokine release by titanium-alloy particles. J Biomed Mater Res 1998;41(3):371–6.
[17] Goodman SB, Gibon E, Yao Z. The basic science of periprosthetic osteolysis. Instr Course Lect 2013;62:201–6.
[18] Campbell PA, Kung MS, Hsu AR, Jacobs JJ. Do retrieval analysis and blood metal measurements contribute to our understanding of adverse local tissue reactions? Clin Orthop Relat Res 2014;472(12):3718–27.
[19] Goodman SB. Wear particles, periprosthetic osteolysis and the immune system. Biomaterials 2007;28(34):5044–8.
[20] Lahdeoja T, Pajarinen J, Kouri VP, Sillat T, Salo J, Konttinen YT. Toll-like receptors and aseptic loosening of hip endoprosthesis-a potential to respond against danger signals? J Orthop Res 2010;28(2):184–90.
[21] Beidelschies MA, Huang H, McMullen MR, Smith MV, Islam AS, Goldberg VM, et al. Stimulation of macrophage TNFalpha production by orthopaedic wear particles requires activation of the ERK1/2/Egr-1 and NF-kappaB pathways but is independent of p38 and JNK. J Cell Physiol 2008;217(3):652–66.
[22] Athanasou NA. The pathobiology and pathology of aseptic implant failure. Bone Joint Res 2016;5(5):162–8.
[23] VanOs R, Lildhar LL, Lehoux EA, Beaule PE, Catelas I. In vitro macrophage response to nanometer-size chromium oxide particles. J Biomed Mater Res B Appl Biomater 2014;102(1):149–59.

[24] Caicedo MS, Samelko L, McAllister K, Jacobs JJ, Hallab NJ. Increasing both CoCrMo-alloy particle size and surface irregularity induces increased macrophage inflammasome activation in vitro potentially through lysosomal destabilization mechanisms. J Orthop Res 2013;31(10):1633−42.
[25] Xia Z, Kwon YM, Mehmood S, Downing C, Jurkschat K, Murray DW. Characterization of metal-wear nanoparticles in pseudotumor following metal-on-metal hip resurfacing. Nanomedicine 2011;7(6):674−81.
[26] Glyn-Jones S, Pandit H, Kwon YM, Doll H, Gill HS, Murray DW. Risk factors for inflammatory pseudotumour formation following hip resurfacing. J Bone Joint Surg Br 2009;91(12):1566−74.
[27] Schmalzried TP, Peters PC, Maurer BT, Bragdon CR, Harris WH. Long-duration metal-on-metal total hip arthroplasties with low wear of the articulating surfaces. J Arthroplasty 1996;11(3):322−31.
[28] Grammatopoulos G, Pandit H, Kwon YM, Gundle R, McLardy-Smith P, Beard DJ, et al. Hip resurfacings revised for inflammatory pseudotumour have a poor outcome. J Bone Joint Surg Br 2009;91(8):1019−24.
[29] Posada OM, Tate RJ, Grant MH. Effects of CoCr metal wear debris generated from metal-on-metal hip implants and co ions on human monocyte-like U937 cells. Toxicol Vitro 2015;29(2):271−80.
[30] Miller RA, Ro JY, Schwartz MR. Adverse tissue reactions after total hip arthroplasty. Ann Diagn Pathol 2017;27:83−7.
[31] Kroemer G, Galluzzi L, Vandenabeele P, Abrams J, Alnemri ES, Baehrecke EH, et al. Classification of cell death: recommendations of the nomenclature committee on cell death 2009. Cell Death Differ 2009;16(1):3−11.
[32] Kerr JF, Wyllie AH, Currie AR. Apoptosis: a basic biological phenomenon with wide-ranging implications in tissue kinetics. Br J Cancer 1972;26(4):239−57.
[33] Bursch W, Karwan A, Mayer M, Dornetshuber J, Frohwein U, Schulte-Hermann R, et al. Cell death and autophagy: cytokines, drugs, and nutritional factors. Toxicology 2008;254(3):147−57.
[34] Zhao H, Jaffer T, Eguchi S, Wang Z, Linkermann A, Ma D. Role of necroptosis in the pathogenesis of solid organ injury. Cell Death Dis 2015;6:e1975.
[35] Wu W, Liu P, Li J. Necroptosis: an emerging form of programmed cell death. Crit Rev Oncol Hematol 2012;82(3):249−58.
[36] Ricciardi BF, Nocon AA, Jerabek SA, Wilner G, Kaplowitz E, Goldring SR, et al. Histopathological characterization of corrosion product associated adverse local tissue reaction in hip implants: a study of 285 cases. BMC Clin Pathol 2016;16:3.
[37] Rana SV. Metals and apoptosis: recent developments. J Trace Elem Med Biol 2008;22(4):262−84.
[38] Simonsen LO, Harbak H, Bennekou P. Cobalt metabolism and toxicology--a brief update. Sci Total Env 2012;432:210−15.
[39] Rovetta F, Stacchiotti A, Faggi F, Catalani S, Apostoli P, Fanzani A, et al. Cobalt triggers necrotic cell death and atrophy in skeletal C2C12 myotubes. Toxicol Appl Pharmacol 2013;271(2):196−205.
[40] Hayot M, Rodriguez J, Vernus B, Carnac G, Jean E, Allen D, et al. Myostatin up-regulation is associated with the skeletal muscle response to hypoxic stimuli. Mol Cell Endocrinol 2011;332(1−2):38−47.
[41] Lopes VR, Loitto V, Audinot JN, Bayat N, Gutleb AC, Cristobal S. Dose-dependent autophagic effect of titanium dioxide nanoparticles in human HaCaT cells at non-cytotoxic levels. J Nanobiotechnol 2016;14:22.
[42] Feng PH, Huang YL, Chuang KJ, Chen KY, Lee KY, Ho SC, et al. Taiwan cardioPulmonary Research G: dysfunction of methionine sulfoxide reductases to repair damaged proteins by nickel nanoparticles. Chem Biol Interact 2015;236:82−9.

[43] Nygaard M, Bastholm L, Elling F, Soballe K, Borgwardt A. Can ultrastructural particle location predict aseptic loosening? a biopsy study of nonloose hip implants one year postoperative using three bearing material combinations. J Long Term Eff Med Implant 2007;17(4):321–34.
[44] Berstock JR, Baker RP, Bannister GC, Case CP. Histology of failed metal-on-metal hip arthroplasty; three distinct sub-types. Hip Int 2014;24(3):243–8.
[45] Vasudevan A, DiCarlo EF, Wright T, Chen D, Figgie MP, Goldring SR, et al. Cellular response to prosthetic wear debris differs in patients with and without rheumatoid arthritis. Arthritis Rheum 2012;64(4):1005–14.
[46] Cobelli N, Scharf B, Crisi GM, Hardin J, Santambrogio L. Mediators of the inflammatory response to joint replacement devices. Nat Rev Rheumatol 2011;7(10):600–8.
[47] Landgraeber S, Jager M, Jacobs JJ, Hallab NJ. The pathology of orthopedic implant failure is mediated by innate immune system cytokines. Mediators Inflamm 2014;2014:185150.
[48] Magone K, Luckenbill D, Goswami T. Metal ions as inflammatory initiators of osteolysis. Arch Orthop Trauma Surg 2015;135(5):683–95.
[49] Nich C, Goodman SB. Role of macrophages in the biological reaction to wear debris from joint replacements. J Long Term Eff Med Implant 2014;24(4):259–65.
[50] Yadav J, Samelko L, Gilvar P, McAllister K, Hallab NJ. Osteoclasts lose innate inflammatory reactivity to metal and polymer implant debris compared to monocytes/macrophages. Open Orthop J 2013;7:605–13.
[51] Purdue PE. Alternative macrophage activation in periprosthetic osteolysis. Autoimmunity 2008;41(3):212–17.
[52] Kou PM, Babensee JE. Macrophage and dendritic cell phenotypic diversity in the context of biomaterials. J Biomed Mater Res A 2011;96(1):239–60.
[53] Nich C, Takakubo Y, Pajarinen J, Ainola M, Salem A, Sillat T, et al. Macrophages-key cells in the response to wear debris from joint replacements. J Biomed Mater Res A 2013;101(10):3033–45.
[54] Jamsen E, Kouri VP, Olkkonen J, Cor A, Goodman SB, Konttinen YT, et al. Characterization of macrophage polarizing cytokines in the aseptic loosening of total hip replacements. J Orthop Res 2014;32(9):1241–6.
[55] Lundqvist M. Nanoparticles: tracking protein corona over time. Nat Nanotechnol 2013;8(10):701–2.
[56] Corbo C, Molinaro R, Parodi A, Toledano Furman NE, Salvatore F, Tasciotti E. The impact of nanoparticle protein corona on cytotoxicity, immunotoxicity and target drug delivery. Nanomed (Lond) 2016;11(1):81–100.
[57] Lawrence H, Mawdesley AE, Holland JP, Kirby JA, Deehan DJ, Tyson-Capper AJ. Targeting toll-like receptor 4 prevents cobalt-mediated inflammation. Oncotarget 2016;7(7):7578–85.
[58] Hirayama T, Tamaki Y, Takakubo Y, Iwazaki K, Sasaki K, Ogino T, et al. Toll-like receptors and their adaptors are regulated in macrophages after phagocytosis of lipopolysaccharide-coated titanium particles. J Orthop Res 2011;29(7):984–92.
[59] Willert HG, Buchhorn GH, Fayyazi A, Flury R, Windler M, Koster G, et al. Metal-on-metal bearings and hypersensitivity in patients with artificial hip joints. A clinical and histomorphological study. J Bone Joint Surg Am 2005;87(1):28–36.
[60] Campbell P, Ebramzadeh E, Nelson S, Takamura K, De Smet K, Amstutz HC. Histological features of pseudotumor-like tissues from metal-on-metal hips. Clin Orthop Relat Res 2010;468(9):2321–7.
[61] Silverman EJ, Ashley B, Sheth NP. Metal-on-metal total hip arthroplasty: is there still a role in 2016? Curr Rev Musculoskelet Med 2016;9(1):93–6.

[62] Duggan PJ, Burke CJ, Saha S, Moonim M, George M, Desai A, et al. Current literature and imaging techniques of aseptic lymphocyte-dominated vasculitis-associated lesions (ALVAL). Clin Radiol 2013;68(11):1089−96.

[63] Natu S, Sidaginamale RP, Gandhi J, Langton DJ, Nargol AV. Adverse reactions to metal debris: histopathological features of periprosthetic soft tissue reactions seen in association with failed metal on metal hip arthroplasties. J Clin Pathol 2012;65 (5):409−18.

[64] Nawabi DH, Nassif NA, Do HT, Stoner K, Elpers M, Su EP, et al. What causes unexplained pain in patients with metal-on metal hip devices? A retrieval, histologic, and imaging analysis. Clin Orthop Relat Res 2014;472(2):543−54.

[65] Vendittoli PA, Mottard S, Roy AG, Dupont C, Lavigne M. Chromium and cobalt ion release following the Durom high carbon content, forged metal-on-metal surface replacement of the hip. J Bone Joint Surg Br 2007;89(4):441−8.

[66] Mistry JB, Chughtai M, Elmallah RK, Diedrich A, Le S, Thomas M, et al. Trunnionosis in total hip arthroplasty: a review. J Orthop Traumatol 2016;17 (1):1−6.

[67] Haynes DR, Crotti TN, Potter AE, Loric M, Atkins GJ, Howie DW, et al. The osteoclastogenic molecules RANKL and RANK are associated with periprosthetic osteolysis. J Bone Joint Surg Br 2001;83(6):902−11.

[68] Langton DJ, Joyce TJ, Jameson SS, Lord J, Van Orsouw M, Holland JP, et al. Adverse reaction to metal debris following hip resurfacing: the influence of component type, orientation and volumetric wear. J Bone Joint Surg Br 2011;93 (2):164−71.

[69] Kwon YM, Ostlere SJ, McLardy-Smith P, Athanasou NA, Gill HS, Murray DW. Asymptomatic" pseudotumors after metal-on-metal hip resurfacing arthroplasty: prevalence and metal ion study. J Arthroplasty 2011;26(4):511−18.

[70] Mittal S, Revell M, Barone F, Hardie DL, Matharu GS, Davenport AJ, et al. Lymphoid aggregates that resemble tertiary lymphoid organs define a specific pathological subset in metal-on-metal hip replacements. PLoS One 2013;8(5):e63470.

[71] Haughom BD, Erickson BJ, Hellman MD, Jacobs JJ. Do complication rates differ by gender after metal-on-metal hip resurfacing arthroplasty? a systematic review. Clin Orthop Relat Res 2015;473(8):2521−9.

[72] Kwon YM, Glyn-Jones S, Simpson DJ, Kamali A, McLardy-Smith P, Gill HS, et al. Analysis of wear of retrieved metal-on-metal hip resurfacing implants revised due to pseudotumours. J Bone Joint Surg Br 2010;92(3):356−61.

[73] Williams DH, Greidanus NV, Masri BA, Duncan CP, Garbuz DS. Prevalence of pseudotumor in asymptomatic patients after metal-on-metal hip arthroplasty. J Bone Joint Surg Am 2011;93(23):2164−71.

[74] Davis DL, Morrison JJ. Hip arthroplasty pseudotumors: pathogenesis, imaging, and clinical decision making. J Clin Imaging Sci 2016;6:17.

[75] Case CP, Langkamer VG, James C, Palmer MR, Kemp AJ, Heap PF, et al. Widespread dissemination of metal debris from implants. J Bone Joint Surg Br 1994;76(5):701−12.

[76] Keegan GM, Learmonth ID, Case CP. A systematic comparison of the actual, potential, and theoretical health effects of cobalt and chromium exposures from industry and surgical implants. Crit Rev Toxicol 2008;38(8):645−74.

[77] Chang EY, McAnally JL, Van Horne JR, Van Horne JG, Wolfson T, Gamst A, et al. Relationship of plasma metal ions and clinical and imaging findings in patients with ASR XL metal-on-metal total hip replacements. J Bone Joint Surg Am 2013;95 (22):2015−20.

[78] Pahuta M, Smolders JM, van Susante JL, Peck J, Kim PR, Beaule PE. Blood metal ion levels are not a useful test for adverse reactions to metal debris: a systematic review and meta-analysis. Bone Joint Res 2016;5(9):379–86.

[79] Case CP, Langkamer VG, Lock RJ, Perry MJ, Palmer MR, Kemp AJ. Changes in the proportions of peripheral blood lymphocytes in patients with worn implants. J Bone Joint Surg Br 2000;82(5):748–54.

[80] Huk OL, Catelas I, Mwale F, Antoniou J, Zukor DJ, Petit A. Induction of apoptosis and necrosis by metal ions in vitro. J Arthroplasty 2004;19(8 Suppl 3):84–7.

[81] Davies AP, Sood A, Lewis AC, Newson R, Learmonth ID, Case CP. Metal-specific differences in levels of DNA damage caused by synovial fluid recovered at revision arthroplasty. J Bone Joint Surg Br 2005;87(10):1439–44.

[82] Hart AJ, Skinner JA, Winship P, Faria N, Kulinskaya E, Webster D, et al. Circulating levels of cobalt and chromium from metal-on-metal hip replacement are associated with CD8+ T-cell lymphopenia. J Bone Joint Surg Br 2009;91 (6):835–42.

[83] Machado C, Appelbe A, Wood R. Arthroprosthetic cobaltism and cardiomyopathy. Heart Lung Circ 2012;21(11):759–60.

[84] Bradberry SM, Wilkinson JM, Ferner RE. Systemic toxicity related to metal hip prostheses. Clin Toxicol (Phila) 2014;52(8):837–47.

[85] Tower SS. Arthroprosthetic cobaltism: neurological and cardiac manifestations in two patients with metal-on-metal arthroplasty: a case report. J Bone Joint Surg Am 2010;92(17):2847–51.

[86] Visuri T, Borg H, Pulkkinen P, Paavolainen P, Pukkala E. A retrospective comparative study of mortality and causes of death among patients with metal-on-metal and metal-on-polyethylene total hip prostheses in primary osteoarthritis after a long-term follow-up. BMC Musculoskelet Disord 2010;11:78.

[87] Visuri T, Pukkala E, Pulkkinen P, Paavolainen P. Decreased cancer risk in patients who have been operated on with total hip and knee arthroplasty for primary osteoarthrosis: a meta-analysis of 6 Nordic cohorts with 73,000 patients. Acta Orthop Scand 2003;74(3):351–60.

[88] Wagner P, Olsson H, Lidgren L, Robertsson O, Ranstam J. Increased cancer risks among arthroplasty patients: 30 year follow-up of the Swedish Knee Arthroplasty Register. Eur J Cancer 2011;47(7):1061–71.

[89] Makela KT, Visuri T, Pulkkinen P, Eskelinen A, Remes V, Virolainen P, et al. Risk of cancer with metal-on-metal hip replacements: population based study. BMJ 2012;345:e4646.

[90] Ziaee H, Daniel J, Datta AK, Blunt S, McMinn DJ. Transplacental transfer of cobalt and chromium in patients with metal-on-metal hip arthroplasty: a controlled study. J Bone Joint Surg Br 2007;89(3):301–5.

[91] Engh CA, MacDonald SJ, Sritulanondha S, Korczak A, Naudie D, Engh C. Metal ion levels after metal-on-metal total hip arthroplasty: a five-year, prospective randomized trial. J Bone Joint Surg Am 2014;96(6):448–55.

[92] Jomova K, Valko M. Advances in metal-induced oxidative stress and human disease. Toxicology 2011;283(2–3):65–87.

[93] Colognato R, Bonelli A, Ponti J, Farina M, Bergamaschi E, Sabbioni E, et al. Comparative genotoxicity of cobalt nanoparticles and ions on human peripheral leukocytes in vitro. Mutagenesis 2008;23(5):377–82.

[94] Scharf B, Clement CC, Zolla V, Perino G, Yan B, Elci SG, et al. Molecular analysis of chromium and cobalt-related toxicity. Sci Rep 2014;4:5729.

[95] Fujishiro T, Moojen DJ, Kobayashi N, Dhert WJ, Bauer TW. Perivascular and diffuse lymphocytic inflammation are not specific for failed metal-on-metal hip implants. Clin Orthop Relat Res 2011;469(4):1127–33.
[96] Descotes J. Importance of immunotoxicity in safety assessment: a medical toxicologist's perspective. Toxicol Lett 2004;149(1–3):103–8.
[97] Granchi D, Ciapetti G, Stea S, Cavedagna D, Bettini N, Bianco T, et al. Evaluation of several immunological parameters in patients with aseptic loosening of hip arthroplasty. Chir Organi Mov 1995;80(4):399–408.
[98] Savarino L, Granchi D, Ciapetti G, Stea S, Donati ME, Zinghi G, et al. Effects of metal ions on white blood cells of patients with failed total joint arthroplasties. J Biomed Mater Res 1999;47(4):543–50.
[99] Akbar M, Brewer JM, Grant MH. Effect of chromium and cobalt ions on primary human lymphocytes in vitro. J Immunotoxicol 2011;8(2):140–9.
[100] Wang JY, Tsukayama DT, Wicklund BH, Gustilo RB. Inhibition of T and B cell proliferation by titanium, cobalt, and chromium: role of IL-2 and IL-6. J Biomed Mater Res 1996;32(4):655–61.
[101] Granchi D, Cenni E, Ciapetti G, Savarino L, Stea S, Gamberini S, et al. Cell death induced by metal ions: necrosis or apoptosis? J Mater Sci Mater Med 1998;9(1):31–7.
[102] Wyles CC, Van Demark 3rd RE, Sierra RJ, Trousdale RT. High rate of infection after aseptic revision of failed metal-on-metal total hip arthroplasty. Clin Orthop Relat Res 2014;472(2):509–16.
[103] Nakamura S, Yasunaga Y, Ikuta Y, Shimogaki K, Hamada N, Takata N. Autoantibodies to red cells associated with metallosis--a case report. Acta Orthop Scand 1997;68(5):495–6.
[104] Coleman RF, Herrington J, Scales JT. Concentration of wear products in hair, blood, and urine after total hip replacement. Br Med J 1973;1(5852):527–9.
[105] Cadosch D, Chan E, Gautschi OP, Filgueira L. Metal is not inert: role of metal ions released by biocorrosion in aseptic loosening--current concepts. J Biomed Mater Res A 2009;91(4):1252–62.
[106] Wawrzynski J, Gil JA, Goodman AD, Waryasz GR. Hypersensitivity to orthopedic implants: a review of the literature. Rheumatol Ther 2017;4(1):45–56.
[107] Evans EM, Freeman MA, Miller AJ, Vernon-Roberts B. Metal sensitivity as a cause of bone necrosis and loosening of the prosthesis in total joint replacement. J Bone Joint Surg Br 1974;56-B(4):626–42.
[108] Post ZD, Orozco FR, Ong AC. Metal sensitivity after TKA presenting with systemic dermatitis and hair loss. Orthopedics 2013;36(4):e525–8.
[109] Nam D, Li K, Riegler V, Barrack RL. Patient-reported metal allergy: a risk factor for poor outcomes after total joint arthroplasty? J Arthroplasty 2016;31(9):1910–15.
[110] Granchi D, Cenni E, Giunti A, Baldini N. Metal hypersensitivity testing in patients undergoing joint replacement: a systematic review. J Bone Joint Surg Br 2012;94(8):1126–34.
[111] Sabokbar A, Mahoney DJ, Hemingway F, Athanasou NA. Non-canonical (rankl-independent) pathways of osteoclast differentiation and their role in musculoskeletal diseases. Clin Rev Allergy Immunol 2016;51(1):16–26.
[112] Granchi D, Pellacani A, Spina M, Cenni E, Savarino LM, Baldini N, et al. Serum levels of osteoprotegerin and receptor activator of nuclear factor-kappaB ligand as markers of periprosthetic osteolysis. J Bone Joint Surg Am 2006;88(7):1501–9.

[113] Eastwood SE, John A, Jones SA, Hodgson H, Mason D, Waddington R, et al. Osteoclastogenesis-related cytokines and peri-prosthetic osteolysis in revision metal-on-metal total hip replacements. Hip Int 2015;25(4):355–60.
[114] Holland P, Santini AJ, Davidson JS, Pope JA. Five year survival analysis of an oxidised zirconium total knee arthroplasty. Knee 2013;20(6):384–7.
[115] Vertullo CJ, Lewis PL, Graves S, Kelly L, Lorimer M, Myers P. twelve-year outcomes of an oxinium total knee replacement compared with the same cobalt-chromium design: an analysis of 17,577 prostheses from the australian orthopaedic association national joint replacement registry. J Bone Joint Surg Am 2017;99(4):275–83.
[116] Maurer-Ertl W, Friesenbichler J, Holzer LA, Leitner L, Ogris K, Maier M, et al. Recall of the asr xl head and hip resurfacing systems. Orthopedics 2017;40(2):e340–7.

CHAPTER ELEVEN

Neurology and psychiatry

Thamizharasan Sampath[1,*], Sandhiya Thamizharasan[2], Monisha Saravanan[3] and Prakash Srinivasan Timiri Shanmugam[4]

[1]ACSMCH, DRMGR Educational & Research Institute, Chennai, Tamil Nadu, India
[2]SDC, Saveetha Institute of Medical and Technical Sciences, Chennai, Tamil Nadu, India
[3]IQVIA, Bangalore, Karnataka, India
[4]HCL America Inc., Sunnyvale, CA, United States
*Corresponding author

Abstract

Neurons are the primary units involved in the transmission of impulses from various parts of the body to the brain and vice versa. With the advancement of brain–computer interface technology, several brain chips or implants are implanted directly into the brain to restore any lost function. Despite having the potential to improve the patient's sensory capabilities and restore lost functionalities, these implants should be handled with care during implantation and it also requires continuous monitoring postimplantation. This chapter provides an insight into the benefits of neurological implants as well as their toxic effects and their treatments.

Keywords: Neurology; brain disorders; neural implant; novel treatment; neurotoxicity

Highlights

- This chapter provides information on various implants used to treat neural problems.
- The text explains the importance of neural implants and their treatment outcome.
- This chapter covers the toxicological impact of neural implants.
- This section also provides a brief description on failure and nonadherence of implants.

List of abbreviations

AMPA α-amino-3-hydroxy-5-methyl-4-isoxazole propionic acid receptors
AP action potential

Toxicological Aspects of Medical Device Implants.
DOI: https://doi.org/10.1016/B978-0-12-820728-4.00011-3
© 2020 Elsevier Inc.
All rights reserved.

BCM	Bienenstock–Cooper–Munro
BMI	biomedical implant
BSDS	brain state-dependent stimulation
DBS	deep brain stimulation
ECoG	electrocorticography
EEG	electroencephalography
EMG	electromyography
FES	field electrical stimulation
ICMS	intracortical microstimulation
IPG	implanted pulse generator
MoM	metal on metal
NGC	nerve guidance conduit
NMDAR	*N*-methyl D-aspartate receptor
NP	nanoparticles
OCD	obsessive–compulsive disorder
PAS	paired associative stimulation
SCI	spinal cord injury
SCP	slow cortical potential
SNM	sacral neural modulation
STDP	spike-timing-dependent plasticity
STN	subthalamic nucleus
UMEA	Utah microelectrode array
VNS	vagal nerve stimulation
TBS	theta burst stimulation
TMS	transcranial magnetic stimulation

11.1 Introduction

Neural implants are technical systems that are clinically used to stimulate various parts and structures of the nervous system with the aid of implanted electrical circuits or record the electrical activity of nerve cells. Their application in current clinical practice has given rise to the fields known as "neuromodulation" and "neuroprosthetics." The concept of controlling technical devices and neural prostheses by "thoughts" currently drives research in the field of brain–machine interfaces, where a large variety of different materials and approaches compete to become the first reliable solution for a clinical application. Unfortunately, enthusiasm about the technological opportunities masks the risk and adverse effects that come along with implantation. Therefore benefits and adverse effects have to be carefully considered in any medical and surgical treatment, and ultimately the patient must give the final consent for implantation to occur. All neural implants have to fulfill basic requirements to become approved as a medical device. They must not harm the body and should stay stable and functional over a certain lifetime that is in most cases in the range of decades. Packages made of ceramics or titanium are the state of the art to protect the implant electronics from moisture and ions. These packages are implanted in most cases in a place that is quite far away from the neuronal target tissue to prevent any undesired interaction or damage [1]. The key challenge for any neural implant is the proper design of the neurotechnical interface. Multiple electrical contact sites have to get in close contact with nerve tissue to selectively stimulate subsets of nerve cells. Nerves are delicate, and structures of soft tissue get easily damaged by hard materials used in implants especially when forces due to movements occur. Polymers have been found in the optimal material class when requirements of little response to implantation, long-term stability in a hostile environment, low material stiffness, and good electrical insulation of metallic conductors have to be combined in a single material.

11.1.1 Background

From the experience gained by the early experiments in the 1960s, miniaturization technologies, material sciences and the progress in medical and especially neuroscientific knowledge evolved and paved the way to these novel applications in therapies of neurological diseases and rehabilitation of lost functions in clinical practice. Neuromodulation, namely the stimulation of central nervous system structures to modulate nerve excitability and the release of neurotransmitters, alleviates the effects of many neurological diseases. Deep brain stimulation helps patients suffering from Parkinson's disease to suppress tremor and movement disorders. It is also a treatment option for severe psychiatric diseases like depression and obsessive—compulsive disorder. Vagal nerve stimulation has been applied first to treat epilepsy but has now expanded to psychiatric diseases, and many more applications are under development in preclinical and clinical trials. The most commonly implanted device in the neuromodulation sector is the spinal cord stimulator, used to alleviate chronic pain and to treat incontinence [1]. More than 130,000 patients have benefitted from these implants that derive from cardiac pacemakers, first developed decades ago. Neural implants aim to restore lost functions of the body, either sensory, motor, or vegetative. An early example can be dated back to about 1970 when Giles Brindley implanted the first electrodes around the sacral nerves of spinal cord injured persons to manage their bladder function. Other implants have been developed in parallel to help patients suffering from stroke or from spinal cord injury [2]. Motor implants to restore grasping, stance and gait as well as ventilation by electrical stimulation of the diaphragm have been developed and introduced into preclinical studies or even as commercial products to the market. However, the number of patients that benefit from these systems is relatively low, in part due to some technical shortcomings, but mainly as a result of the limited performance of the implants in patients due to their individual course of injury [3]. In combination with a limited market, it is economically quite unattractive for companies to develop and approve a new device, as the reimbursement is uncertain and the sale volume is (too) low. Sensory implants to restore normal hearing, so-called "cochlear implants," are one of the main success stories of neural prostheses. More than 150,000 patients have been implanted with these technical systems that stimulate the nerve cells in the inner ear at several sites when the sensory cells (hair cells) are no longer present, for example, due to aging, diseases (meningitis or Meniere's disease), or by certain drug treatments.

11.2 Types of neural implants

Electric implants are those that are capable of stimulating specific target organs with the help of electrical energy. The stimulation might cause beneficial effects to the human body such as pain relief and revoking a lost functionality of the damaged body part. There exist different kinds of electrical implants like cardiac pacemaker, nerve, and muscle stimulators. Researchers proved that small electrical implants help to relieve symptoms related to Parkinson's disease and in partial treatment of incontinence. It also provides benefits in treating obsessive–compulsive disorder (OCD), epilepsy, mood disorder, addiction, and spinal cord injury.

11.2.1 Deep brain stimulator

A recently emerging technique called deep brain stimulation (DBS) is used to reduce the symptoms of Parkinson's disease such as muscle tremor, stiffness, and walking problems. Electrodes are implanted into the brain and are controlled by a pulse generator positioned at the chest level. It delivers a continuous electrical stimulus to the cortex. This technique has also been studied in patients with depression or OCD as a means of therapy. Researchers believe that these electrical pulses contribute toward resetting the malfunctioning area of the brain responsible for depression [4]. A DBS device contains an electrode lead with four or six cylindrical electrodes at equally spaced depths attached to an implanted pulse generator (IPG), which is surgically positioned below the collarbone. DBS technique has many advantages, such as the fact that it is reversible. It is also potentially much less dangerous than lesioning and is highly successful in many cases. Neurosurgeons have started implanting neurostimulators connected to deep brain electrodes positioned in the thalamus, subthalamus, or globus pallidus of the brain to treat Parkinson's disease, tremors, dystonia, and pain. The concept of the stimulator is to produce warning signals before the tremors start so that the IPG stimulator only needs to generate signals occasionally rather than continuously, thus operating in a similar fashion to a heart pacemaker. AI tools based on artificial neural networks have been shown to successfully predict the onset of tremors [5].

11.2.2 Spinal cord stimulator

A spinal cord stimulator (SCS) or dorsal column stimulator is a type of implantable neuromodulation device that is used to send electrical signals to select the location of the spinal cord (dorsal columns) for the treatment of certain severe pain conditions. SCS implants are the treatment option for patients who have a pain condition that has not responded to more conservative therapy. The stimulation of spinal nerves has a predominant role in restoring locomotion of the paraplegics and is capable of reducing chronic back pain. SCS utilizes a device implanted in the body through a needle positioned at the back near the spine [6]. The pulse generator that delivers short electric pulses via the inserted needle is placed underneath the skin, whose intensity can be controlled by the patient.

11.2.3 Vagus nerve stimulator

The primary function of an electrical implant falls into three categories: to replace the interrupted signals, to record and supply signals in the form of feedback, and to serve as an obstructive device for unwanted signals. For instance, patients suffering from urinary incontinence: emptying of the bladder without being instructed to do so can be treated by bladder stimulators to block the signal to restore the mechanism. A device similar to pacemaker has been implanted to stimulate the vagus nerve in the neck to tackle epilepsy and depression.

The human body is prone to various adverse effects while conventional medicine is employed. However, bioelectronics tends to manipulate the neural network of the body eliminating the need for drugs such as narcotics and analgesics. The conventional way of treating rheumatoid arthritis employs drugs targeting tumor necrosis factor (TNF) and suppressing its signals from reaching the brain. It delivers a temporary relief from the symptoms caused by the disease. The bioelectronic approach uses stimulation of the vagus nerve to switch off the release of TNF. They indirectly communicate to the spleen to release neurotransmitters [7]. The knock-on effect of the T-cells increases their activity to reduce the release of TNF from macrophages. This procedure is known as vagus nerve stimulation (VNS).

11.2.4 Implants for mood disorders

Brain implants that deliver electrical impulses tuned to a person's feelings and behavior are being tested by the US military's research arm, the Defense Advanced Research Projects Agency, and have initiated preliminary trials of "closed-loop" brain implants that use algorithms to detect patterns associated with mood disorders. These implant devices can shock the brain back to a healthy state without any input from a neurophysician. The closed-loop technique explains how mood is encoded in the brain over time. With the implanted electrode, an algorithm is used to "decode" that person's changing moods from their brain activity. Some broad patterns emerged, particularly in brain areas that have been associated with the change of mood [8].

Rather than detecting a particular mood disorder or mental illness, scientists want to map the brain activity associated with behaviors that are present in multiple disorders such as difficulties with concentration and empathy. They also reported the tests of algorithms they developed to stimulate the brain when a person is distracted from a set task, such as matching images of numbers or identifying emotions on faces. The delivering electrical pulses to areas of the brain involved in decision-making and emotion significantly improved the performance of test participants. The team also mapped the brain activity that occurred when a person began failing or slowing at a defined set task because they were forgetful or distracted, and found that they were able to reverse it with stimulation. The algorithm provides electrical impulses based on that mood mapping to maintain neural homeostasis [9]. The researchers believe that closed-loop stimulation has more long-term promise. However, this still gives researchers insight into a person's emotions in real time. If these implants can start to manipulate a person's emotions over time, that person may change for better or bad. Those with genetic neurological disorders such as Huntington's disease may be some of the first candidates or candidates most likely to show positive responses to the neural implants.

11.2.5 Implants for epilepsy

When the first signals of a seizure were detected, the device delivered a naturally occurring brain chemical (a neurotransmitter) that stopped the seizure from progressing. There are many different types of epileptic seizure but in most people with epilepsy, the seizure occurs because neurons in the brain become hyperexcited and start firing, signaling to neighboring neurons to start firing too. The resulting seizure can affect consciousness and motor control [10].

Most people with epilepsy are treated with medication, but even where seizure control is good, these antiepileptic medications can have unpleasant and serious adverse effects. Moreover, in 3 out of every 10 epilepsy patients, the drugs do not work in effectively controlling seizures. In this technique, the researchers used a neurotransmitter that acts as the "brake" at the source of the seizure, essentially signaling to the neurons to stop firing and end the seizure. The drug is delivered to the hyper firing region of the brain by a neural probe incorporating a small ion pump and electrodes to monitor neural activity. The work represents another advance in the development of soft, flexible electronics that interface well with brain tissue. These thin, organic films do lesser damage in the brain, and their electrical properties are well suited for these types of applications. Although there are many different types of seizures, in most patients with epilepsy, neurons in the brain start firing and signal to neighboring neurons to fire as well, in a snowball effect that will affect consciousness or motor control [11]. When the neural signal of a seizure is detected by the electrodes, the ion pump is triggered, creating an electric field that pushes the drug across an ion exchange membrane and out of the device, a process named as electrophoresis. The amount of drug will be controlled by tuning the strength of the electric field.

11.2.6 Neuro surgical implants

There is more than one type of implants used in the treatment of a brain tumor. Some are surgical while the other is a part of radiation therapy [12]. The primary treatment option for brain cancer is surgery and the following are surgical implants:

Shunt: Here a thin tube (called a shunt) is placed into a ventricle of the brain, through a tiny hole in the skull. This device moves excess fluid from the brain to another part of the body, such as the abdominal cavity, where it is absorbed into the bloodstream. A filter catches stray tumor cells that may be in the cerebral spinal fluid (CSF). This implant procedure can help relieve pressure in the skull.

Placement of an Ommaya reservoir: During this brain cancer surgery, a tiny reservoir attached to a tube under the scalp is implanted. The tubing leads into a ventricle of the brain where the cerebral spinal fluid circulates, allowing us to deliver chemotherapy to the brain and CSF, or to remove fluid for biopsy. The reservoir can be removed when it is no longer needed.

11.2.7 Brachytherapy (radiation implants)

Brachytherapy is a kind of treatment for cancers; it puts radiation appropriately close to the disease tissue. Little radioactive inserts are put into or close to the cerebrum tumor amid surgery. They are otherwise called seeds or pellets. This type of treatment is additionally called interstitial radiation. Brachytherapy is not utilized as regularly as outside radiation to treat cerebrum tumors [13].

11.2.8 Sacral neuromodulation

Sacral neuromodulation is a proven treatment method for bladder and bowel control. More than 220,000 patients worldwide have received sacral neuromodulation treatment for bladder control and bowel control. Tiny lead is placed parallel to the sacral nerve (targeting S3). Implantable neurostimulator triggers mild electrical impulses that are delivered through the lead electrodes. Clinician and patient assistants are used to set the parameters of the electrical pulses. SNM is delivered through the InterStim system [14]. The implanted neurostimulator and lead electrically trigger the sacral nerve that is thought to facilitate neural communication between the bladder and brain and the bowel and brain. Different from oral medications that target the muscular component of bladder control, sacral neuromodulation offers control of symptoms via direct modulation of the nervous system. This implant system for bladder and bowel control helps to control symptoms of overactive bladder, non-obstructive urinary retention, and chronic fecal incontinence through direct stimulation of the nerve activity. Sacral neuromodulation represents the nerve component. The sacral neuromodulation is thought to help normalize neural activity from the bladder to the brain, enabling patients to experience improved urinary function [15].

11.2.9 Median nerve stimulation

For patients with severe disorders of consciousness, median nerve stimulation has been used to enhance oxygen perfusion to the brain and increase blood–brain barrier permeability for medications intended to help stabilize the acute injury environment. Median nerve stimulation (MNS) has also been found to elevate dopamine levels, resulting in accelerated awakening from a deep coma. DeFina et al. published an advanced care protocol for the rehabilitation of patients in minimally conscious and vegetative states from traumatic brain injury that involves sequential administration of a number of medications followed by specific interventions and treatments aimed at facilitating neuroplasticity (traditional occupational, physical, and speech therapy plus median nerve stimulation). Patients during this study also completed a 1-year course of pharmaceutical grade nutrients ("neutraceuticals") that resulted in a greater improvement in disability beyond standard treatment in literature controls [16].

11.2.10 Robotic therapy

Another area of growing interest is rehabilitative robotic therapy, primarily for its ability to deliver highly intense and repetitive motor practice. There is great evidence in some clinical applications, robotic therapy is noninferior to conventional therapy. However, as it stands today, robotic therapy has some limitations in its applications, largely because of its inability to individualize goal-directed rehabilitation paradigms fitted to unique patient needs. Despite this challenge, robotic interfaces are actively becoming more sophisticated, and a wide range of strategies are now being used to facilitate whole body functions [17]. For example, an advanced rehabilitative robot with the ability to evaluate individualized statistics regarding gait and balance stability has been demonstrated. This specific robot also contains a mode with locomotive capabilities that can go upstairs, as well as a training mode with epidural stimulation, repetitive training, and pharmacologic excitation built in. The latter mode has been shown to achieve voluntary overground walking, stair walking, and precise foot placement after a stroke. An EEG-based lower extremity exoskeleton and virtual reality leg simulations have been shown to improve somatic sensation and enable new voluntary motor control in the legs of spinal cord injury patients, promoting some patients up to an incomplete paraplegia classification. The adaptive physiological mechanisms improve and reduce the cost. Robotic therapy will likely become increasingly integral to rehabilitative strategies due to its ability to be applied in both a clinic and home setting [18].

11.3 Neurophysiology and mechanism of implants

11.3.1 Brain—machine and neural interface

Neural or brain—machine interfaces are electrode computer constructs the extract and decode information from the nervous system to generate functional outputs. These have been developed to bypass motor lesions and to facilitate neural plasticity and motor learning to enhance recovery after injury.

Interfaces generally contain four components: (1) a method of receiving signals from the nervous system, (2) a way to decode the signals to predict user intent, (3) an output to influence the subject's environment, and (4) a feedback system to assist the user refine the output. Means of receiving nervous system signals range from invasive [intracortical microelectrodes and larger scale sub or epidural electrodes (ECoG-EMG)]. The targeted outputs have included cursors on a virtual typing screen, prosthetic arms, wheelchairs, exoskeletons, the spinal cord, and a patient's own extremities [19].

Although initially designed due to the belief/concept that the human nervous system will not self-regenerate, biomedical implants have also led to exciting and innovative ways to understand, integrate, and interact with the nervous system. Current understanding of nervous system function recognizes an intricate arrangement of connections within units and circuits that express to a larger performing network, as compared to classic models that viewed the brain as a collection of independent anatomical modules with complex functions. It has been shown that functionally coupled remote brain locations display near synchronous discharges that represent emergent properties of their same networks [20]. This dispersion of information likely denotes why motor information can be found widely distributed throughout the cortex, and how random samples of neurons can provide enough information to reconstruct specific movements in great detail. However, it has also been shown that no matter how well tuned a single neuron is to a behavioral task, that an individual cell only contains very little information and can differ greatly over a short period of time. Interestingly, once an ensemble of neurons reaches a particular size, its collective predictive ability plateaus, suggesting that there is redundancy in the neuronal network and that there are a critical number of neurons required to decode motor information. These concepts have led to population algorithms or decoders that exploit the concept that individual neurons encode various parameters with different weights and may differ from trial to trial. However, useful information is maintained within a population instead of individual neurons. The advantage of population decoding systems is that they work even when individual neurons badly encode motor behavior [21].

The biomedical implants develop to encode signals that are more robust across different positional dynamics than trajectory-based biomedical implants (BMIs). For gait decoding, there is solid evidence that motor cortex BMIs may perform better when estimating gait phases or locomotor behaviors as opposed to continuous kinematic variables of leg movement. More interestingly, bimanual arm control appears to have its own representation in the cortex and does not seem to be expressed easily by a superposition of unilateral movements. The human arm has 7 degrees of freedom, and the hand has more than 20. As it turns out, natural grasp postures and reaching to grasp movements exist in a much smaller subspace than physically possible movements. This provides a strategy for neural interfaces to recapitulate potentially more complex appearing movements while expressing fewer degrees of freedom [22].

11.3.2 Neural plasticity

In recent years, neural interfaces have been designed to enhance neural plasticity and facilitate recovery (rehabilitative BMIs) in addition to bypassing lesions (assistive BMIs). The transition from assistive biomedical implant to rehabilitative BMIs has come with the realization that patients with a chronic neurologic injury may not be at a static level of functioning as thought early, and that underlying networks even in chronic injury can be modified over time. Rehabilitative BMIs pair goal-oriented tasks with expected treatment outcomes and work to activate lesioned circuits to create plasticity for long-lasting improvements. This approach takes advantage of a principle called spike-timing-dependent plasticity or Hebbian plasticity [23]. This is the concept that synaptic strength is redistributed to favor functionally relevant pathways that are coincidently active, inferring that both the sign and magnitude of synaptic modification are determined by the precise timing of APs. The best-known example of Hebbian plasticity is long term potentiation (LTP) and long term depression (LTD) in memory circuits. For modeling of complex, larger scale circuits, the Bienenstock–Cooper–Munro model may be more representative of behavior. This theory incorporates both presynaptic and postsynaptic firing rates and applies a sliding threshold for LTP/LTD based on postsynaptic activity as the metric for stabilization.

A related idea employed in some rehabilitative BMIs is paired associative stimulation, or the act of pairing stimulation sites to promote plasticity. An example of a commonly used central stimulation strategy is transcranial magnetic stimulation. Transcranial magnetic stimulation (TMS) involves applying rapidly changing magnetic fields to the scalp through a magnetic stimulator. Continuous low frequency repetitive stimuli ($\leq$1 Hz rTMS) decreases the excitability of target areas while bursts of intermittent high frequency stimuli enhance excitability. These techniques have been used to trigger modulation across cortico-subcortical and cortico-cortical networks through the trans-synaptic spread, resulting in distant but specific changes along with functional networks. If time and placement are correct, corresponding sensory inputs can be potentiated. Functional electrical stimulation of paralyzed muscles or electrical stimulation of the nervous system distal to the injury timed with voluntary effort has been shown to fasten recovery in both spinal cord injury and stroke [24].

11.3.3 Neural prostheses

The first assistive implant for patients with severe motor impairment was developed for patients with locked-in syndrome, a condition where a patient is cognitively aware of his or her environment but not able to move or make sounds. An EEG-based system designed to translate motivational slow cortical potentials into a binary selection of letters or words on a screen. Since then, EEG-based systems have advanced to move cursors on a screen in up to three-dimensions open and close a hand orthosis provide limited field electrical stimulation (FES)-control of upper and lower extremities, and ambulate a lower extremity exoskeleton; however, their potential is hindered due to inherently poor reliability, latency, and generally nonintuitive nature [25].

They have demonstrated brain control of a robotic arm to perform three-dimensional reach and grasp movements in two patients, including the ability to drink coffee from a bottle. Since then, intracortical BMIs have enabled brain-controlled typing, driven seven degrees of freedom in a prosthetic limb at over 90% accuracy, restored voluntary movement and grasp via real-time FES to the subject with a paralyzed hand, coordinated cervical intraspinal simulation to enact reach and grasp in the upper extremities, restored functional hand movement to a patient with quadriplegia, and alleviated gait defects with hemicord injuries through brain-controlled spinal epidural stimulation. Additionally, ICEs distributed in more diffuse frontoparietal areas have enabled simultaneous bimanual control of arms [26].

To date, the recording modalities stable enough to drive assistive BMIs over a long period of time are implanted electrodes. Even here, the major problem with chronically implanted intracortical sensors is signal longevity. Microelectrode arrays (MEAs) face gliosis that starts in the first few months and can lead to failure at an average of 1 year. Eventually, the progressive meningeal fibrosis can elevate a microarray out of the cortex region. Immune reactions and reactive oxygen species lead to the degradation of the materials over time. In the most commonly used MEA known as the Utah array, failure can be due to cracking of parylene, corrosion of platinum, and delamination of silicone elastomer. Other intracortical recording techniques have been developed to minimize cortical damage and have recorded stable signals for years [27].

11.3.4 EcoG systems

This concern for longevity is one of the reasons ECoG-based systems have become popular, as there is supportive evidence that functional potential may have greater longevity and stability than spikes. Currently, a fully implantable ECoG system has been used to design a typing interface for a locked-in patient with ALS by decoding hand motor intention. FPs recorded from the surface of the human motor cortex contain high gamma activity (70–300 Hz) and time features that can be used to code continuous force, isometric force, and muscle activity in finger flexors with higher levels of accuracy [28]. Recently, a high-density ECoG array over the motor cortex is used to get control of individual fingers on a prosthetic limb by a human subject with epilepsy. ECoG-based systems have also been used as a mechanism to provide treatment to chronic stroke patients who would otherwise not able to participate. A patient gained volitional control of a feedback device and engaged himself in repetitive, high-intensity exercises of finger pointing and wrist extension without the need for a physician. He could simultaneously monitor his own ability to modulate his brain activity and receive immediate rewards for success, eventually enhancing the function of the targeted muscle. Additionally, there is now evidence that epidural arrays can provide similar information to subdural arrays regarding finger kinematics, thus potentially giving a less invasive and equally viable option for such clinical applications [29].

Furthermore, implantation of the electrodes will contain the risks associated with the angiographic deployment of a stent, including thrombosis, stroke hemorrhage, and infection. Notably, many of these limitations and risks are shared with other implantable electrode systems. Although these patients achieved enough voluntary control of their upper extremities to help with some activities of daily living, their extremities did not reach antigravity strength and there were serious limitations due to limb spasticity. EMG-based FES systems also do not work on patients who cannot voluntarily contract any muscles, and they need the use of preprogrammed stimulation patterns that can be nonintuitive. In addition, for clinical viability, any interface needs to be reliable for a very long period of time, and, unfortunately, this remains a problem for virtually every studied neural implant except DBS electrodes. Future microelectrode arrays could address concerns about durability through improved insulation materials, inert electrode alloys, and/or incorporation of antiinflammatory material along the lines of drug-eluting stents [30].

11.3.5 Neurorehabilitation and electrical stimulation

Using electrical techniques to generate stepping in combination with extensive goal-directed physical therapy, patients with chronic and complete spinal cord injury (SCI) have now shown the ability to develop positive functional plasticity and regain some voluntary control of lower extremity movement. Other subjects with complete SCIs have regained the ability to selectively move their hips, knees, and ankles, as well as regain some coordination of flexor and extensor muscles. Furthermore, some of these patients learned how to stand independently and activate lower limb musculature during partial weight-bearing stepping. In addition to attaining better lower extremity control, improvements in cardiovascular, temperature, bladder, and bowel control have been noted, as well as enhanced sexual function in some. In other subjects, subthreshold epidural stimulation between L2 and S1, or direct stimulation of the pudendal nerve, has been shown to initiate micturition [31].

The mechanism by which complete and chronic SCI patients regain voluntary motor control of their lower extremities is currently unclear. The fact that positive, lasting plasticity (up to years after training) can be induced suggests that there are likely subclinical surviving descending tracts in the injured spinal cord that are amenable to modulation and strengthening. When used for SCI rehabilitation, epidural stimulation is often combined with monoamine therapy to increase the baseline excitatory state of distal functional elements and prime them for activation. Neurons are known to release serotonin (5HT), norepinephrine, and dopamine during locomotion within most laminae of lumbosacral segments. These monoamines are thought to operate through volume neurotransmission (i.e., perisynaptic signal diffusion), and, along with epidural stimulation, have helped promote locomotion in both animal models and human patients with incomplete and complete spinal cord injuries [32]. After repeated stimuli, areas of movement representation have been seen to shift several microns and increase in size with a corresponding increase in spine density in pyramidal cell layers III and V. Stimulation to other areas of the brain has also gained interest for goals other than motor recovery. For example, deficits in learning and memory after traumatic brain injury (TBI) have been improved by theta burst stimulation of the fornix and hippocampus. There is also human data supporting the use of subthreshold cortical stimulation for recovery after an ischemic infarct; however, recent data from phase III trials have been negative [33].

New closed-loop stimulation paradigms are also being developed for patients who cannot participate in traditional therapy, including brain state-dependent stimulation (BSDS). Researchers published an experiment where TMS of the motor cortex and haptic feedback to the hand were controlled by sensorimotor desynchronization during motor imagery in one healthy and one stroke subject with chronic hand paresis. They found that BSDS increased the excitability of the stimulated motor cortex in both patients, an effect not observed in non-BSDS protocols. Both transcranial direct current and magnetic stimulation therapies are in the early stages.

There are many reasons to be optimistic about the potential for human nervous system repair. For the first time in history, we are seeing patients with chronic and complete spinal cord injuries voluntarily move their legs. Advances in modern neurobiological, neuroengineering, and neurorehabilitation strategies have provided hope for better outcomes, and the synergistic potential of integrated strategies is only beginning to be realized. In fact, there is a substantial amount of evidence reviewed here that suggests multidisciplinary approaches might not only be helpful but will be critical for any technique to realize its full therapeutic capability. Although the essential nature of many rehabilitation strategies remains a subject of debate, well-timed, goal-directed therapy and some form of associated positive feedback mechanism appear to be necessary components of therapeutic paradigms aimed at generating axonal sprouting and lasting functional improvement [34]. Until the complete neurological repair is achievable, optimizing the timing of a variety of treatments and tailoring therapies to different phases of injury and recovery remains the gold standard approach. In American hospitals, standard of care during the acute phase of neurological injury aims to stabilize the injury and prevent further loss of tissue through (1) the initiation of hypothermia after cardiac arrest, (2) the maintenance of neural perfusion pressures after TBI or SCI, (3) the recannulation of occluded vessel(s) after stroke by thrombectomy or thrombolysis, or (4) surgery to evacuate mass lesions or decompress edematous tissue. Furthermore, generating axonal regrowth on its own does not ensure restoration of function. Also notable in clinical applications is the relative paucity of biomarkers that might help drive prognosis and diagnose phases of injury/recovery, as well as the large discrepancy between known mechanisms of injury repair and viable options for intervention. Now that outcomes may start improving, it would be interesting to monitor known markers through improved recovery periods, as well as to search for new ones in the hopes of helping inform the timing and selection of therapeutic applications. Perhaps by combining new developments in the neurobiology lab with the essential elements of neurological rehabilitation, neural simulation, and the concept of a multidisciplinary intervention on micro- and macroscopic levels, success will be found where previously promising therapies have failed [35].

11.4 Toxicological effects of neural implants

The use of neural implants for neurodiagnostic and neurotherapeutic purposes provides superior benefits than the conventional approaches, it may be potentially toxic in the central nervous system. In this respect, nanotechnological research focuses on nanoneurotoxicity and nanoneurosafety concepts. Despite these efforts, nanoparticles may cause neurotoxicity, neuroinflammation, and neurodegeneration by penetrating the brain-olfactory route and blood–brain barrier. Indeed, due to their unique structures, nanomaterials can easily cross biological barriers, thus avoiding drug-delivery problems [36]. Despite the advancement of nanotechnology for designing therapeutic agents, the toxicity of these nanomaterials is still a concern. The activation of neurons by astrocytic glutamate is a result of NPs-mediated astrocyte-neuron crosstalk. Increased extracellular glutamate levels due to enhanced synthesis and reduced reuptake may induce neuronal damage by abnormal activation of extrasynaptic *N*-methyl D-aspartate receptor subunits. Moreover, *N*-methyl D-aspartate receptor (NMDAR) is the key factor that mediates the disturbances in intracellular calcium homeostasis, mitochondrial dysfunction, and generation of reactive oxygen species in NPs exposed neurons. Although some NPs cause neuronal death by inducing NMDARs, others may be neurotoxic through the α-amino-3-hydroxy-5-methyl-4-isoxazole propionic acid receptors or protect the neurons via blocking NMDARs. However, mechanisms of dual effects of NPs, neurotoxicity, or neuroprotection are not precisely known. Some NPs present neuroprotective effects either by selectively inhibiting the extrasynaptic subunit of NMDARs or by attenuating oxidative stress. NPs-related proinflammatory activation of microglia contributes to the dysfunction and cytotoxicity in neurons. Therefore investigation of the interaction of neural implants with the neuronal signaling molecules and neuronal receptors is necessary for the better understanding of the neurotoxicity or neurosafety [37].

11.4.1 Side effects of DBS electric implants

Deep brain stimulation involves implanting electrodes within affected areas of the brain. These electrodes produce electrical impulses that regulate abnormal impulses. The amount of stimulation in the deep brain is controlled by a pacemaker-like device placed under the skin in the upper chest. A wire that travels under your skin connects this device to the electrodes in your brain [38]. Deep brain stimulation is approved to treat a number of conditions, such as the following:

- Dystonia
- Epilepsy
- Essential tremor
- Obsessive–compulsive disorder
- Parkinson's disease.

Deep brain stimulation is also being studied as a potential treatment for the following:

- Addiction
- Chronic pain
- Cluster headache
- Dementia
- Depression (major)
- Huntington's disease
- Multiple sclerosis
- Stroke recovery
- Tourette syndrome
- Traumatic brain injury.

Although deep brain stimulation is minimally invasive and considered safe, any type of surgery has the risk of complications. Also, the brain stimulation itself can cause side effects. Deep brain stimulation involves creating small holes in the skull to implant the electrodes, and surgery to implant the device that contains the batteries under the skin in the chest. Complications of surgery may include the following:

- Misplacement of lead
- Bleeding in the brain
- Stroke
- Infection
- Breathing problems
- Nausea
- Heart problems
- Seizure.

Post implant side effects of deep brain stimulation may include the following:

- Seizure
- Infection
- Headache
- Confusion

- Difficulty concentrating
- Stroke
- Hardware complications, such as an eroded lead wire
- Temporary pain and swelling at the implantation site.

A few weeks after the surgery, the device will be turned on and the process of finding the best settings will begin. Some implant settings may cause side effects, but these often improve with further adjustments of your device.

- Numbness or tingling sensations
- Muscle tightness of the face or arm
- Speech problems
- Balance problems
- Lightheadedness
- Vision problems, such as double vision
- Unwanted mood changes, such as anger and depression.

VNS may influence voice changes, sore throat, neck pain, discomfort at the site of implantation, difficulty in breathing, and dysphagia. Adverse events in SNS patients include pain at the implant site, new pain, suspected lead migration, infection, transient sensation of electric shock, and pain at the lead site, with more than 50% of patients requiring surgical revision of the implant or leads within 5 years. Patients who did not have a functioning auditory nerve received an auditory brainstem implant in the DCN. The majority of successfully implanted patients reported a reduction in tinnitus perception or even completes suppression during stimulation. Side effects of stimulation that have been described include facial pain and ocular vibration. Electrical stimulation of the IC in patients with unilateral deafness showed some side effects including the perception of unpleasant sounds, paresthesia, dizziness, facial twitches, and temperature changes. DBS has been performed in obsessive–compulsive disorder patients and is associated with a risk of hypomania. Human functional magnetic resonance imaging studies have demonstrated the involvement of the amygdala and hippocampus in tinnitus, and these areas could, therefore, be considered as possible DBS targets. Side effects such as negative emotions have appeared in some patients during stimulation and make these areas less suitable for the treatment of tinnitus with DBS [39].

11.4.2 Adverse effects of sacral neuromodulation

The most common adverse effects recorded during clinical studies of patients with sacral neuromodulation include pain at implant sites, lead migration, infection, technical or device problems, adverse changes in bowel or voiding function, and undesirable stimulation or sensations. Complications can occur with the SNS evaluation, including the movement of the wire, technical problems with the device, and some temporary pain. Patients must be instructed on operating the test device and given other precautions related to the evaluation as well as activity restrictions [40].

11.4.3 Blood–brain barrier disruption in intracortical implants

Chronically implanted microelectrodes in the neural tissue exhibit inflammatory responses that are time varying and have been shown to depend on multiple factors. Among these factors, blood–brain barrier (BBB) disruption has been published as one of the significant factors resulting in implant failure. A series of events that include BBB and cell-membrane disruption occurs during electrode implantation that triggers multiple reactions responsible for microglial and astroglial activation, hemorrhage, edema, and release of proinflammatory neurotoxic cytokines that causes neuronal degeneration and dysfunction [41]. Typically, microwire arrays and silicon probes are inserted slowly into the neural tissue whereas the silicon Utah MEAs (UMEA) are inserted at a high speed using a pneumatic inserter. They have reported the sequence of electrode-implant induced cortical injury at various acute time points in UMEAs implanted in the brain tissue by quantifying the expression profile for factor genes mediating the inflammatory response and tight junction and adherens junction proteins that form the BBB and are critical to the functioning of the BBB. This information provides an insight into the physiological events related to neuroinflammation and BBB-disruption occurring at acute time-points following the insertion of UMEAs [42].

11.4.4 Adverse effects of brachytherapy

The patient may be awake during this procedure. Thin cylinders (catheters) might be set into tiny gaps in your skull. The radioactive seeds or nanoparticles are sent through the catheters into the tumor. The catheters may be evacuated immediately or they might be left set up until the point that the seeds are evacuated. The nanoparticles may emit a low dimension of radiation and the patient may need to wear a head protector or should stay in the protected room [43]. Few adverse effects of brachytherapy includes the following:

- Contamination
- Seizures
- Cerebral pain
- Death of close-by tissue
- Brain swelling.

11.4.5 Biocompatibility and neurotoxicity of metals used for neural repairs

Metals play a significant role in the neurological structure and function. Metals such as titanium, platinum, tungsten, stainless steel, and magnesium are widely used in neuromodulation device, recording electrodes, cochlear implant, and coils. Metal dyshomeostasis has been correlated in the pathology of neurodegenerative diseases including Alzheimer's disease, amyotrophic lateral sclerosis, Huntington disease, Menkes, occipital horn syndrome, and Parkinson's and Prion disease. Metals including aluminum, copper, lead, manganese, mercury, and thallium are known nervous system toxins. Oxidative stress may be a vital factor in the development or progression of neurodegenerative disorders. Neurological symptoms, including cognitive decline, memory difficulties, tremor, incoordination, polyneuropathy, vertigo, hearing loss, and visual changes have been reported from cobalt and chromium toxicity post hip replacement. Nerve injury, especially the large-size nerve damage, is a serious condition affecting millions of people. Entubulation of two ends of the injured nerve by using an implantable device, for example, nerve guidance conduit, to guide the regeneration of nerve tissue is a promising approach for treating the large-size nerve defect. Magnesium and its alloys used in implants are biodegradable, conductive, and own good mechanical properties. Mg^{2+} ion, one of the main degradation products of Mg and its alloys, was reported to enhance the proliferation of neural stem cells and their neurite production. Thus Mg and its alloys are potential materials for the fabrication of nerve repair implants. However, the biocompatibility of magnesium alloys to cells, especially nerve cells is not clear. Mg alloys degraded in cell culture media and artificial cerebrospinal fluid. Neurocognitive abnormalities may be mediated by either static brain damage caused by chromium and cobalt toxicity or could represent a dynamic process, that is an early onset dementia triggered by metallosis [44].

Corrosion of metals: Corrosion of metal implants is an important clinical problem. Structural failure or reduced implant integrity may result in increased local and systemic concentrations of metals leading to patient morbidity. Corrosion is the major concern in younger patients, who may be exposed to systemic metal toxicity for longer periods of time. All metallic implant inside the body is subjected to electrochemical degradation. The combination of various ions in an aqueous environment, including calcium, magnesium, bicarbonate, sodium, chloride, and plasma proteins creates a thermodynamic force for oxidation–reduction reactions. A protective oxide layer, surface modification techniques, and materials provide some protection reducing the rate of corrosive attack. Those working in the fields of orthopedic, psychiatry, and primary care should be needed to assess the neuropsychiatric state of their patients after MoM implant operations. Other than revision surgery, there is no effective adsorption or chelation therapy for chromium and cobalt, and there is a need to develop such therapies that could be safely developed to avoid the need for further surgery. In the meantime, to preserve the neurocognitive function, implant should be removed as soon as possible after toxicity is detected [45].

There is a possibility of identification of the neuropathological substrate to dementia in such patients. Till date, there is no neuroimaging study or any autopsy brain tissue analysis on these patients and this would be a future area of research, as would studies looking at the mediating process linking any toxicity with neurocognitive impairment including studies on allergic immune response and protein accumulation in the brain or direct neurotoxicity.

11.4.6 Diagnosis and treatment of metallosis-induced toxicity

Metallosis is the putative medical condition involving deposition of metal debris due to aseptic fibrosis, local necrosis, or loosening of the prosthesis secondary to metallic corrosion and release of wear debris. It has been reported with a wide range of metallic implants including titanium, stainless steel, and cobalt–chromium alloys but may also occur with metal on neural and polyethylene joint replacements. Diagnosis depends upon clinical history, examination, and investigations. Symptoms and signs of metallosis may include pain, grey discoloration of the tissues surrounding the joint, increasing noise from the replacement, a sense of joint instability, and effusion although implant loosening, periprosthetic fracture, osteonecrosis, infection, tendinitis, impingement, lesion, and referred pain may cause similar symptoms. Investigations including serum metal levels, hip aspiration, and imaging may be useful. Rising serum cobalt and chromium levels may be an early indicator of implant failure. Cobalt levels in hair, blood, urine, and placenta are often elevated in patients with metal-on-metal replacements. The diagnosis may be evaluated by the aspiration of dark gray or black synovial fluid. Radiological findings may include misalignment and loss of joint space, suggesting wear or fracture of the prosthesis liner, amorphous densities in the periprosthetic tissues, and hyperdense rounded images with a higher contour (metal deposits). Elevated blood levels of cobalt and chromium can persist for at least a year following revision, especially in patients with high levels of exposure. Nickel is a common contact allergen but, based on the low release rates of nickel, sensitization caused by stainless steel is unlikely. Nickel-free implants have been developed. Serum and urine levels of chromium and nickel have been found to be elevated in patients with scoliosis who had undergone spinal instrumentation [46,47].

The discovery of new alloys and improvement in metallurgy has expanded both the therapeutic and diagnostic indications for metal-containing implants. Concerns regarding systemic and local metal ion toxicity, other implants containing cobalt and chromium, have resulted in regulatory bodies including the US Food and Drug Administration, UK Medicines and Health Care Products and Regulatory Authority, and Therapeutic Goods Administration publishing clinical algorithms to detect potential implant failure and metal toxicity. There is currently no consensus statement outlining the relationship between symptoms, peak metal ion levels, or the length of exposure. For other metal implants and newer alloys, little toxicity data exist. Important preoperative consideration for the anesthetist when assessing a patient for surgery who has new neurological, cardiac, thyroid, renal, or hematological impairment should include a thorough history, particularly noting the presence of metal implants. If clinical history and examination are insufficient to explain the patient's symptoms and they have a metal prosthesis, then an attempt should be made to identify the type, components, and duration of implant insertion. For patients with older implants, known to contain cobalt or chromium, or have clinical features of metallosis, then consideration should be given to a toxicological evaluation to exclude metal toxicity as an underlying cause of the organ impairment [48].

11.4.7 Foreign body response as a cause of implant failure

The nervous tissue response to implantable microelectrodes is a complex process characterized by a sequence of biochemical alterations and chemical reactions occurring at the level of the tissue–material interface. These biochemical and chemical alterations may develop in an undesired immune response. Once surgically implanted, microelectrodes must remain intact for several years to ensure the efficacy of the therapy and device functionality [49]. To provide successful integration, reliability, and durability once implanted in the brain tissue, microelectrodes must fulfill the following requirements:

Biocompatibility: The surface of the microelectrode must be nontoxic for neural cells without causing any side effects to the surrounding tissues.

Biomimicry: The surface has to mimic the physical, chemical, and mechanical characteristics of the extracellular matrix to enhance neurite outgrowth toward the electrode surface and to avoid activation and recruitment of glial cells and fibroblasts that can contribute to the encapsulation of the electrodes.

Biostability: Microelectrodes need to maintain their physical integrity, electrochemical stability, and functionality and resist the highly corrosive tissue microenvironment without undergoing any structural modification.

11.4.8 Astrocytes damage

Astrocytes are another type of neuroglia that is damaged after implantation. Astrocytes perform various functions, including biochemical support of endothelial cells that form the BBB, supplying nutrients to the nervous tissue, maintenance of extracellular ion balance, having a significant role in the repair and scar process of the nervous system. In analogy to microglia, astrocytes exist in a proinflammatory phenotype and an antiinflammatory phenotype. PI astrocytes are activated by PI microglia and secret neurotoxins creating a hostile environment for neuronal and oligodendrocytes regeneration. PI astrocytes are activated by Il-1β, TNF-α, and complement component from microglia, responding immediately to electrode implantation and changes in neuronal activity, accumulating in the vicinity of the microelectrode during the first week after implantation. At this level, astrocytes alter the neuronal viability causing neuronal loss, reduction of fiber density and overexpression of glial fibrillary protein, and vimentin, which are critical for their change in morphology and extension of the protrusions at the injury site [50].

11.4.9 Acute vascular damage and hemorrhage

Insertion of the electrode leads to acute disruption of the BBB and hemorrhages from disrupted small brain blood vessels. The disruption of BBB leads to the deposition of plasma proteins foreign material to the CNS including albumin (40 mg/mL), globulins (10 mg/mL), fibrin/fibrinogen (3 mg/mL), plasmin, thrombin complement, and red blood cells (hemosiderin). The vascular damage is accompanied by fluid displacement, dragging of the blood vessels, and eventual vessel severing. The most severe form of vascular damage is the vessel rupture, which is accompanied by hemorrhage. For example, Ward reports traumatic insertion of Cyberkinetic probes accompanied by hemorrhages. Such damage causes BBB rupture, infiltration of leukocytes and platelets, and extravasation of serum proteins, notably albumin, which can cause direct activation of astrocytes and microglia. The variability in intracortical hemorrhaging resulting from microelectrode insertion was first demonstrated under double photon imaging. It was shown that penetrating a single large intracortical blood vessel resulted in. They examined the short- or long-term effect of bleeding on neuronal and glial cell densities. Signs of heavy bleeding were visible at both 1 and 12 weeks after surgery. Tissue around the electrode tracks was damaged and very few, if any, neurons or glial cells could be observed [51].

11.4.10 Ethical concern of neural implant

Evidently, the implant technology described in this section has enormous potential for application in a broad spectrum of different fields. Restricting this neural technology to therapeutic purposes would also limit the need for a philosophical argument. At the same time, extending the scope for its significant application would open up numerous possibilities. For example, employing such methods or techniques to relieve depression raises the possibility of recreational use. Perhaps the most significant option would potentially be their use to overcome negative character, and not merely bad habits, a scenario fictionalized in a movie too. If signals could then be transmitted remotely from a brain to a computer and back again, who will be responsible for that person's actions, particularly if they were to commit a crime. It also keeps thorny ethical concerns, not least because the technique could give researchers a degree of access to a person's brain or inner feelings in real time [52].

11.5 Conclusion and future directions

Researchers have long been developing ways to improve the quality of life for patients who suffer from spinal cord injury, stroke, epilepsy, and other neurological disorders classically categorized as permanent. Several disciplines, namely neurobiology, neuroengineering, and neurorehabilitation, have all made great output. However, understanding the path to achieve complete neurological recovery for human patients remains remote and complex. Nonetheless, patients are now starting to show recovery beyond that which was previously thought impossible. Several biocompatible materials have been commercially used for fabricating implantable devices. Bioresorbable materials disintegrate gradually in vivo and their derivatives get absorbed completely in the body fluid with no residue and with minimal toxic effects, thus eliminating the need for retrieval operations [53].

This chapter discussed the most recent advances in the biology of neurological injury, molecular mechanisms of neural repair, physiology of neurological recovery, neurophysiology underlying brain–machine and neural interface training, state of the art in neural and brain–machine interfaces, neurorehabilitation strategies, and ideas for how to integrate future research. As the development of immunotherapies, electrical stimulation, neural interfaces, stem cells, gene therapies advance, their reparative potential may only be realized by integrating them into a rehabilitation framework that includes conscious intention and positive neural feedback. Special attention must be given to timing, sequence, and dose of therapy. Hopefully, these concepts will help the user in the next frontier of nervous system recovery [54]. The pharmacological, psychosocial, psychological models, and interventions have been there since the last few decades to address nonadherence. Hence, new powerful, long acting, lesser side effects, and novel psychotropic implant can be developed and could soon revolutionize the treatment in psychiatry.

References

[1] Hassle C, Boretius T, Stieglitz T. Polymers for neural implants. J Polym Sci 2011;49:18–23.

[2] Ko WH. Early history and challenges of implantable electronics. J Emerg Technol Comput Syst 2012;8:1–9.

[3] Chatterjee S, Saxena M, Padmanabhan D, Jayachandra M, Pandya HJ. Futuristic medical implants using bioresorbable materials and devices. Biosens Bioelectron 2019;142.

[4] Aguilar ZP. Nanomedical devices. Nanomaterials for medical applications. Elsevier; 2013, ISBN: 9780123850898. p. 235–92. Available from: https://doi.org/10.1016/B978-0-12-385089-8.00006-6.
[5] Daroff RB, et al. Deep brain stimulation. Bradley's neurology in clinical practice. 7th ed. Philadelphia, PA: Saunders Elsevier; 2016. Available from: https://www.clinicalkey.com.
[6] Edwards CA, et al. Neurostimulation devices for the treatment of neurologic disorders. Mayo Clin Proc 2017;92:1427.
[7] Holtzheimer PE, et al. Subcallosal cingulate deep brain stimulation for treatment-resistant depression: a multisite, randomised, sham-controlled trial. Lancet Psychiatry 2017;4(11):839–49.
[8] Reardon S. AI-controlled brain implants for mood disorders tested in people. Nature 2017;551:549–50. Available from: https://doi.org/10.1038/nature.2017.23031.
[9] Implants Used in Brain Cancer Treatment, (2019), https://onco.com/about-cancer/cancer-types/brain-tumor/treatment/implants/.
[10] Noblett K, Siegel S, Mangel J, et al. Results of a prospective, multicenter study evaluating quality of life, safety, and efficacy of sacral neuromodulation at 12 months in subjects with symptoms of OAB. Neurourol Urodyn 2014;. Available from: https://doi.org/10.1002/nau.22707.
[11] Johnson M. Transcutaneous electrical nerve stimulation. Proven Treat Option Bladder Control Bowel Control 2012. Available from: https://doi.org/10;2012.
[12] Staskin DR, Peters KM, MacDiarmid S, Shore N, de Groat WC. Percutaneous tibial nerve stimulation: a clinically and cost effective addition to the overactive bladder algorithm of care. Curr Urol Rep 2012;13(5):327–34. Available from: https://doi.org/10.1007/s11934-012-0274-9.
[13] Herbison GP, Arnold EP. Sacral neuromodulation with implanted devices for urinary storage and voiding dysfunction in adults. Cochrane Database Syst Rev 2009;2009 (Suppl. 2):CD004202. Available from: https://doi.org/10.1002/14651858.CD004202.
[14] Okada T, Suzuki H. Toll like receptor4 as a possible therapeutic target for delayed brain injuries after aneurismal subarachnoid hemorrhage (in eng). Neural Regen Res 2017;12(2):193–6.
[15] Klingler HC, Pycha A, Schmidbauer J, Marberger M. Use of peripheral neuromodulation of the S3 region for treatment of detrusor overactivity: a urodynamic-based study. Urology 2000;56(5):766–71. Available from: https://doi.org/10.1016/S0090-4295(00)00727-5.
[16] van Zwieten G, Smit JV, Jahanshahi A, Temel Y, Stokroos RJ. Tinnitus: is there a place for brain stimulation. Surgical Neurol Int 2016;7(Suppl. 4):S125–9. Available from: https://doi.org/10.4103/2152-7806.176134.
[17] Krucoff MO, Rahimpour S, Slutzky MW, Edgerton VR, Turner DA. Enhancing nervous system recovery through neurobiologics, neural interface training, and neurorehabilitation. Front Neurosci 2016;10:584. Available from: https://doi.org/10.3389/fnins.2016.00584.
[18] Bennett C, Samikkannu M, Mohammed F, Dietrich WD, Rajguru SM, Prasad A. Blood brain barrier (BBB)-disruption in intracortical silicon microelectrode implants. Biomaterials 2018;164:1–10.
[19] Engin AB, Engin A. Chapter 9 - Nanoparticles and neurotoxicity: dual response of glutamatergic receptors. Progress in brain research, vol. 245. Elsevier; 2019. p. 281–303.
[20] Fei J, Wen X, Lin X, Saijilafu, Wang W, Ren O, et al. Biocompatibility and neurotoxicity of magnesium alloys potentially used for neural repairs. Mater Sci Eng C 2017;78:1155–63 ISSN 0928-4931.

[21] Langley A. Modern metal implant toxicity and anaesthesia. Australasian anaesthesia; 2015.

[22] Deep brain stimulation for movement disorders fact sheet. National Institute of Neurological Disorders and Stroke. <https://www.ninds.nih.gov/Disorders/Patient-Caregiver-Education/Fact-Sheets/Deep-Brain-Stimulation-Movement-Disorders-Fact/> [accessed 19.10.18].

[23] Patient-specific modeling of deep brain stimulation. In: Krames ES, et al., editors. Neuromodulation. 2nd ed. London, UK: Elsevier Academic Press; 2018. <https://www.clinicalkey.com/>.

[24] Shah RS, et al. Deep brain stimulation: technology at the cutting edge. J Clin Neurol 2010;6:167.

[25] Deep Brain Stimulation. American Association of Neurological Surgeons. <https://www.aans.org/Patients/Neurosurgical-Conditions-and-Treatments/Deep-Brain-Stimulation/>; 2018.

[26] Jones RSG, daSilva AB, Whittaker RG, Woodhall GL, Cunningham MO. Human brain slices for epilepsy research: pitfalls, solutions and future challenges. J Neurosci Methods 2016;260:221–32. Available from: https://doi.org/10.1016/j.jneumeth.2015.09.021.

[27] Neurosurgery. In: Brunicardi FC, et al., editors. Schwartz's principles of surgery. 10th ed. New York, NY: McGraw-Hill Education; 2018. 2015. <https://accessmedicine.mhmedical.com/>.

[28] Kozai TDY, Jaquins-Gerstl AS, Vazquez AL, Michael AC, Cui XT. Brain tissue responses to neural implants impact signal sensitivity and intervention strategies. ACS Chem Neurosci 2015;6:48–67. Available from: https://doi.org/10.1021/cn500256e.

[29] Kelly SK, Shire DB, Jinghua C, Doyle P, Gingerich MD, Cogan SF, et al. A hermetic wireless subretinal neurostimulator for vision prostheses. IEEE Trans Biomed Eng 2011;58:3197–205.

[30] Hadler C, Wissel K, Brandes G, Dempwolf W, Reuter G, Lenarz T, et al. Photochemical coating of KaptonR with hydrophilic polymers for the improvement of neural implants. Mater Sci Eng C 2017;75:286–96. Available from: https://doi.org/10.1016/j.msec.2017.2.

[31] Feng XL, Chen A, Zhang Y, Wang J, Shao L, Wei L. Central nervous system toxicity of metallic nanoparticles. Int J Nanomed 2015;10:4321–40.

[32] AskMayoExpert. Deep brain stimulation. Rochester, MN: Mayo Foundation for Medical Education and Research; 2018.

[33] Chen R, Romero G, Christiansen MG, Mohr A, Anikeeva P. Wireless magnetothermal deep brain stimulation. Science 2015;347:1477–80. Available from: https://doi.org/10.1126/science.1261821.

[34] Peters KM, Killinger KA, Ibrahim AM, Villaba PS. The relationship between subjective and objective assessments of sacral neuromodulation effectiveness in patients with urgency-frequency. Neurourol Urodyn 2008;27:775–8. Available from: https://doi.org/10.1002/nau.20592.

[35] Gerhardsson L, Lundh T, Minthon L, Londos E. Metal concentrations in plasma and cerebrospinal fluid in patients with Alzheimer's disease. Dement Geriatr Cogn Disord 2008;25(6):508–15. Available from: https://doi.org/10.1159/000129365.

[36] Green B, Griffiths E, Almond S. Neuropsychiatric symptoms following metal-on-metal implant failure with cobalt and chromium toxicity. BMC Psychiatry 2017;17(1). Available from: https://doi.org/10.1186/s12888-016-1174-1.

[37] Liu JY, et al. Neuropathology of the blood-brain barrier and pharmaco-resistance in human epilepsy. Brain 2012;135(Pt10):3115–33.

[38] Rezai AR, et al. Improved function after deep brain stimulation for chronic, severe traumatic brain injury. Neurosurgery 2016;79:204.

[39] Kozai T, Langhals N, Hooi F, Kipke, D. Time course of blood brain barrier disruption due to microelectrode insertion into cerebral cortex. In: Presented at the biomedical engineering society, annual meeting, Pittsburgh, PA, October 7 – 10; 2009.
[40] Venkatraghavan L. Anesthesia for patients who undergo deep brain stimulator implantation. <https://www.uptodate.com/contents/search/ > ; 2018.
[41] Lyons MK. Deep brain stimulation: current and future clinical applications. Mayo Clin Proc 2011;86:662.
[42] Chang SY, et al. Development of the Mayo investigational neuromodulation control system: toward a closed-loop electrochemical feedback system for deep brain stimulation. J Neurosurg 2013;119:1556.
[43] Medtronic DBS System for Epilepsy. Food and Drug Administration. <https://www.fda.gov/MedicalDevices/ProductsandMedicalProcedures/DeviceApprovalsandClearances/Recently-ApprovedDevices/ucm606550.htm/>; 2018.
[44] Hallab N, Jacobs JJ, Black J. Hypersensitivity to metallic biomaterials: a review of leukocyte migration inhibition assays. Biomaterials 2000;21(13):1301–14.
[45] Merritt K, Brown SA. Biological effects of corrosion products from metals. In: Fraker A, Griffin C, editors. Corrosion and degradation of implanted materials: second symposium. ASTM STP 859. Philadelphia: American Society for Testing and Materials; 1985. p. 105–16.
[46] Feng X, Chen A, Zhang Y, Wang J, Shao L, Wei L. Application of dental nanomaterials: potential toxicity to the central nervous system. Int J Nanomed 2015;10:3547–65.
[47] Carossino AM, Carulli C, Ciuffi S, Carossino R, Zappoli Thyrion GD, Zonefrati R, et al. Hypersensitivity reactions to metal implants: laboratory options. BMC Musculoskelet Disord 2016;17(1):486.
[48] Panigutti MA, Merritt K, Bruner RJ, et al. Correlation of allergy, metal levels, implant alloy, and implant damage in patients undergoing revision joint arthroplasties. Trans Soc Biomater 1992;15:7.
[49] Pacheco KA. Allergy to surgical implants. Clin Rev Allergy Immunol 2019;56 (1):72–85.
[50] Polikov VS, Tresco PA, Reichert WM. Response of brain tissue to chronically implanted neural electrodes. J Neurosci Methods 2005;148(1):1–18.
[51] Xu J, Guo H, Nguyen AT, Lim H, Yang Z. A bidirectional neuromodulation technology for nerve recording and stimulation. Micromachines 2018;9:E538. Available from: https://doi.org/10.3390/mi9110538.
[52] Williams DF. On the nature of biomaterials. Biomaterials 2009;30:5897–909. Available from: https://doi.org/10.1016/j.biomaterials.2009.07.027.
[53] Zhang W, Li Z, Gilles M, Wu D. Mechanical simulation of neural electrode-brain tissue interface under various micromotion conditions. J Med Biol Eng 2014;34:386–92.
[54] Donoghue JP, Nurmikko A, Black M, Hochberg LR. Assistive technology and robotic control using motor cortex ensemble-based neural interface systems in humans with tetraplegia. J Physiol 2007;579(3):603–11.

Further reading

Rezai AR, Phillips M, Baker KB, Sharan AD, Nyenhuis J, Tkach J, et al. Neurostimulation system used for deep brain stimulation (DBS): MR safety issues and implications of failing to follow safety recommendations. Investig Radiol 2004;39:300–3.

Index

Note: Page numbers followed by "*f*" and "*t*" refer to figures and tables, respectively.

9780128207284